Ruminant Immunology

Editor

CHRISTOPHER CHASE

VETERINARY CLINICS OF NORTH AMERICA: FOOD ANIMAL PRACTICE

www.vetfood.theclinics.com

Consulting Editor
ROBERT A. SMITH

November 2019 • Volume 35 • Number 3

ELSEVIER

1600 John F. Kennedy Boulevard • Suite 1800 • Philadelphia, Pennsylvania, 19103-2899

http://www.vetfood.theclinics.com

VETERINARY CLINICS OF NORTH AMERICA: FOOD ANIMAL PRACTICE Volume 35, Number 3
November 2019 ISSN 0749-0720, ISBN-13: 978-0-323-68345-6

Editor: Colleen Dietzler
Developmental Editor: Laura Kavanaugh

Veterinary Clinics of North America: Food Animal Practice (ISSN 0749-0720) is published in March, July, and November by Elsevier Inc., 360 Park Avenue South, New York, NY 10010-1710. Subscription prices are $256.00 per year (domestic individuals), $434.00 per year (domestic institutions), $100.00 per year (domestic students/residents), $283.00 per year (Canadian individuals), $572.00 per year (Canadian institutions), $335.00 per year (international individuals), $572.00 per year (international institutions), and $165.00 per year (international and Canadian students/residents). To receive student/resident rate, orders must be accompanied by name of affiliated institution, date of term, and the signature of program/residency coordinator on institution letterhead. *Clinics* subscription prices. All prices are subject to change without notice. **POSTMASTER:** Send address changes to *Veterinary Clinics of North America: Food Animal Practice*, Elsevier Health Sciences Division, Subscription Customer Service, 3251 Riverport Lane, Maryland Heights, MO 63043. Customer Service (orders, claims, online, change of address): Elsevier Health Sciences Division, Subscription **Customer Service, 3251 Riverport Lane, Maryland Heights, MO 63043. Tel: 1-800-654-2452 (U.S. and Canada); 314-447-8871 (ouside U.S. and Canada). Fax: 314-447-8029. E-mail: journalscustomerservice-usa@elsevier.com (for print support); journalsonlinesupport-usa@elsevier.com (for online support).**

Reprints. For copies of 100 or more, of articles in this publication, please contact the Commercial Reprints Department, Elsevier Inc., 360 Park Avenue South, New York, NY 10010-1710. Tel.: 212-633-3874; Fax: 212-633-3820; E-mail: reprints@elsevier.com.

Veterinary Clinics of North America: Food Animal Practice is covered in *Current Contents/Agriculture, Biology and Environmental Sciences, MEDLINE/PubMed (Index Medicus), and Excerpta Medica.*

Contributors

CONSULTING EDITOR

ROBERT A. SMITH, DVM, MS
Diplomate, American Board of Veterinary Practitioners; Veterinary Research and Consulting Services, LLC, Greeley, Colorado, USA

EDITOR

CHRISTOPHER CHASE, DVM, MS, PhD
Professor of Veterinary and Biomedical Sciences, South Dakota State University, Brookings, South Dakota, USA

AUTHORS

HEBA ATALLA, PhD
Department of Pathobiology, Ontario Veterinary College, University of Guelph, Guelph, Ontario, Canada

MICHAEL A. BALLOU, PhD
Professor, Department of Veterinary Sciences, Texas Tech University, Lubbock, Texas, USA

PAUL R. BROADWAY, PhD
USDA-ARS Livestock Issues Unit, Lubbock, Texas, USA

JEFFERY A. CARROLL, PhD
USDA-ARS Livestock Issues Unit, Lubbock, Texas, USA

CHRISTOPHER CHASE, DVM, MS, PhD
Professor of Veterinary and Biomedical Sciences, South Dakota State University, Brookings, South Dakota, USA

MARCIO C. COSTA, DVM, DVSc, PhD
Department of Veterinary Biomedicine, University of Montreal, Saint-Hyacinthe, Quebec, Canada

EMILY M. DAVIS, MS
Department of Veterinary Sciences, Texas Tech University, Lubbock, Texas, USA

MEHDI EMAM, DVM
PhD Candidate, Department of Pathobiology, Ontario Veterinary College, Department of Animal Biosciences, Center for Genetic Improvement of Livestock, University of Guelph, Guelph, Ontario, Canada

KLIBS N. GALVÃO, DVM, MVPM, PhD
Diplomate, American College of Veterinary Theriogenology; Department of Large Animal Clinical Sciences, College of Veterinary Medicine, University of Florida, Gainesville, Florida, USA

LISA GAMSJÄGER, Mag.med.vet
Diplomate, American College of Veterinary Internal Medicine; PhD Student, Department of Production Animal Health, University of Calgary Faculty of Veterinary Medicine, Calgary, Alberta, Canada

SANDRA M. GODDEN, DVM, DVSc
Professor, Department of Veterinary Population Medicine, College of Veterinary Medicine, University of Minnesota, St Paul, Minnesota, USA

DIEGO E. GOMEZ, DVM, MSc, MVSc, PhD
Diplomate, American College of Veterinary Internal Medicine; Department of Large Animal Clinical Sciences, College of Veterinary Medicine, University of Florida, Gainesville, Florida, USA

MARIANA GUERRA-MAUPOME, DVM, PhD
Graduate Research Assistant, Department of Veterinary Microbiology and Preventive Medicine, Iowa State University, Ames, Iowa, USA

HEATHER D. HUGHES, PhD
SciWrite Consulting, Canyon, Texas, USA

BENJAMIN A. KASL, DVM
Department of Veterinary Sciences, Texas Tech University, Lubbock, Texas, USA

RADHEY S. KAUSHIK, BVSc, MVSc, PhD
Professor, Department of Biology and Microbiology, South Dakota State University, Brookings, South Dakota, USA

ALEXANDRA LIVERNOIS, PhD
Department of Pathobiology, Ontario Veterinary College, University of Guelph, Guelph, Ontario, Canada

JASON E. LOMBARD, DVM, MS
Dairy Specialist, Veterinary Epidemiologist, National Animal Health Monitoring System (NAHMS), USDA:APHIS:VS:CEAH, Fort Collins, Colorado, USA

BONNIE MALLARD, PhD
Department of Pathobiology, Ontario Veterinary College, Department of Animal Biosciences, Center for Genetic Improvement of Livestock, University of Guelph, Guelph, Ontario, Canada

FIONA P. MAUNSELL, BVSc, PhD
Clinical Assistant Professor, Department of Large Animal Clinical Sciences, College of Veterinary Medicine, University of Florida, Gainesville, Florida, USA

JODI L. McGILL, MSc, PhD
Assistant Professor, Department of Veterinary Microbiology and Preventive Medicine, Iowa State University, Ames, Iowa, USA

MARLENE PAIBOMESAI, PhD
Ontario Ministry of Agriculture and Rural Affairs, Guelph, Ontario, Canada

JOHN T. RICHESON, PhD
Department of Agricultural Sciences, West Texas A&M University, Canyon, Texas, USA

JUAN C. RODRIGUEZ-LECOMPTE, DVM, MSc, PhD
Department of Pathology and Microbiology, Atlantic Veterinary College, University of Prince Edward Island, Charlottetown, Prince Edward Island, Canada

JAMISON R. SLATE, BS, MSc
Graduate Research Assistant, Department of Veterinary Microbiology and Preventive Medicine, Iowa State University, Ames, Iowa, USA

DAVID R. SMITH, DVM, PhD
Diplomate, American College of Veterinary Preventive Medicine (Epidemiology); Endowed Professor, Department of Pathobiology and Population Medicine, Mississippi State University College of Veterinary Medicine, Mississippi State, Mississippi, USA

M. CLAIRE WINDEYER, BSc, DVM, DVSc
Associate Professor, Department of Production Animal Health, University of Calgary Faculty of Veterinary Medicine, Calgary, Alberta, Canada

AMELIA R. WOOLUMS, DVM, MVSc, PhD
Diplomate, American College of Veterinary Internal Medicine; Diplomate, American College of Veterinary Microbiology; Professor, Department of Pathobiology and Population Medicine, College of Veterinary Medicine, Mississippi State University, Mississippi State, Mississippi, USA

ALAN J. YOUNG, PhD
Professor, Department of Veterinary and Biomedical Sciences, South Dakota State University, Brookings, South Dakota, USA

Contents

Vaccination is a critical tool in modern animal production and key to maintaining animal health. Adjuvants affect the immune response by increasing the rate, quantity, or quality of the protective response generated by the target antigens. Although adjuvant technology dates back to the nineteenth century, there was relatively little improvement in adjuvant technology before the late twentieth century. With the discovery of molecular pathways that regulate the timing, quantity, and quality of the immune response, new technologies are focused on bringing safer, more effective, and inexpensive adjuvants to commercial use.

Infectious diseases are the outcome of complex interactions between the host, pathogen, and environment. After exposure to a pathogen, the host immune system uses various mechanisms to remove the pathogen. However, environmental factors and characteristics of pathogens can compromise the host immune responses and subsequently alter the outcome of infection. In this article, genetic and epigenetic factors that shape the individual variation in mounting protective responses are reviewed. Different approaches that have been used by researchers to investigate the genetic regulation of immunity in ruminants and various sources of genetic information are discussed.

This article discusses key concepts important for mucosal immunity. The mucosa is the largest immune organ of the body. The mucosal barrier (the tight junctions and the "kill zone") along with the mucosa epithelial cells maintaining an anti-inflammatory state are essential for the mucosal firewall. The microbiome (the microorganisms that are in the gastrointestinal, respiratory, and reproductive tract) is essential for immune development, homeostasis, immune response, and maximizing animal productivity. Mucosal vaccination provides an opportunity to protect animals from most infectious diseases because oral, gastrointestinal, respiratory, and reproductive mucosa are the main portals of entry for infectious disease.

Colostrum management is the single most important management factor in determining calf health and survival. Additional benefits of good colostrum management include improved rate of gain and future productivity. Successful colostrum management requires producers to provide calves with a sufficient volume of clean, high-quality colostrum within the first few hours of life. This article reviews the process of colostrogenesis and colostrum composition, and discusses key components in developing a successful colostrum management program. In addition, the article discusses approaches for monitoring and proposes new goals for passive immunity in dairy herds.

A growing body of evidence has shown that calves can mount an immune response when vaccinated in the face of maternal antibodies (IFOMA), albeit inconsistently and often in ways that differ from seronegative calves or older cattle. Several previous reviews have endeavored to explain bovine neonatal immunology and have documented the issue of vaccinating young calves. However, as preweaning vaccination becomes more common in both beef and dairy production systems, so too has research on the impacts of such vaccination programs. This article aims to briefly review the challenges and opportunities for vaccinating calves IFOMA.

Vaccination is a critical component of cattle health management. Effective cattle vaccine programs should consider the timing of vaccination in relation to expected disease challenge, risk for wild-type exposure of various bovine pathogens, and host factors during vaccination. Nearly all consulting veterinarians recommend vaccination of stressed, high-risk calves on feedlot arrival. However, this recommendation fails to consider several factors associated with vaccine efficiency. Further research evaluating vaccine interactions in stressed cattle and potential additive effects of endotoxin from multiple bacterin administration may reveal new evidence-based vaccination guidelines for cattle in the various segments of beef and dairy production systems.

Herd immunity is an important concept of epidemic theory regarding the population-level effect of individual immunity to prevent transmission of pathogens. Herd immunity exists when sufficient numbers of animals in a group or population have immunity against an agent such that the likelihood of an effective contact between diseased and susceptible individuals is reduced. Understanding herd immunity requires consideration of infection dynamics, modes of transmission, as well as the acquisition of immunity by individuals in the population. Loss of herd immunity may also explain age-associated epidemics of disease related to loss of passively acquired maternal immunity.

VETERINARY CLINICS OF NORTH AMERICA: FOOD ANIMAL PRACTICE

SERIES OF RELATED INTEREST

Veterinary Clinics of North America: Exotic Animal Practice
Available: https://www.vetexotic.theclinics.com/

THE CLINICS ARE NOW AVAILABLE ONLINE!
Access your subscription at:
www.theclinics.com

Preface

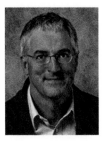

Christopher Chase, DVM, MS, PhD
Editor

Few fields have seen such growth in information as immunology. It has been over 15 years since the last issue of *Veterinary Clinics of North America: Food Animal Practice* contained an issue on ruminant immunology. The aim of this issue was not to provide proscriptive vaccine protocols but to guide the reader to the current concepts and approaches to understand how to optimize the immune system in these times when we are decreasing reliance on antimicrobials. Two-thirds of the subjects in this issue were not more than abstract ideas in 2003. The concept that too much innate immunity often contributes to disease processes is touched on in a number of articles. The emergence of the interaction between the immune system, the mucosa, and the microbiome has become the new frontier of study. There are 4 articles that provide basic to applied information (microbiome, mucosal immunity, gamma delta T cells, and nutraceutical) on maximizing these intricate interactions. Two other topics on vaccine responsiveness (genetics and adjuvants) are also included. We have included applied articles in this issue on maternal immunity (both induction and interference), herd immunity, and vaccine dos and don'ts to give to the reader some additional guidance in developing vaccine protocols. Finally, we have included an article on the bovine pathogen, *Mycoplasma bovis*. This pathogen, which is a frequent secondary invader, has emerged as a primary pathogen in cattle. The lack of efficacious vaccines and poor responsiveness to antimicrobial therapy make further understanding of the immune response to *M bovis* essential. We hope you enjoy this issue.

Christopher Chase, DVM, MS, PhD
Department of Veterinary and Biomedical Sciences
South Dakota State University
PO Box 2175, SAR Room 125
North Campus Drive
Brookings, SD 57007, USA

E-mail address:
Christopher.Chase@SDSTATE.edu

Vet Clin Food Anim 35 (2019) xiii
https://doi.org/10.1016/j.cvfa.2019.08.007
0749-0720/19/© 2019 Published by Elsevier Inc.

Adjuvants
What a Difference 15 Years Makes!

Alan J. Young, PhD

KEYWORDS

- Vaccine • Immunostimulant • Immunity • Adjuvant • Ruminants
- Antibody generation • Antisera

KEY POINTS

- Adjuvants are a necessary component to boost immunity to killed vaccines.
- Adjuvants boost the immune response by assisting in normal immunologic processes.
- Traditional adjuvants work through chemical means to regulate antigen delivery to the immune system and boost immunologic responses.
- Modern adjuvants target specific pathways of the immune system to reduce tissue side effects while boosting and modifying the immune response.

INTRODUCTION

Since its introduction, vaccination has been 1 of the great "success stories" of immunology. In humans, widespread application of vaccines has been responsible for the eradication of smallpox, as well as significant improvements in public health and reduction of diseases.[1] In the veterinary world, vaccination has successfully eradicated Rinderpest, and resulted in greater efficiency of production of animal protein, increased profitability, and reduced need for antibiotic use.[2] With the worldwide reduction of antibiotic use in animal agriculture, vaccination strategies will continue to be critical to maintaining a sustainable animal agriculture industry. Although a great deal of the focus on the development of new vaccines lies in determining appropriate protein antigen "targets" and antigen formulations to protect against disease, adjuvants play a critical role in vaccine effectiveness.[3–5] Adjuvants are components added to vaccines to "nonspecifically" boost the rate, magnitude, format, or quality of the immune response. They are a key aspect of modern vaccine development and have been a major focus of vaccine research and development over the past 2 decades. Despite these advances, many questions remain regarding the precise molecular

Disclosure: A.J. Young is Chief Technical Officer and Founder of Medgene Labs, an Immunological Services Provider based in Brookings, South Dakota. Funded by USDA AES Animal Health Project SD00A676 to A. J. Young.
Department of Veterinary and Biomedical Sciences, South Dakota State University, Box 2175, ARW168F, Brookings, SD 57006, USA
E-mail address: alan.young@sdstate.edu

mechanisms underlying adjuvant function, and further research will help to uncover new areas where adjuvant formulations can further target vaccine function to meet the needs of modern agriculture.

This review discusses the role of adjuvants in vaccination, molecular mechanism of action, commercially relevant adjuvants for use in ruminants, and future needs with direct focus on the US Animal Agriculture industry and regulatory framework. It is important to clarify that, just as with the component antigens found in commercial vaccines, trade secrets are closely held regarding the development of adjuvant technology in veterinary vaccines. With few exceptions, the technologies discussed in this review focus on those general adjuvant formulations that are in use in the field, commercially available "standalone" adjuvants, and adjuvants under experimental development in the literature. The goal is to provide a greater understanding of the capabilities and limits of adjuvant formulations in terms of practical field use, especially as related to the health of production ruminants. Key aspects of the history of adjuvant development and importance geared to specific vaccine formulations, an overall outline of known adjuvant "functions" in boosting vaccine effectiveness, known adjuvant mechanisms of action, and new developments in adjuvant research are discussed.

WHAT ARE ADJUVANTS, AND HOW DO THEY WORK?

The beginning of the modern age of vaccination is generally traced back to the work of Jenner, when he recognized that the process of exposing individuals to the cowpox virus resulted in protection from the lethal effects of smallpox infection.[6] In this early stage, pustules of the cowpox virus were used to directly inoculate individuals who then developed mild local reactions that resulted in "immunity" to infection against later exposure to the smallpox agent. Despite this breakthrough, this technology was not generally used until Pasteur discovered that the observation could be extended to many more agents, particularly in the veterinary world.[7] Pasteur had been doing experiments on chickens and their susceptibility to the causative agent of chicken cholera, and noticed that when chickens were inoculated with "old" cultures, these cultures not only lacked the virulence of fresh isolates, but chickens that had been exposed to these early "attenuated" organisms were then protected against later infection with the virulent agent. In effect, Pasteur had developed the first modified live attenuated vaccine. Through the work of Pasteur and Jenner, the basic concepts of vaccination had been developed and formed the basis of the field of vaccination for control of infectious disease.

Briefly, the process of vaccination is designed to provide "safe" exposure to infectious agents to prepare the immune system for later encounter with the virulent agent. This capitalizes on the 2 primary aspects of the immune system: specificity for individual agents and memory to provide lasting protection against these agents. The work of Jenner used a closely related virus—cowpox—to "prime" the immune system into recognizing not only the cowpox virus but also the closely related smallpox virus.[6] The work of Pasteur used a weakened "strain" to provide a weakened exposure to the immune system, expanding and enhancing the immune response for later encounter with the more deadly organism.[7] Both are examples of "modified live" or "attenuated" vaccines. Currently, live vaccines are commercially available to treat a variety of cattle diseases, including many agents associated with bovine respiratory disease complex.[8,9] These attenuated vaccines have the advantage that they actively "simulate" a virulent infection, replicate (to a limited extent) in the vaccinated animal, generate both a cellular and antibody-based response (as appropriate), and induce both specific and innate immune protective mechanisms. It is this ability to mimic natural infection that can lead to the "early" onset of immunity associated with live vaccines compared with killed or subunit approaches. Unfortunately, the development and licensing of "safe" attenuated live vaccines is a complex process and can potentially exacerbate outbreaks in the field through reversion to virulence or field recombination with circulating strains that ultimately results in greater disease.[10] The simpler and more widespread means of developing specific vaccines for use in animals therefore involves the use of "killed" or "inactivated" products, which require the use of adjuvants to be fully effective. This includes both licensed products as well as traditional autogenous vaccine production.

Although Jenner and Pasteur laid the groundwork for vaccination as a means of widespread specific disease protection, it was not until the work of Gaston Ramon, a veterinarian, that the importance of adjuvants was recognized.[3,4] Ramon recognized that production of specific horse antisera was increased when animals developed an abscess at the injection site. When he injected nonspecific inflammatory stimulants such as starch, breadcrumbs, or tapioca, he significantly increased antibody production. In complementary work, Alexander Glenny and others are credited with identifying the immune-enhancing effects of aluminum salts.[5,11] As a result of this work, aluminum salts were added to human vaccines in 1932 and remained the only adjuvant in licensed human products for 70 years. A key component of this recognition of the importance of adjuvants in vaccination and the enhancement of the immune response was that the results, as defined by increased protection or other increased response, were independent of any understanding of the molecular mechanisms. Simply put, they increased the immune response as measured by vaccination outcome, but specific information on the method whereby they accomplished this task was completely unknown. Despite the great degree of knowledge that has been acquired in the past 15 years, adjuvant-induced enhancement mechanisms remain unclear and the adjuvant formulations in widespread commercial use have not changed significantly. A current challenge is to use our knowledge of these mechanisms of action to bring more effective, targeted adjuvants to the veterinary vaccine market.

MECHANISMS OF ADJUVANT FUNCTION

Although it had been recognized for some time that a key component of adjuvant function was a general increase in local inflammation, specific mechanisms associated with this enhancement remained unclear. The 1970s saw an explosion in our understanding of immunology, including identification of the role(s) of B cells and T cells, mechanisms associated with antibody and T cell receptor specificity, identification of the regulatory and signaling function of cytokines, and the importance of antigen-presenting cells (dendritic cells) in regulating the immune response.[12–14] The key components associated with adjuvant function are discussed in the following.

Physical Regulation of Antigen Release

In general, traditional formulations such as alum or Freund adjuvants are believed to boost immune response through a combination of physical, chemical, and molecular means.[4] Most adjuvants promote immune responses through a combination of these factors, which together act to increase, prolong, and enhance exposure of the immune system and hence optimize the vaccine. The first, and most recognized means to enhance immune activation is through establishing a local "antigen depot" at the site of injection, which leads to an extended release of antigen to stimulate the local lymph node over an extended period, rather than through a "burst" of antigen exposure.[15] This prolonged antigen exposure was generally accomplished through the use of oil-based adjuvants. However, newer technologies to produce molecular "hydrogels" similar to that promoted through aluminum salts have also shown efficacy.[16–18] At a simple level, the "antigen-depot" effect is believed to simulate the well-known enhancement of immune responses associated with multiple "prime/boost" 2-dose vaccination protocols.

Enhanced Response to Antigen Exposure

In an effort to explain the basis of how the immune response is initiated, Matzinger and colleagues[19] proposed the "Danger Hypothesis".[20] This hypothesis stated that specific signals within the innate immune system determine whether a foreign body initiates tissue damage or is an innocuous agent that can effectively be ignored. Although this hypothesis largely restated the long-held recognition that the innate and acquired immune systems cooperatively respond to protect the organism, it did lead to the identification and characterization of the role of pattern recognition receptors (including the Toll-like receptors [TLRs]) and their role in initiating and regulating immune responses.[11,21–24] Over the past 20 years, a significant amount of basic research has been focused on the use of TLR stimulants to act as molecular adjuvants that can be used to enhance immune responses in the absence of specific tissue damage. Although their use has proven to be more complex than initially hoped, several of these agents have been shown to effectively boost the production of specific antibody and T cells.

Regulation of the Quality of the Immune Response

Although the identification of pattern recognition receptors helped to explain the initiation of the response, additional work has since been performed to define how the response evolves.[21,25–30] This has led to our understanding of the regulation of the qualitative aspects of the response and notably the well-characterized "polarization" of the response that dictates the relative production of specific antibody subtypes, as well as the relative production of antibody versus T cells.[31] In the late 1900s, it became clear that individual antibody subtypes performed unique role(s) in combating infection, although the mechanisms regulating their generation remained unclear.[32] With the discovery of the role of T cells and dendritic cells in the immune response, researchers isolated specific cell-associated and soluble factors (cytokines) that dictated the generation of IgM, IgG, IgA, or IgE specific antibodies or alternatively the selective production of cytotoxic T cells.[33] Based on this work, translational research to adapt this knowledge to the generation of rationally constructed adjuvants is underway.[34]

UNIQUE CONSIDERATIONS OF VETERINARY ADJUVANTS

Although it can safely be assumed that development of adjuvants for veterinary and human use follow the same general principles, the ultimate targeting and focus of development of veterinary adjuvants is subject to constraints different from those used in human medicine. In humans, the primary focus of adjuvant development is to enhance the response to the vaccine, limit associated pathology in the vaccinated individual, and provide protection lasting years after vaccination. Cost is rarely a factor in determination of effective adjuvants for human use. In contrast, adjuvants for use in food animals provide greater latitude in terms of duration of immunity and local tissue responses but are subject to much greater cost restrictions than those developed for human medicine. This has therefore led to the interesting situation whereby more vaccines are currently licensed for use in animal species than in humans.[9] Unfortunately, many of the new technologies published in research journals are unsuitable for use in food animals because of excessive cost, although future research may lead to optimized methods to produce these adjuvants for ruminants. At the present time, commercial adjuvants found in veterinary vaccines generally fall into several categories, including aluminum-based salts, oil-based adjuvants, saponins, immunostimulants, and nanoparticle-based delivery systems.[3,5,31] The mechanism of action, availability, and limitation of these adjuvants for commercial vaccine production are discussed in the following.

BASIC OUTLINE OF THE IMMUNE RESPONSE RELATED TO ADJUVANT TARGETING

The overall function of any adjuvant is to enhance the final immune response to a given vaccine. In general, this enhancement can occur due to a shortening in the time of onset, an increase in total response (antibody or T cells), or influence the quality of the response in terms of antibody isotype, cellular response, or a combination of both. The potential "checkpoints" that can be affected by adjuvant are outlined in terms of a simplified immune response to injected vaccine.

Modified live vaccines generally behave in a manner similar to the live, virulent organism and are therefore slightly different and generally do not require strong adjuvants. The focus of this review, therefore, is on the application of adjuvants to killed, nonreplicating vaccines. When a vaccine is injected, the target antigen is initially encountered at the injection site. The first encounter is generally with the innate immune system, either through complement activation or (more commonly) with antigen-presenting cells such as macrophages or dendritic cells. Uptake of the antigen is regulated by nonspecific recognition processes, and the resulting response, including secretion of intracellular signals, initiates the local inflammatory response. The antigen is then transported to the regional lymph node by the dendritic cell or free in the draining lymph, where it concentrates in the lymphoid regions of the node.[35] Dendritic cells "digest" the protein antigen, which is then presented to T cells as short peptides. These activated T cells then serve to "regulate" the resulting B cell response. B cells, in contrast, recognize whole, unprocessed antigen based on the 3-dimensional conformation. Once activated, responding B cells are stimulated and guided by interaction with T cells to produce large amounts of IgM antibody. Eventually, depending on the type of T cell response that is generated, some of the B cells begin to shift to production of IgG, IgA, or IgE antibody associated with memory. These antibodies are then released from the lymph node, where they can be detected as a serum antibody. This antibody, therefore, is associated with protection from infection and generally recognized as a "serum neutralizing" antibody. If a second vaccine dose is given, the same process takes place, with the exception that large amounts of IgG, IgA, or IgE are produced more rapidly after injection.

The primary steps in this process that can be adjusted through the use of adjuvant include (1) provision of a long-term source of vaccine antigen at the injection site through an "antigen-depot" effect; (2) specific enhancement of targeting of antigen to dendritic cells or B cells to promote earlier and stronger immune responses; (3) regulation of signaling of dendritic cells or T cells to affect the quality of the resulting response through specific generation of T cells or B cells secreting IgG, IgA, or IgE, respectively; and (4) focusing on the generation of strong immunologic memory to potentiate the immune response. Currently licensed or developing technologies relevant to adjuvant function in ruminants are discussed in the context of each adjuvant formulation (**Table 1**).

Table 1
Outline of adjuvant methodologies in use or in development for ruminants

	Examples	Mechanism of Action		
		Antigen Depot	Immune Activation	APC Targeting
Adjuvants in use				
Aluminum salts	Alum Aluminum hydroxide Aluminum phosphate Potassium alum	✓		
Emulsions				
Oil/water	Emulsigen (MVP) Montanide ISA 15A VG (Seppic)	✓	✓	
Water/oil	Freund incomplete Freund complete MF59 Montanide ISA 61 VG (Seppic) Montanide ISA 50 V2 (Seppic)	✓	✓	
Water/oil/water	Montanide ISA 201 VG (Seppic) Montanide ISA 206 VG (Seppic) ELANCO Montanide ISA 207 VG (Seppic)	✓	✓	✓
Saponins	Quil A QS-21			✓
In development				
Immunostimulants	CpG Poly I:C CAF09 IL-18 (DNA vaccines) Flagellin		✓	✓
Molecular adjuvants	CD40L C3b motifs			✓
Delivery systems	Nanoparticles Microparticles Liposomes Exosomes			✓

Abbreviation: APC, antigen-presenting cell.

ADJUVANT FORMULATIONS IN WIDESPREAD COMMERCIAL USE
Aluminum Salts

The first adjuvants licensed for use were derived from aluminum compounds and remain a staple in human vaccinology.[5,11,31,36] Basically, aluminum salts were found to increase the titer of antibody when combined with nonreplicating antigen, and due to the relatively simple formulation, continue to be used in both human and veterinary medicine. The 3 primary compounds that have been found to have adjuvant activity are aluminum hydroxide, aluminum phosphate, and alum, which differ in their basic chemistry, usefulness, and ability to boost vaccine responses.[37,38] Despite their widespread and historical use in the field, their precise mechanism of action remains unclear. However, potential mechanisms include creating an antigen depot, increased uptake by antigen-presenting cells, and activation of the innate immune system through proinflammatory pathways.[39] The antigen-depot effect, unlike emulsion-based adjuvants, seems to be based on the ability of aluminum hydroxide–based adjuvant particles to adsorb antigens to the surface, while retaining all antigenic characteristics.[39] Following uptake by antigen-presenting cells, the antigen is released slowly where it prolongs antigen exposure to the immune system and specifically activates a known molecular component of inflammation termed the "NLRP3 inflammasome".[40] In addition to these activities, aluminum hydroxide is widely used in veterinary vaccines for its capacity to bind and inactivate bacterial endotoxins, thereby reducing risk of negative reactions in autogenous vaccine products.[41] One key limitation to aluminum salt adjuvants is their sensitivity to freezing, whereby adjuvanticity and endotoxin-absorbing characteristics are eliminated.[3] In addition, these adjuvant formulations may have adverse tissue reactions, such as erythema, nodules, contact hypersensitivity, and granulomas.[39] More importantly, despite their relative safety and long history of use, aluminum salts tend to be relatively weak adjuvants relative to emulsion-based approaches.

Emulsion-Based Adjuvants

Following the characterization of aluminum salt adjuvants, emulsions were found to induce highly effective immune responses. The most widely recognized adjuvant used in research is Freund adjuvant, formulated as Freund incomplete adjuvant (FIA), which is an emulsification of oil and water, or Freund complete adjuvant (FCA), which contains *Mycobacteria bovis*.[42] In the absence of the mycobacteria, Freund adjuvants are largely believed to affect antigen release and exposure to the immune system, and the formation of "antigen depot". Although Freund adjuvant is not licensed for commercial use in veterinary species due to the significant local tissue effects, oil and water emulsions modeled on this formulation are in widespread use in vaccines for agricultural animals using a variety of oils and emulsification techniques (see **Table 1**). The most common emulsions used as adjuvants are oil in water (O/W), water in oil (W/O), and water-in-oil-in-water (W/O/W) emulsions. Their characteristics and use are described in the following, however the most important considerations in the development of these adjuvants are (1) droplet size of the water or oil droplets; (2) antigen concentration in each phase of the emulsion, particularly the W/O/W emulsions; and (3) choice of oils and surfactants to promote good emulsification that is stable for extended periods of time.

Oil in Water

O/W emulsions are formed when oil droplets are contained within a continuous water phase. Antigen is generally dissolved within the water phase, with the oil phase promoting antigen-presenting cell activation. Briefly, the oil droplets are believed to stimulate the activation of innate immune cells to recruit immune cells to the site of injection, increasing inflammatory activation and therefore the overall immune response.[43] Commercially, several formulations are available and in use for veterinary species, including MF59, the Montanide ISA adjuvants from Seppic, and Emulsigen (MVP Laboratories). The primary value of these types of adjuvants seems to lie in stimulation of strong immune responses against viral antigens, particularly compared with aluminum-based adjuvants.[44]

Water in Oil

W/O emulsions involve a dispersion of water droplets in an excess of oil, whereby soluble antigen is largely contained within the water droplets surrounded by the oil, and therefore slowly released to the surrounding tissue and immune system as the oil dissipates.[45] This significantly increases the duration of release of antigen to the immune system, potentiating the exposure and increasing the immune response. Freund adjuvants, both FIA and FCA, fall into this category, and because of their highly effective mechanism of action, they are a "standard" in research for defining target antigen efficacy. There are also commercially available W/O emulsions based on mineral oil or squalene that are available for research purposes, or already licensed for use in food animals (Seppic, France). These adjuvants demonstrate highly effective immune responses, without the associated tissue damage of FCA.[46,47]

Water/Oil/Water

To optimize the characteristics of O/W and W/O emulsions, investigators have developed W/O/W emulsions.[48] In these emulsions, water droplets are formed inside oil droplets, which are then dispersed in a solid aqueous solvent. Antigen is therefore dispersed both inside the inner water droplets encased with oil, providing the "antigen-depot" effect of W/O emulsions, and within the aqueous outer phase, providing immediate antigen delivery. The end result is that antigen delivery occurs in 2 "phases," similar to a traditional prime/boost injection, and the oil droplets also stimulate innate immune cell interactions. These emulsions are more difficult to formulate, and therefore only a few W/O/W emulsions are available on the market, including Montanide ISA 201 and 206 products from Seppic. Although these emulsions are also somewhat less stable than simpler W/O and O/W formulations, they have been shown to demonstrate significant effectiveness and provide protection with a variety of antigens of livestock.[49–51]

IMMUNOSTIMULANTS

One key aspect of adjuvant activity is to mimic the innate inflammation associated with infection to promote strong T cell and antibody responses. Over the past 20 years, it has become clear that this so-called danger signal is a result of interaction of cell-surface receptors on cells with "patterns" associated with pathogens or tissue destruction, so-called pattern recognition receptors.[21,27,28,30,36,52] These agents that are recognized by the pattern recognition receptors include fungal, bacterial, and viral components, as well as byproducts of cell and tissue destruction. One of these families of receptors, the TLRs, has been highly researched in veterinary science for adjuvant activity. When stimulated by their ligands, these receptors promote cellular activation, increased phagocytic activity, and production of soluble factors that provide downstream stimulation for T and B cells. Despite the explosion in research regarding the use of TLR agonists in veterinary vaccine development, relatively few have shown promise as standalone adjuvants. Bacterial CpG oligonucleotides, recognized by TLR9, have been used in numerous vaccine development trials and reported to stimulate strong cellular immune responses.[53–56] Specific oligonucleotide sequences similar to those found in bacteria are required to bind to the TLR9 receptor and have been shown to be effective adjuvants. Despite this fact, CpG has not been widely incorporated into commercial products. Flagellin, a TLR5 agonist, has also been used in the development of cattle vaccines and demonstrated to promote strong IgA responses in cattle.[23] This interesting observation allows the possibility of developing injectable vaccines that would specifically target mucosal immunity. Additional TLR agonists that have been used in veterinary vaccine trials and have demonstrated some efficacy include byproducts of normal infection, including poly I:C (which mimics zymogen-activated plasma), CAF09, and peptidoglycans. To date, these agents have not been developed as commercial adjuvants.

MOLECULAR ADJUVANTS

As more information became available regarding the molecular processes that regulate the stepwise activation of immune cells, and their ultimate function, specific techniques to stimulate these processes in acquired immune cells were investigated. Briefly, most of these techniques involved either the specific engineering of activation motifs within the target antigen or inclusion of stimulating molecules within the final formulation. One of the earliest discoveries was that protein sequences associated with complement activation in the target antigen enhanced antibody production by B cells.[57–59] In addition, sequences targeting antigen directly to the antibody receptor on B cells also enhance B cell activation and antibody production. Although this technique showed promise, inclusion of these sequences in commercial vaccines has yet to be realized. A final target for this approach is soluble molecules that directly stimulate surface activation molecules of T cells and B cells. In general, these are believed to lower the signaling threshold of immune cells, reducing the level of antigen required and enhancing immunity. One example is the inclusion of the CD40L molecule in vaccine formulations. The CD40/CD40L interaction on B cells is responsible for promoting B cell activation and class switching of immunoglobulins. In several studies, the addition of CD40L to vaccinated antigen has been demonstrated to enhance B cell responsiveness, as well as the development of specific T cells.[34,60] Although these approaches are prolific in basic research, they have not been used to date in veterinary vaccines.

DELIVERY SYSTEMS

A final approach to increase immune responses is to target the enhanced delivery of targets to antigen-presenting cells. Briefly, this involves enhancing the uptake of target antigen by antigen-presenting cells to initiate the immune response through physical means. The first method that was developed to accomplish this was the generation of "virus-like particles", or VLPs.[61–64] VLPs are basically small, virus-like particles that contain surface proteins similar to a target virus but do not possess any nucleic acids. These particles have been found to enhance targeting of antigen to the immune system and thereby increase immune responses. More recently, bacterial versions of these VLPs have been developed, termed "bacterial ghosts."[65,66] Investigators have also simulated the effects of these VLPs and bacterial ghosts through chemical particles that encapsulate antigen, thereby increasing uptake and antigenicity.[67] These techniques include the use of polymers, such as poly(lactic-co-glycolic acid), inulin, or lipids, to form nanoparticles that contain antigen.[68–72] Regardless of the methodology, the efficacy of this approach depends entirely on the relatively small size (frequently <50 nm) of the particles, their ability to effectively carry antigen to the phagocytic cells, and their degradability by innate immune cells. The primary limitation of chemical encapsulation of antigen lies in the large amount of antigen loss encountered during formulation, which renders the technology expensive and less suited for veterinary applications. Methods to directly target encapsulation with limited antigen loss will lead to increased usage of this technology.

FUTURE DIRECTIONS/NEEDS

As more information becomes available regarding the mechanism of adjuvant function, the focus should be on developing advanced "programming" of adjuvant formulations to support the development of next-generation approaches. Key aspects that should be an area of focus are to develop effective adjuvants to target current problems. First, adjuvants should be developed that support single-dose vaccination strategies for inactivated vaccines. Although current adjuvants do, to some extent, support single-dose approaches, booster vaccinations also provoke significantly increased responses, illustrating a need for improvement. Adjuvants that accomplish these same antibody titers with a single dose should be a focus. A second focus should be on extending the duration of immunity with single-dose adjuvants to support the development of lasting immunologic memory. This is particularly true of cattle, because the expected lifespan is significantly longer than other agricultural species, and cattle would therefore benefit from less-frequent need for vaccination. A final, and more difficult focus, would be development of adjuvant technologies to produce immunity in the face of maternal antibody. Specific vaccination technologies to provide neonatal protection during the period that colostral or maternal immunity is waning, in the face of maternal antibody, would be of significant value in all agricultural species. Techniques to develop this approach would necessarily involve the use of technology developed to vaccinate against antiself epitopes, and would therefore borrow extensively from human tumor biology.

REFERENCES

1. Voigt EA, Kennedy RB, Poland GA. Defending against smallpox: a focus on vaccines. Expert Rev Vaccines 2016;15(9):1197–211.
2. Greenwood B. The contribution of vaccination to global health: past, present and future. Philos Trans R Soc Lond B Biol Sci 2014;369(1645):20130433.
3. Burakova Y, Madera R, McVey S, et al. Adjuvants for animal vaccines. Viral Immunol 2018;31(1):11–22.
4. Apostolico Jde S, Lunardelli VA, Coirada FC, et al. Adjuvants: classification, modus operandi, and licensing. J Immunol Res 2016;2016:1459394.
5. Di Pasquale A, Preiss S, Tavares Da Silva F, et al. Vaccine adjuvants: from 1920 to 2015 and beyond. Vaccines (Basel) 2015;3(2):320–43.
6. Riedel S. Edward Jenner and the history of smallpox and vaccination. Proc (Bayl Univ Med Cent) 2005;18(1):21–5.
7. Collins WJ. M. Pasteur's experiments with chicken-cholera. Lancet 1880; 116(2988):913.
8. Meeusen EN, Walker J, Peters A, et al. Current status of veterinary vaccines. Clin Microbiol Rev 2007;20(3):489–510.
9. USDA-APHIS. Veterinary biological products: licensees and permittees. Ames (IA): USDA; 2019.
10. Jang G, Kim JA, Kang WM, et al. Endemic outbreaks due to the re-emergence of classical swine fever after accidental introduction of modified live LOM vaccine on Jeju Island, South Korea. Transbound Emerg Dis 2019;12(10):13121.
11. Powell BS, Andrianov AK, Fusco PC. Polyionic vaccine adjuvants: another look at aluminum salts and polyelectrolytes. Clin Exp Vaccine Res 2015;4(1):23–45.
12. Matthyssens G, Hozumi N, Tonegawa S. Somatic generation of antibody diversity. Ann Immunol (Paris) 1976;127(3–4):439–48.
13. Yanagi Y, Yoshikai Y, Leggett K, et al. A human T cell-specific cDNA clone encodes a protein having extensive homology to immunoglobulin chains. Nature 1984;308(5955):145–9.
14. Steinman RM, Cohn ZA. Identification of a novel cell type in peripheral lymphoid organs of mice. I. Morphology, quantitation, tissue distribution. J Exp Med 1973; 137(5):1142–62.

15. McKee AS, Marrack P. Old and new adjuvants. Curr Opin Immunol 2017;47: 44–51.
16. Giang Phan VH, Duong HTT, Thambi T, et al. Modularly engineered injectable hybrid hydrogels based on protein-polymer network as potent immunologic adjuvant in vivo. Biomaterials 2019;195:100–10.
17. Noh HJ, Noh YW, Heo MB, et al. Injectable and pathogen-mimicking hydrogels for enhanced protective immunity against emerging and highly pathogenic influenza virus. Small 2016;12(45):6279–88.
18. Adams JR, Haughney SL, Mallapragada SK. Effective polymer adjuvants for sustained delivery of protein subunit vaccines. Acta Biomater 2015;14:104–14.
19. Matzinger P. An innate sense of danger. Semin Immunol 1998;10(5):399–415.
20. Pradeu T, Cooper EL. The danger theory: 20 years later. Front Immunol 2012; 3:287.
21. Werling D, Jungi TW. TOLL-like receptors linking innate and adaptive immune response. Vet Immunol Immunopathol 2003;91(1):1–12.
22. Basto AP, Leitao A. Targeting TLR2 for vaccine development. J Immunol Res 2014;2014:619410.
23. Tahoun A, Jensen K, Corripio-Miyar Y, et al. Functional analysis of bovine TLR5 and association with IgA responses of cattle following systemic immunisation with H7 flagella. Vet Res 2015;46:9.
24. Bilgen N, Kul BC, Offord V, et al. Determination of genetic variations of toll-like receptor (TLR) 2, 4, and 6 with next-generation sequencing in native cattle breeds of Anatolia and Holstein Friesian. Diversity (Basel) 2016;8(4):23.
25. Jann OC, King A, Corrales NL, et al. Comparative genomics of Toll-like receptor signalling in five species. BMC Genomics 2009;10:216.
26. Bagheri M, Zahmatkesh A. Evolution and species-specific conservation of toll-like receptors in terrestrial vertebrates. Int Rev Immunol 2018;37(5):217–28.
27. Ishengoma E, Agaba M. Evolution of toll-like receptors in the context of terrestrial ungulates and cetaceans diversification. BMC Evol Biol 2017;17:54.
28. Liu G, Zhang L, Zhao Y. Modulation of immune responses through direct activation of Toll-like receptors to T cells. Clin Exp Immunol 2010;160(2):168–75.
29. Mukherjee S, Huda S, Babu SPS. Toll-like receptor polymorphism in host immune response to infectious diseases: a review. Scand J Immunol 2019;90(1):e12771.
30. Jungi TW, Farhat K, Burgener IA, et al. Toll-like receptors in domestic animals. Cell Tissue Res 2011;343(1):107–20.
31. Del Giudice G, Rappuoli R, Didierlaurent AM. Correlates of adjuvanticity: a review on adjuvants in licensed vaccines. Semin Immunol 2018;39:14–21.
32. Cyster JG, Allen CDC. B cell responses: cell interaction dynamics and decisions. Cell 2019;177(3):524–40.
33. Junttila IS. Tuning the cytokine responses: an update on interleukin (IL)-4 and IL-13 receptor complexes. Front Immunol 2018;9:888.
34. Martin C, Waghela SD, Lokhandwala S, et al. Characterization of a broadly reactive anti-CD40 agonistic monoclonal antibody for potential use as an adjuvant. PLoS One 2017;12(1):e0170504.
35. Young AJ. The physiology of lymphocyte migration through the single lymph node in vivo. Semin Immunol 1999;11(2):73–83.
36. Gavin AL, Hoebe K, Duong B, et al. Adjuvant-enhanced antibody responses in the absence of toll-like receptor signaling. Science 2006;314(5807):1936–8.
37. Bowersock TL, Martin S. Vaccine delivery to animals. Adv Drug Deliv Rev 1999; 38(2):167–94.

38. Gupta RK. Aluminum compounds as vaccine adjuvants. Adv Drug Deliv Rev 1998;32(3):155–72.
39. He P, Zou Y, Hu Z. Advances in aluminum hydroxide-based adjuvant research and its mechanism. Hum Vaccin Immunother 2015;11(2):477–88.
40. Harte C, Gorman AL, McCluskey S, et al. Alum activates the bovine NLRP3 inflammasome. Front Immunol 2017;8:1494.
41. Shi Y, HogenEsch H, Regnier FE, et al. Detoxification of endotoxin by aluminum hydroxide adjuvant. Vaccine 2001;19(13–14):1747–52.
42. Dvorak AM, Dvorak HF. Structure of Freund's complete and incomplete adjuvants. Relation of adjuvanticity to structure. Immunology 1974;27(1):99–114.
43. O'Hagan DT, Ott GS, De Gregorio E, et al. The mechanism of action of MF59 - an innately attractive adjuvant formulation. Vaccine 2012;30(29):4341–8.
44. Wack A, Baudner BC, Hilbert AK, et al. Combination adjuvants for the induction of potent, long-lasting antibody and T-cell responses to influenza vaccine in mice. Vaccine 2008;26(4):552–61.
45. Herbert WJ. The mode of action of mineral-oil emulsion adjuvants on antibody production in mice. Immunology 1968;14(3):301–18.
46. Khorasani A, Madadgar O, Soleimanjahi H, et al. Evaluation of the efficacy of a new oil-based adjuvant ISA 61 VG FMD vaccine as a potential vaccine for cattle. Iran J Vet Res 2016;17(1):8–12.
47. Faburay B, Lebedev M, McVey DS, et al. A glycoprotein subunit vaccine elicits a strong Rift Valley fever virus neutralizing antibody response in sheep. Vector Borne Zoonotic Dis 2014;14(10):746–56.
48. Bozkir A, Hayta G. Preparation and evaluation of multiple emulsions water-in-oil-in-water (w/o/w) as delivery system for influenza virus antigens. J Drug Target 2004;12(3):157–64.
49. Petermann J, Bonnefond R, Mermoud I, et al. Evaluation of three adjuvants with respect to both adverse effects and the efficacy of antibody production to the Bm86 protein. Exp Appl Acarol 2017;72(3):303–15.
50. Khalifa ME, El-Deeb AH, Zeidan SM, et al. Enhanced protection against FMDV in cattle after prime-boost vaccination based on mucosal and inactivated FMD vaccine. Vet Microbiol 2017;210:1–7.
51. Aziz-Boaron O, Leibovitz K, Gelman B, et al. Safety, immunogenicity and duration of immunity elicited by an inactivated bovine ephemeral fever vaccine. PLoS One 2013;8(12):e82217.
52. Coscia MR, Giacomelli S, Oreste U. Toll-like receptors: an overview from invertebrates to vertebrates. Invertebrate Surviv J 2011;8(2):210–26.
53. Nichani AK, Mena A, Kaushik RS, et al. Stimulation of innate immune responses by CpG oligodeoxynucleotide in newborn lambs can reduce bovine herpesvirus-1 shedding. Oligonucleotides 2006;16(1):58–67.
54. Nichani AK, Mena A, Popowych Y, et al. In vivo immunostimulatory effects of CpG oligodeoxynucleotide in cattle and sheep. Vet Immunol Immunopathol 2004;98(1–2):17–29.
55. Ioannou XP, Griebel P, Mena A, et al. Safety of CpG oligodeoxynucleotides in veterinary species. Antisense Nucleic acid Drug Dev 2003;13(3):157–67.
56. Ioannou XP, Griebel P, Hecker R, et al. The immunogenicity and protective efficacy of bovine herpesvirus 1 glycoprotein D plus Emulsigen are increased by formulation with CpG oligodeoxynucleotides. J Virol 2002;76(18):9002–10.
57. Barrington RA, Zhang M, Zhong X, et al. CD21/CD19 coreceptor signaling promotes B cell survival during primary immune responses. J Immunol 2005;175(5):2859–67.

58. Diaz de Stahl T, Dahlstrom J, Carroll MC, et al. A role for complement in feedback enhancement of antibody responses by IgG3. J Exp Med 2003;197(9):1183–90.
59. Gonzalez SF, Kuligowski MP, Pitcher LA, et al. The role of innate immunity in B cell acquisition of antigen within LNs. Adv Immunol 2010;106:1–19.
60. Pujol J, Bouillenne F, Farnir F, et al. Generation of a soluble recombinant trimeric form of bovine CD40L and its potential use as a vaccine adjuvant in cows. Vet Immunol Immunopathol 2015;168(1–2):1–13.
61. Watanabe S, Iizuka T, Hatama S, et al. Production of highly immunogenic virus-like particles of bovine papillomavirus type 6 in silkworm pupae. Vaccine 2017; 35(43):5878–82.
62. Celma CC, Stewart M, Wernike K, et al. Replication-deficient particles: new insights into the next generation of bluetongue virus vaccines. J Virol 2017;91(1) [pii:e01892-16].
63. Forzan M, Maan S, Mazzei M, et al. Generation of virus like particles for epizootic hemorrhagic disease virus. Res Vet Sci 2016;107:116–22.
64. Alshaikhahmed K, Roy P. Generation of virus-like particles for emerging epizootic haemorrhagic disease virus: towards the development of safe vaccine candidates. Vaccine 2016;34(8):1103–8.
65. Hajam IA, Dar PA, Appavoo E, et al. Bacterial ghosts of *Escherichia coli* drive efficient maturation of bovine monocyte-derived dendritic cells. PLoS One 2015; 10(12):e0144397.
66. Marchart J, Rehagen M, Dropmann G, et al. Protective immunity against pasteurellosis in cattle, induced by *Pasteurella haemolytica* ghosts. Vaccine 2003; 21(13–14):1415–22.
67. Mahony D, Mody KT, Cavallaro AS, et al. immunisation of sheep with bovine viral diarrhoea virus, E2 protein using a freeze-dried hollow silica mesoporous nanoparticle formulation. PLoS One 2015;10(11):e0141870.
68. Cruz LJ, Tacken PJ, Eich C, et al. Controlled release of antigen and Toll-like receptor ligands from PLGA nanoparticles enhances immunogenicity. Nanomedicine (Lond) 2017;12(5):491–510.
69. Cooper PD. Vaccine adjuvants based on gamma inulin. Pharm Biotechnol 1995; 6:559–80.
70. Cooper PD, Steele EJ. The adjuvanticity of gamma inulin. Immunol Cell Biol 1988; 66(Pt 5–6):345–52.
71. Kumar S, Kesharwani S, Kuppast B, et al. Discovery of inulin acetate as a novel immune-active polymer and vaccine adjuvant: synthesis, material characterization, and biological evaluation as a Toll-like receptor-4 agonist. J Mater Chem B 2016;4:7950–6.
72. Kumar S, Tummala H. Development of soluble inulin microparticles as a potent and safe vaccine adjuvant and delivery system. Mol Pharm 2013;10(5):1845–53.

Genetic and Epigenetic Regulation of Immune Response and Resistance to Infectious Diseases in Domestic Ruminants

Mehdi Emam, DVM[a,b],*, Alexandra Livernois, PhD[a],
Marlene Paibomesai, PhD[c], Heba Atalla, PhD[a], Bonnie Mallard, PhD[a,b]

KEYWORDS

- Genetic • Epigenetic • Disease • Resistance • Resilience • Tolerance
- Immunocompetence • Ruminants

KEY POINTS

- Infection with a pathogen does not always result in disease, but infectious diseases are the outcome of interactions among 3 factors: host, pathogen, and environment. Several layers of sophisticated interactions between host and pathogens have been a major limiting factor in decoding and identifying the genetic rules of disease resistance.

- Different research groups have used different strategies to dissect this complex network and to understand the genetic rules of diseases resistance. These strategies can be grouped based on the genetic information examined (eg, candidate genes, pedigree-based genetic information, and genome-wide studies) and the phenotypic information available (eg, single-disease, immunocompetence, and reductionist models).

- Recent technological advances are helping researchers to generate big data sets of the host-pathogen-environment interactions. Nonetheless, defining the relevant phenotypes seems to be the main challenge to reveal the genetic blueprint of disease resistance.

- The possibility of negative genetic correlations in resistance to 2 pathogens (eg, intracellular vs extracellular organisms), even those causing the same disease (eg, the many diverse organisms causing bovine mastitis or pneumonia), or negative associations between resistance to a pathogen with important production traits, are other challenges to the single-disease approach, as well as other approaches to selecting for health.

Continued

Disclosures: None.
[a] Department of Pathobiology, Ontario Veterinary College, University of Guelph, 50 Stone Road East, Guelph, Ontario N1G 2W1, Canada; [b] Department of Animal Biosciences, Center for Genetic Improvement of Livestock, University of Guelph, 50 Stone Road East, Guelph, Ontario N1G 2W1, Canada; [c] Ontario Ministry of Agriculture and Rural Affairs, 1 Stone Road W, Guelph, Ontario N1G 4Y2, Canada
* Corresponding author. Department of Pathobiology, Ontario Veterinary College, University of Guelph, 50 Stone Road East, Guelph, Ontario N1G 2W1, Canada.
E-mail address: semam@uoguelph.ca

Vet Clin Food Anim 35 (2019) 405–429
https://doi.org/10.1016/j.cvfa.2019.07.002
0749-0720/19/© 2019 Elsevier Inc. All rights reserved.

Continued

- An alternative method to scrutinize these complex interactions is to simplify the main interaction network into subsystems that can be examined in detail using in vitro methods. In any subsystems, the genetic control requires the contribution of a smaller number of genes, which may simplify the genetic pathways examined. Although reductionist models can reveal potential genes and pathways important for further examination to host defense, they may not fully reflect the intricacies of in vivo disease resistance.

INTRODUCTION

During disease outbreaks, some individuals in a population are more resistant to infection than others. Resistant individuals may survive, whereas others in the population may die or have less severe signs of disease, or may completely eliminate the infection without showing clinical signs of disease. Infection with a pathogen does not always result in disease, but, when it does, infectious diseases are the outcome of interactions among 3 factors: host, pathogen, and environment.[1–3] Each of these factors has been examined in many studies that aimed to reduce the occurrence (increase resistance or resilience) or soften the impact of infection on the host (increase tolerance) (**Box 1**). Among the factors mentioned earlier, the host (or specifically the host immune system) has gained tremendous recognition because of its direct role in protecting the host against pathogens and also the possibility of genetic improvement of this system. However, several layers of sophisticated interactions between host and pathogens have been a major limiting factor in decoding and identifying the genetic rules of disease resistance.[4] The first layer is the functional complexity of the immune system. The immune system is an intricate network of cells and molecules that applies various strategies to protect the host against a broad range of pathogens.[5,6] These strategies range from nonspecific physical barriers to specific cytotoxic activity of lymphocytes. Innate defenses classically initiate immune responses; adaptive immune responses follow if innate mechanisms are not successful to eliminate the pathogen. Cells of the innate

---

Box 1
Resistance, resilience, and tolerance

These terms have varied definitions in the literature, but, for the purpose of this article, the following definitions are applied. Disease resistance is defined as the ability of the host to control the infection passively (eg, absence of a target receptor) or actively (ie, mounting the protective immune responses).[5] The resistant animals can clear the pathogen, entirely. Resilience is the ability of the host to recover after a disease.[144] Resistance and resilience are closely related but not interchangeable. Resilience is always an active phenomenon, whereas resistance could be passive because of the absence of the target receptor. Resilience can also be defined through the overall performance of the host in the face of general environmental challenges, not only in the face of disease. These challenges include, but are not limited to, weaning, handling, moving to a new feedlot, and disease. Livestock may cope with these challenges via physiologic, behavioral, and also immune responses. Various studies have shown that the performance of immune response at the time of challenge can be a good indicator of the overall resilience of the animal in future.[49] The current livestock management practices make it possible to measure all components of resilience to predict the overall performance in future. Tolerance is the ability of the host to cope with the presence of the pathogen. Tolerant animals can maintain their production in the face of pathogenic infection.[5]

immune system mainly recognize microbe-associated molecular patterns via pathogen recognition receptors. Following recognition, they attempt to destroy the pathogen, which is followed by sending activating signals to the adaptive immune system. Cells of the adaptive immune system generate pathogen-specific responses. Although immune responses generally follow the pathways mentioned earlier, multifunctionality of cells and molecules, numerous subpopulations of cells, redundancy in responses, and various exceptions to the general rules are a few examples that increase the complexity of immune system.[4,7] For instance, $\gamma\delta$ T cells, a subpopulation of T cells, belong to the adaptive immune system but can also act like cells of innate defense. These cells are prominent (50%–60% of lymphocytes) in circulating blood in the early life in ruminants, but their population decreases with age (5%–25% of circulating T lymphocytes). Nonetheless, the percentage of $\gamma\delta$ T cells among lymphocytes, even in adult ruminants, is higher than in humans and mice (1%–5%). These cells originate from lymphocyte progenitors but are not antigen (Ag) specific and do not need to recognize Ags in the context of major histocompatibility complex (MHC) molecules. Bovine $\gamma\delta$ T cells have both inflammatory and regulatory activities. Cattle $\gamma\delta$ T cells respond within a few hours of viral infection (similar to innate responses) by producing large amounts of interferon-γ (IFN-γ; a proinflammatory cytokine) or interleukin (IL)-10 (a regulatory cytokine) following exposure to antigen-presenting cells.[8,9] The proportion and functional capacity of these cells show individual variation among cattle genetically selected for immune responsiveness.[10]

Another layer of immunologic complexity relates to the genetic control of immune responses. Approximately, 20% of the bovine genome (ARS-UCD1.2, ENSEMBL 95) is annotated with the immune response.[11] This portion is composed of 5369 genes that are directly involved in mounting immune responses. High-throughput technologies have shown expression of up to 71.4% of the bovine genome in one cell type, the macrophage, after exposure to a pathogen. Compared with the unchallenged control, approximately 245 to 574 genes are differentially expressed.[12] Given the possible nonadditive effects (epistatic and dominance) and epigenetic mechanisms, the genetic control of immune response is astonishingly complex.

A third layer of genetic complexity is caused by the pathogen evolving during an infection. For instance, viral pathogens are well known to escape the immune response through genetic mutations (eg, antigenic shift and drift in influenza viruses) or stabilize themselves in the host via inserting their genome in the host genome, (eg, bovine leukemia virus). This phenomenon potentially results in multistrain infection in 1 host or 1 population during an outbreak.

In this article, recent advances in genetic and epigenetic regulation of immunocompetence and disease resistance in domesticated ruminants are discussed. Moreover, because of the importance of climate change, recent studies of gene-by-environment effects on the regulation of host defense are also discussed.

GENETIC REGULATION OF IMMUNOCOMPETENCE AND DISEASE RESISTANCE

Recent technological advances have helped researchers to generate big data sets of the host-pathogen-environment interactions. Nonetheless, defining the relevant phenotypes seems to be the main challenge in revealing the genetic blueprint of disease resistance.[13,14] Various research groups have used different strategies to dissect this complex network and to understand the genetic rules of diseases resistance. These strategies can be grouped based on the genetic information (candidate genes, pedigree-based, and genome-wide studies) and the phenotypic information (single-disease, immunocompetence, and reductionist models) (**Table 1**). The advantages and pitfalls of each strategy are discussed here.

Source of Genetic Information: Candidate Gene, Genome-Wide, or Pedigree

The main difference between a candidate-gene versus a genome-wide approach is the goal of the study: the candidate gene approach is hypothesis driven, whereas the genome-wide approach is discovery based. The hypothesis in the candidate-gene approach is based on a previously established biological link or association between the candidate gene and the health trait. In most cases, the candidate gene has a strong biological and well-defined role in the pathway of pathogenesis or the protective immune response. However, this information, which is the basis of the new hypothesis on the gene of interest, has usually been proved in other species or the magnitude of its effect has not been measured on the specific disease (type I studies) or immune response (type II studies) (see **Table 1**).

Genes of the MHC are arguably the most studied health trait genes in ruminants, as well as other species. One of the first reports of an MHC polymorphism and its association with immune response was from a study in guinea pigs published in 1975.[15] The genetic polymorphism within the bovine MHC known as the bovine lymphocyte antigen (BoLA) system was first reported in 1979.[16] Since then, the association of BoLA with many infectious and metabolic diseases, as well as characteristics of immunity, has been the subject of numerous studies.[17–23] Despite the extensive studies on BoLA, the findings have rarely been commercially used in breeding programs because of the inverse association with different pathogens and between types of immune responses.[23] An exception was specific BoLA DRB-3 and DQB alleles being used to reduce bovine dermatophilosis from 0.76 to 0.02 in Brahman-Zebu cattle on the island of Martinique.[24] This approach worked well because the disease was highly prevalent in a well-contained population of cattle.

The genome-wide association and pedigree-based studies are descriptive studies designed to discover novel associations (type V and VI studies) or to estimate breeding values for individuals in the population (type III and IV studies) (see **Table 1**). The genome-wide genetic information can be combined with pedigree information to increase the reliability of breeding value estimates by accounting for polygene effects. These estimates are known as genomic breeding values,[25] which are currently being used by breeding companies, such as the Semex Alliance, to improve accuracy of selection for various traits, including for Immunity+. However, the findings of genome-wide association studies should be validated (eg, using candidate gene studies), and the findings of pedigree-based studies only hold within the population

Table 1
Classification of studies on genetic control of immune response and resistance to infectious disease based on genetic and phenotypic information

		Genetic Polymorphism		
		Candidate Gene	Pedigree	Genome-wide
Phenotype	Single Disease	Type I	Type III	Type V
	Immunocompetence	Type II	Type IV	Type VI

The pedigree information can be used alone, or it can be added to the genome-wide study to account for polygenic effects. The pedigree information can also be used to select samples in candidate gene approaches to maximize the diversity of the samples.

or the breed of the studied population, depending on the structure of the sample population.[26]

In genetic association studies, single nucleotide polymorphisms (SNPs) have been the primary source of genetic information used to identify variation between individuals. Over the past decade, technological advances in sequencing and bioinformatics have provided other sources of genetic information, mainly structural polymorphisms at the genomic, epigenomic, and transcriptomic levels (**Box 2**).[27] These structural variants are novel and remain expensive to detect. Therefore, the studies on ruminants using structural polymorphism are limited. Copy number variation (CNV) and splicing variants are two types of novel polymorphisms that have been reported in cattle, water buffalo, sheep, and goat.[28–31] Studies on the association of the structural variants mentioned earlier with health traits in ruminants are rare. However, there is a limited number of reports on the association of CNVs with bovine clinical mastitis, somatic cell score, and resistance to gastrointestinal nematodes in cattle and resistance to retroviral infection in sheep.[32–35] The methods to detect structural variants and the challenges in their application in breeding have been reviewed by Bickhart and Liu.[36]

Source of Phenotypic Information: Single Disease or Immunocompetence

In the single-disease approach, the goal is to identify alleles (type I studies) or to estimate genetic variance components (type III and V studies) by comparing animals classified as resistant, resilient, or tolerant to a disease or syndrome following infection (natural or experimental challenge) with animals classified as susceptible. Any type of investigation of the genetic regulation of immune response and disease resistance needs a large sample size. The sample size required to achieve adequate statistical power can be ambiguously estimated using the predicted number of quantitative trait loci (QTLs) that control the trait, minor allele frequency of QTLs, the threshold to detect QTL effects, effective population size, and estimated environmental effects.[37,38] Although environmental effects can be controlled or removed in experimental challenges, this type of study in large ruminants (ie, to investigate the genetic control of disease resistance) is less feasible because of the space needed for the containment facility and the high cost to study a large sample population. These limitations have led some researchers to choose case-control studies following natural infection as the most feasible approach to study the genetic control of health traits in ruminants.[39] The most critical step in case-control studies is to accurately define the phenotype and assign the samples to the appropriate class. During natural infections, the time of occurrence of the infection, the dose of infection, and any prior exposure to the pathogen are often unknown factors. Therefore, animals might be classified

---

Box 2
Novel sources of genetic variation

Copy number variation (CNV). CNV is a type of structural variation defined as a segment of DNA (more than 1 kb) with more than 1 copy in the genome. These segments have undergone inversion, deletion, or duplication mutations, but the sequences of these segments are very similar to each other. These segments are called copy number polymorphism when their frequency in the population is more than 1%.[145]

Spicing variants. During messenger RNA (mRNA) maturation, intron segments are removed from pre-mRNA, and exons are joined together. Through this process, alternative combination of exons and residues of introns can result in different variants of a mature mRNA, called splicing variants. The association of splicing variants and mastitis has been reported in cattle.[146,147]

incorrectly. For instance, one individual might be classified as resistant but was not exposed to the pathogen, or the animal might have been previously exposed and developed immunologic memory. These types of errors can potentially introduce prominent experimental "noise," resulting in an inability to detect QTLs with small effects or rare alleles. However, when the mortality of a disease is very high (eg, highly pathogenetic avian influenza) or the genetic defect is lethal (eg, bovine leukocyte adhesion deficiency [BLAD]) the study noise does not obscure identifying cases and controls. Therefore, identification of genetic regulation at the level of causal mutation is feasible. For instance, BLAD was found to be caused by a mutation on the cluster of differentiation (CD) 18 gene that encodes an adhesion molecule (β2 integrin) on the leukocytes surface causing major defect in phagocytosis, chemotactic response, and other normal functions of neutrophils.[40] In investigating the genetic regulation of diseases with lower mortality or morbidity rate, the study noise must be carefully considered in case-control studies and modified designs are being proposed for complex diseases, such as bovine mastitis.[41]

Genetic regulation of resistance to complex diseases, such as clinical and subclinical mastitis, Johne disease, lameness, calf diarrhea, bovine leukosis, bovine tuberculosis, and helminth infestations, are the subject of numerous investigations by using the single-disease approach. The heritabilities of these traits are low compared with production and immune response traits (**Table 2**). Therefore, the genetic gain will be slow depending on selection intensity.[42]

Table 2
Heritabilities of health traits in cattle

Health Trait	Heritability	References
Disease Resistance		
Clinical mastitis	0.02–0.04	Govignon-Gion et al,[148] 2016; Koeck et al,[149] 2014
Subclinical mastitis	0.04–0.06	Narayana et al,[150] 2018
Johne disease	0.04–0.06	Brito et al,[151] 2018; Kirkpatrick & Lett,[152] 2018
Lameness	0.01–0.09	Chapinal et al,[153] 2013; Koeck et al,[149] 2014
Bovine leukosis	0.08	Abdalla et al,[154] 2013
Bovine tuberculosis	0.10	Raphaka et al,[51] 2018
Nematode infestation	0.06–0.23	Passafaro et al,[155] 2015
Immunocompetence		
Cell-mediated immune response	0.18	Mallard et al,[156] 2018
Natural antibody	0.27–0.31	de Klerk et al,[65] 2018
Specific antibody response	0.46	Emam et al,[157] 2014
Cellular Traits		
Percentage of CD4+ lymphocytes	0.46	Denholm et al,[73] 2017
Percentage of CD8+ lymphocytes	0.41	Denholm et al,[73] 2017
Percentages of monocytes	0.15	Denholm et al,[73] 2017
Percentages of monocytes	0.42	Denholm et al,[73] 2017
In vitro nitric oxide response of bovine monocyte-derived macrophages	0.78	Emam et al[75]

Additional challenges to the single-disease approach, as well as other approaches to selecting for health, are introduced by the possibility of negative genetic correlations in resistance to 2 pathogens, even those causing the same disease (eg, the many diverse pathogens that cause bovine mastitis or pneumonia), or negative associations between resistance to a pathogen and important production traits. Mahmoud and colleagues[43] investigated the genetic correlation between 9 calf and 14 cow pathogens/diseases. In addition to a strong favorable correlation between resistance to the most common causal agents of mastitis (*Escherichia coli* and *Staphylococcus aureus*), they also reported negative correlations between rotavirus and chorioptic scabies, and between *E coli* and daily weight gain in calves.[43] Rupp and colleagues[23] reported similar negative associations in relation to mastitis, somatic cell count, and immune response traits. However, other studies have not shown these negative associations.[44–46] For example, breeding for enhanced immunity in cattle has not been associated with any notable negative impact on production, growth, or reproduction.[47–50] This lack of association may be caused by overall better health minimizing any decreases in feed intake caused by illness or beneficial shared genes that control a range of fitness traits.

It is possible to define customized breeding programs to increase genetic resistance to disease by combining epidemiologic data on the common pathogens in any geographic location with the results of single-disease approaches. Bovine tuberculosis (bTB) is a significant threat to the cattle industry globally and a distressing problem in the United Kingdom, where the carrier of the pathogen, badgers, are protected by law. Nonetheless, Raphaka and colleagues[51] predicted that the risk of transmission of bTB between the herd mates can be reduced by 50% in 6 generations by selecting the top 25% of bTB-resistant sires (heritability of 0.1). Improving resistance to subclinical mastitis by reducing the somatic cell score in dairy cows has been used for decades. In addition, Scandinavian countries have been selecting for improved resistance to clinical mastitis, and more recently this has been added in Canada and the United States as other examples of the commercially available programs to improve health in dairy cattle.[26] In March 2016, Zoetis Inc introduced a Wellness Trait Index (WT$) on their Bovine Clarifide Plus SNP chip into the United States as part of their genomics program. The index includes genomic information on combined health traits, including mastitis, retained placenta, metritis, displaced abomasum, ketosis, lameness, and polled. In Canada, the Canadian Dairy Network offers a similar combined health index.[52] The limitation of these indices relates to the accuracy of disease event recording and the low heritability of these traits. In 2018, the Semex Alliance began to offer a genomics test for immunocompetence as part of their Elevate program. Rather than being based on lowly heritable clinical scoring data, the genomics test for immunity is based on direct measurements of the more highly heritable information on both antibody-mediated and cell-mediated immune responses, which control responses to a wide range of bacterial and viral pathogens.

Improvement of immunocompetence (also known as overall immune responsiveness) is another approach to increase resistance against infectious diseases. The rationale behind the immunocompetence approach is the beneficial direct link between the type and magnitude of an immune response with protection of the host. This approach makes sense because the immune system is the body's defense against infectious disease and cancer. The idea of selection based on immune response traits dates back to Biozzi and colleagues[53] in 1972 and the mouse model they generated. These mice are currently known as the ABH strain.[54] Biozzi selected these mice for many generations for increased antibody and decreased cellular responses to investigate the genetic regulation of susceptibility and resistance to infectious diseases. In livestock, the idea was first introduced in the late twentieth century and continued research led to the first commercially available health index for dairy cattle in 2013, based on their immunocompetence.[6] Improving the overall immune responsiveness provides the opportunity for resistance to a broad range of pathogens when heritable, well-balanced, and broad-based aspects of immunity are contained within the selection index. Simultaneously, responses to vaccines have been reported to improve, and, in ruminants, their colostrum contains higher amounts of immunoglobulin (Ig) to protect their newborns.[48,6,55] Cows classified as having superior immunocompetence have a lower occurrence of various diseases, such as mastitis, metritis, and pneumonia.[6] This finding is true both in research and commercial application.[56] Also, as mentioned earlier, this approach has not been found to adversely affect production or reproductive traits of dairy cattle.[56,57]

The main challenge in the immunocompetence approach is to develop methods to measure immune responses that can reflect the overall performance of this complex system. The immune system is composed of an integrated network of innate and adaptive immune responses. The antibody-mediated and cell-mediated immune responses are the effector mechanisms of the adaptive immune system. Measuring serum antibody as the indicator of antibody-mediated immune response is accurate, inexpensive, and technically simple. However, defining an index to measure antibody-mediated and cell-mediated immune responses, as well as capture innate cellular responses, is much more challenging. The cell-mediated response can be evaluated by measuring T-cell cytotoxicity, interferon-γ, delayed-type hypersensitivity (DTH), or other measures of T-cell effector functions.[58,59] Although there are various methods to capture these T-cell responses, they are generally not as simple, cost-effective, or as accurate as measuring antibody. One of the advantages of measuring DTH is that it involves a variety of important leukocyte populations (neutrophils, macrophages, dendritic cells, and natural killer cells) from the innate system, as well as T and B lymphocytes from the adaptive immune system that are involved in mounting the DTH response.[60] Not surprisingly, the genetic control of this response is complex and involves many genes on various chromosome. The results of genome-wide association studies of serum antibody and DTH responses in dairy cattle show the differences in the genetic control of these two responses. Two major QTLs on chromosomes 21 and 23 are associated with antibody response to a type II antigen, whereas associations of SNPs with DTH are scattered over the entire bovine genome. Both traits are under polygenic control, but the nature of that control differs. To date, studies indicate that the heritability of antibody-mediated response is about 2-fold larger than the heritability of DTH response in dairy Holsteins[58] (see **Table 2**). This difference may simply be caused by the large number of leukocyte populations involved in DTH or the difficulty of accurately measuring this response in vivo. Nonetheless, the heritability estimates for both of these immune response traits are moderately high at 0.18 to 0.46, which is more than those for clinical scores of diseases. This difference is partly caused by the immune system directly controlling host defense and disease outcome, whereas clinical scores are an indirect indicator of the host response. For this reason, in 1999 Wilkie and Mallard[61] proposed that heritable adaptive immune responses measured after exposure to carefully selected nonpathogenic antigens can reflect general immunocompetence and be used in a selection index based on estimated breeding values to improve animal health (**Fig. 1**). From a technical point of view, this method is similar to a highly controlled experimental challenge because the background response, the dose of antigen, and the time duration from exposure to the test antigens to sample collection are fully controlled. Moreover, the added benefit of this test method compared with an experimental disease challenge is that

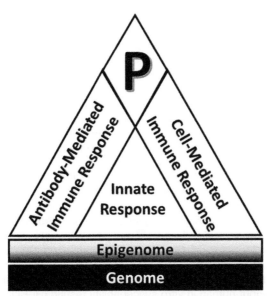

Fig. 1. In 1999, Wilkie and Mallard[61] proposed that the overall performance of the immune system (phenotype [P]) is shaped by adaptive immune responses, including cell-mediated immune responses and antibody-mediated immune responses. Because innate responses initiate adaptive immune responses, adaptive immune responses can reflect the performance of innate defenses. Furthermore, all of these responses are coded by immune response genes in the host genome that can be influenced by the epigenome. (*Adapted from* Wilkie B, Mallard B. Selection for high immune response: an alternative approach to animal health maintenance? Vet Immunol Immunopathol. 1999;72(1-2):231-235. http://www.ncbi.nlm.nih.gov/pubmed/10614513; with permission.)

there is no need for a containment facility because of the nonpathogenic characteristics of the test antigens.[62] These controlled factors result in high heritability of these health traits (see **Table 2**).

Measuring innate host defense can be more challenging than adaptive immune responses because of their varied mechanisms of action, broad specificity, and assorted tissue locations. Measuring innate cellular responses in vivo is very difficult, except for some limited measures in birds (eg, measuring macrophage phagocytosis using carbon clearance test).[63,64] In contrast, humoral innate responses, such as natural antibodies (NAbs), are simpler to measure, and their roles in disease resistance have been well studied in ruminants. NAbs, produced mainly from B1 lymphocytes, are present in the body before exposure to any foreign antigens and are classified as one of the humoral innate responses.[65] NAb provides one of the first barriers to infection. Binding to the pathogen, activating the complement system, and facilitating phagocytosis are the effector mechanisms that are mediated by NAb.[66] Studies on the genetic regulation of IgM and IgG NAbs have shown these as heritability traits in dairy cattle (see **Table 2**). The genes that control specific adaptive antibody responses versus NAb differ, indicating that these are distinct traits, each making unique contributions to defense of the host.[65,67]

Reductionist models
As mentioned previously, disease pathogenesis is the outcome of a highly complex set of interactions between host, pathogen, and environment. An alternative method

to scrutinize these complex interactions is to simplify the main interaction network into subsystems that can be examined in detail using in vitro methods. In any subsystems, genetic control requires the contribution of a smaller number of genes. These genes and their mechanisms of action can, in some cases, be studied in fully controlled in vitro environments in which infectious dose and virulence of the pathogen are set by the investigator.[68] Therefore, the chance of detecting QTLs with smaller effects or discovering causal mutations is higher than with other approaches. The other advantage of the reductionist model is the smaller sample size needed for these types of studies.[37] The downside of using reductionist models to study the complexity of disease resistance is that focusing on a single subsystem in vitro might be misleading. These in vitro models may not represent the in vivo condition, or their effect on the in vivo system might be small. Therefore, the results of the reductionist models should subsequently be evaluated on the in vivo outcome of host-pathogen-environment interactions.

The reductionist concept to study the genetic control of disease resistance was first introduced in 2009 by Ko and colleagues[69] and later was reviewed in a 2014 publication entitled "The Marriage of Quantitative Genetics and Cell Biology: A Novel Screening Approach Reveals People Have Genetically Encoded Variation in Microtubule Stability."[68] Dennis Ko and his colleagues have developed an in vitro model, called high-throughput human in vitro susceptibility testing (Hi-HOST), to screen the response of B lymphocytes followed by a genome-wide association study to investigate host-pathogen interactions. Using the Hi-HOST model, in 2017 they discovered an association between *VAC14*, a gene responsible in the metabolism of phosphoinositide, and resistance to *Salmonella enterica* serovar Typhi.[70] In 2018, an independent study on an African population found the association of the same gene with bacteremia in children.[71,72] These findings represent the potential of the reductionist approach to reveal the genetics rules in resistance to infectious disease.

In dairy cows, the genetic regulation of blood leukocyte proportions was first reported by Denholm and colleagues[73] in 2017, who found the heritability of the percentage of cells from the myeloid and lymphoid lineage in bovine blood ranged from 0.18 to 0.81. However, the researchers did not find any significant associations between these cellular proportions and the infectious diseases they examined.[73] Emam and colleagues[74] studied the effect of host genetics on the function of bovine monocyte-derived macrophages (MDMs) in response to *E coli* and *S aureus*, using a cellular immunogenomic approach in 2018. Using a highly controlled in vitro culture system, they showed a pedigree-based heritability of 0.776 for in vitro nitric oxide production by MDMs against *E coli*.[75] The genome-wide association study on this cellular trait revealed the association of 8 SNPs on chromosome 4, 5, 6, 9, and 27 describing 78% of the phenotypic variation.[76]

Results from reductionist models should be confirmed using other experimental systems. These confirmatory studies can be association studies in an independent population or investigation using genome editing or other appropriate technologies. Inducing disease resistance in ruminants using gene editing has previously been reported. Resistance to *S aureus* in a transgenic cow expressing lysostaphin in epithelial cells of the mammary gland is an example of this approach.[77] At present, new technologies with high efficiency and accuracy in inserting, deleting, or substituting single nucleotides are available. Clustered regularly interspaced short palindromic repeats–associated protein 9 (CRISPR/Cas9) is a tool to edit a specific sequence of the genome with single nucleotide accuracy. Some research groups have reported the successful application of this method in cattle. However, the publications are yet to come because of the long generation interval in cattle and the novelty of the technology.[78] The reductionist models in conjunction with genome editing methods will likely provide the foundation of genetically resistant ruminants in future.

EPIGENETIC CONTROL OF THE IMMUNE SYSTEM IN DOMESTICATED RUMINANTS

Epigenetics is defined as the control of gene expression by mechanisms that do not change the underlying DNA sequence.[79,80] The epigenome can be influenced by environmental factors, including diet, stress, hormones, pathogens, toxins, and drugs, resulting in both permanent and reversible changes to gene expression. The epigenome encompasses all epigenetic modifications, including DNA methylation, histone modifications, and microRNA (miRNA) regulation, which are among the major regulatory elements that dictate chromatin accessibility and gene transcription. The immune system is dynamic and possesses the ability to respond to infection and other stressors while also regulating its own response. Epigenetic modifications regulate gene expression, which drives adaptive and innate immune cell phenotypes, establishing cell memory, cell polarization, and regulation of the immune response.[81]

DNA Methylation

The DNA methylome of the ruminant immune system is influenced by species,[82] tissue and immune cell types,[83–91] disease state,[85,92] stimulation,[93] age,[94] and physiologic event.[83,87,88,93,95–97] Studies investigating the DNA methylation levels and profiles of immune response genes have been performed on immune-associated tissues,[89] specific immune cells,[85,97–99] as well as other non–immune-related tissues[83,86,87,100] in domesticated ruminants species. Studies investigating DNA methylation and the immune system have reported on both the methylation of individual cytokine genes[93,99] and the global DNA methylome.[98] In cattle, CD4+ T-cell polarization depends on expression and secretion of cytokine genes including IFNγ and IL4. Expression and secretion of cytokines by isolated CD4+ T cells showed decreased DNA methylation at the promoter regions of IFNγ and IL4.[93,99] In addition, differential DNA methylation was observed at transcription factors GATA3 and RORC in alveolar macrophages of cattle infected with *Mycobacterium bovis*.[98] In agreement with this observation, examination of MHC-I revealed that DNA methylation of MHC-associated CpG islands are associated with downregulation of MHC-I.[101]

Differentially methylated regions (DMRs) have been identified in cattle using global methylation analysis technologies on different types of immune cells, which are summarized in **Table 3**.[82,85,94,97,98] Evaluation of global DNA methylation can reveal regions of the genome that change in response to a treatment, or that change in a tissue-specific manner. DMRs can differ depending on factors such as the tissue type, comparison of treatments, environmental impacts, and infection. As such, care must be taken when choosing the type of tissue or cell type isolated for DNA methylation analysis. Furthermore, the time of sample collection could affect the presence of DNA methylation or intermediary DNA methylation.[85] Age and diet are also well-known factors that affect global DNA methylation and therefore DMRs.[88,90,91,94] Examination of global DNA methylation in non–immune-related tissues showed an association between decreased DNA methylation at immune-related genes, including TLR4, and increased chromatin accessibility and gene expression in cattle that were fed high-concentrate diets compared with their counterparts that were fed a low-concentrate diet.[95] Overall DNA methylation is associated with transcriptional regulation in ruminants and thus can influence immune cell phenotype and function.

Table 3
Summary of global DNA methylation studies in dairy cattle

Cell Type	Method	Comparison	Number of DMRs	References
CD4+ T lymphocytes	Reduced-representation bisulfite sequencing	M bovis–infected cattle vs noninfected cattle	765 DMR infected vs noninfected cattle	Doherty et al,[98] 2016
Fibroblast	Reduced-representation bisulfite sequencing	Difference between 5 mo and 16 mo of age stimulated with lipopolysaccharide	14,094 DMR (5065 gene regions, 1117 promoters, 1057 gene exons, 2891 gene introns)	Korkmaz & Kerr,[94] 2017
Peripheral blood mononuclear cell	Whole-genome MeDIP-seq	High milk yield and average milk yield	72 DMR high vs average milk yield 252 DMR herd environment	DeChow & Liu,[97] 2018
Alveolar macrophage	Whole-genome bisulfite sequencing	M bovis–infected cattle vs noninfected	0 DMR between infected and noninfected	O'Doherty et al,[85] 2019
Blood cells	Reduced-representation bisulfite sequencing	Creole cattle vs Iberian breeds	334 DMR	Sevane et al,[82] 2019

Abbreviation: MeDIP-seq, methylated DNA immunoprecipitation sequencing.

Histone Modifications

There are limited studies that report on histone modifications in domesticated ruminants, especially in the context of the immune response. Genome-wide assessment of the gene repressor marker, H3K27me3,[102] in bovine peripheral blood lymphocytes identified that this epigenetic mark is predominantly found 2 kb upstream of transcription start sites (TSSs) and in introns.[103] The presence of H3K27me3 at TSSs was generally associated with transcriptional repression for most genes.[103] He and colleagues,[104] investigated the impact of S aureus on H3K27me3 levels in blood mononuclear cells in cattle.[104] Most H3K27me3 was found to be intergenic and 20 kb upstream of TSSs, suggesting it is associated with regulatory factors outside the promoter region, such as enhancers.[104] There was a negative correlation between H3K27me3 and gene expression. In this case, the TSS was a key area of regulation for genes that function in immune-related processes in innate and adaptive immune responses when comparing cows with mastitis with healthy cows.[104] More research is needed to better understand the regulatory role of histone modifications and the histone code in bovine species and how they relate to immunity and immune function.

BOVINE COLOSTRUM AND MILK EXOSOMAL microRNAs

MicroRNAs are abundant in bovine colostrum and milk either free or enclosed within exosomes.[105–107] Notably, immune-related miRNAs are highly expressed in milk, particularly in colostrum, suggesting they are crucial for mammary gland immune regulation as well as promoting development of the calf gut mucosal immune system.[108]

Studies from the Mallard laboratory assessed the bioactivity of bovine colostrum and milk exosomes containing miRNA on gut health. Purified exosomes were noted to have typical phenotypic features similar to those in other body fluids[109] based on size (20–100 nm) and protein markers essential for their interaction with host cells.[110,111] Fluorescently labeled exosomes cocultured with human intestinal epithelial (Caco-2 cells) were taken up and visualized in the vicinity of the nucleus of cultured cells at 2 and 24 hours.[111] Furthermore, colostrum and milk exosomes cocultured with Caco-2 cells were not only noncytotoxic but enhanced cell viability using methylthiazoletetrazolium (MTT) cell proliferation/viability assay. Although both colostrum and milk seem to support Caco-2 cell viability for up to 72 hours, MTT activity was significantly ($P<.0001$) higher in cells cocultured with milk compared with those with colostrum. Furthermore, differences in Caco-2 cells' metabolic activity cocultured with exosomes from cows with different immune response phenotypes was observed. Specifically, metabolic activity after coculture with colostrum and milk exosomes from high immune response cows was significantly greater than those with low immune response exosomes ($P = .0198$). Of note, classification of those cows as high or low immune response was based on estimated breeding values using the patented High Immune Response (HIR) technology. Viability of Caco-2 cells cocultured with either colostrum or milk exosomes from high immune responder cows was significantly greater ($P<.0024$ and $P<.0048$) than that of low responders at 72 hours. A similar observation was reported in porcine milk exosomes.[112]

High-throughput next-generation sequencing of milk exosomal miRNA from average immune responder cows identified 680 mature miRNAs.[110] This study was the first to profile bovine exosomal miRNA isolated by differential ultracentrifugation and report their abundance compared with those identified in bovine milk exosomes by microarray (n = 79[105]) and in porcine milk exosomes (n = 218,[113] n = 491,[114] and n = 234[115]). Similar to the aforementioned studies, immune-related miRNAs, such as miR-148a, let-7 family, miR-21, and miR-26, were highly expressed in the study of cows classified based on their immune response phenotypes.

Important immune-related miRNAs (including miR-148a, miR-155, miR-21, miR-26a, and miR-29b) were also confirmed by quantitative reverse transcription polymerase chain reaction in colostrum and milk exosomes with significantly ($P<.05$) higher expression of miR-155 in colostrum compared with milk exosomes. Further, miR-155, miR-21, miR-26a, and miR-29b were differentially expressed among high and low immune responder cows.[110]

GENE BY ENVIRONMENT EFFECTS ON REGULATION OF IMMUNOCOMPETENCE OF DOMESTICATED RUMINANTS

The environmental component of host-pathogen-environment interactions that dictate disease profiles is discussed next. This area of research is important and topical because the changing climate is affecting livestock health and welfare directly through increased environmental temperatures and drought[116] and indirectly through ecosystem changes that alter the availability of feed resources and the distribution or epidemiology of animal diseases.[117,118] This article defines heat stress (HS) and resilience to climate change and how these factors relate to immunocompetence in domestic ruminants.

Because ruminants are endothermic homeotherms, they can maintain a physiologic body temperature within a certain ambient thermal neutral zone through passive cooling mechanisms (conduction, convection, and radiation).[119] However, when the surrounding ambient temperature is greater than an animal's thermal neutral zone, the animal must expend energy and mobilize body reserves to maintain euthermia through active cooling (sweating and panting).[119,120] In general, cold ambient temperatures are manageable through protective shelters, increasing body size, insulation, and the heat generated through metabolism.[119,120]

Resilience can be defined as the ability of a species to survive and recover from a perturbation.[121] Animals with greater resilience to HS are able to maintain euthermia for longer through heat dissipation before becoming physiologically compromised.[118,122–124] Resilience depends on multiple factors, including region (adaptability), species, breed, sex, and productivity.[117,119] For example, among cattle, an increase in body temperature under HS was less pronounced in Brown Swiss compared with Holstein cows, suggesting that Brown Swiss are more resilient.[125,126] Among dairy animals, goats were identified as the most adapted species to HS in terms of production, reproduction, and disease resistance.[127,128] The question of whether animals more resilient to climate HS can be identified within breed and whether they are more resistant to disease is an area of emerging research.

The temperature-humidity index (THI) has been widely used as an indicator of HS in livestock.[129–131] THI is calculated by combining ambient temperature and humidity (see **Box 1**).[132] Various THI HS thresholds have been estimated, depending on species, breed, and region. For example, estimated THI thresholds for HS in Holstein cows range from 60 (which could correspond with a temperature of 21°C and a relative humidity of 62%; see **Box 1** for calculation of THI) for Holsteins in Germany[133] to 78 for Holsteins in a US subtropical environment.[134] The THI threshold for HS is likely to be higher for animals with lower production rates and for nonlactating animals.[132] Curtis and colleagues[135] used rumen temperature and feed intake to estimate a THI HS threshold of 75.5 for black angus feedlot cattle. Given these diverse ranges for THI thresholds, it is important for studies in various geographic locations to determine the relevant THI thresholds for each study.

Livestock are likely to experience days during the summer months when the THI exceeds their THI HS threshold. HS intensifies when the THI exceeds the threshold for consecutive days because the animal has reduced opportunity to dissipate body heat at night.[136] As an example, analysis of climatic data from a temperate region in southern Ontario, Canada, revealed that livestock frequently experience days, often consecutively, on which the THI HS threshold was likely exceeded (**Fig. 2**).

Stress Responsiveness and Immunocompetence

The environment plays a key role in the nature and outcome of host-pathogen interactions,[137] and it is therefore important to improve understanding of how climate extremes affect animals' responses to pathogens. Furthermore, climate change could induce shifts in the spread and types of diseases to which livestock are exposed.[118] The health and welfare of animals as the climate changes will be dictated in part by their resilience to extreme temperatures as well as their natural resilience to infections agents. As such, it is desirable to select for animals with both enhanced ability to resist disease[49,55,138,139] and superior resilience to HS.

There is evidence for favorable associations between disease resistance and stress responsiveness in livestock.[124] Recently, Aleri and colleagues[49] showed a favorable and significant association between a preferred response to stress and above-average immune competence in Holstein-Friesian and Holstein-Friesian × Jersey heifers. For example, heifers with above-average immune competence had lower serum cortisol concentrations compared with their below-average counterparts, suggesting that they had enhanced ability to cope with management-induced stress.[49] Reduced cortisol production in response to stress is desirable because high

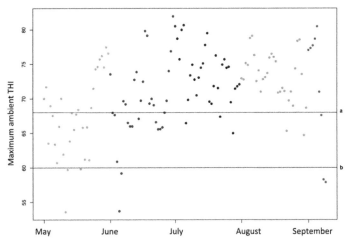

Fig. 2. The THI calculated for the summer months (May to September) of 2018 at a temperate region in southern Ontario, Canada. Suggested THI heat shock thresholds for dairy cows are indicated. [a] Estimated by Zimbelman and colleagues.[132] [b] Estimated by Brügemann and colleagues.[133] (*Data from* Zimbelman RB, Rhoads RP, Collier RJ, Duff GC. A reevaluation of the impact of temperature humidity index (THI) and black globe humidity index (BGHI) on milk production in high producing dairy cows. Proc Southwest Nurr Man Conf. 2009;(January):158-169 and Brügemann K, Gernand E, von Borstel UU, König S. Genetic analyses of protein yield in dairy cows applying random regression models with time-dependent and temperature x humidity-dependent covariates. J Dairy Sci. 2011. https://doi.org/10.3168/jds.2010-4063.)

concentrations can suppress immune function and decrease the ability to cope with stress.[140,141] Because HS also results in increased serum cortisol concentrations,[142,143] it will be informative to investigate associations between immune competence and resilience to HS. For this reason, the Mallard laboratory is investigating the connection between cattle classified based on estimated breeding values of immune responsiveness and their response to HS. Preliminary results indicate substantial individual variation in response to both in vivo and in vitro HS in Holsteins, as well as beef cattle of mixed breeds. Knowledge of the genetic link between resilience to HS and immunocompetence would provide scope for breeding animals that are more resilient to HS and disease for a future with predictions for increased frequency and duration of HS events and changes to the distribution or epidemiology of pathogens.

SUMMARY

Disease resistance has a complex phenotype because of the dynamic interaction between host, pathogen, and environment. Discovering the mechanisms of how the genome shapes this phenotype is an exceptionally complex process with more than 5000 genes controlling host defense. Various strategies that have been used by researchers are limited. Although new technologies and bioinformatic methods are promising to collect and analyze much more complex data, the bottleneck of the investigation seems to be at the starting point: how to accurately translate a biological phenomenon (disease resistance) to a parsable data set. Recently, after decades of researches on the genetic regulation of disease resistance, some technologies became commercially available. However, these technologies are mainly based on association studies and, in some cases, the heritabilities are very low. Therefore, the genetic gain might be limited because of the loss of association over generations or the low heritabilities. Novel strategies and sources of data are required to deepen the current study beyond association, free from study noise, to discover the causal mechanisms with near-perfect heritability to overcome these limitations. Reductionist models, structural variants, and epigenomic research are all examples of novel approaches and source data in an attempt to show the genetic blueprint of disease resistance. It should also be noted that livestock production and health will likely face new challenges with climate change. Emerging or remerging diseases, or the compromised performance of the current traits under environmental stress, such as HS, are just a few examples of the potential future challenges. All these factors warrant further investigation to identify the genetic regulation of disease resistance to improve livestock health now, as well as to be prepared for future challenges.

ACKNOWLEDGMENTS

Contributions from all current and previous staff and students in the Mallard laboratory are gratefully acknowledged. Funding from the Natural Sciences and Engineering Research Council (NSERC), Ontario Ministry of Agriculture and Rural Affairs (OMAFRA) are highly appreciated. This paper is also a contribution to the Food from Thought research program supported by the Canada First Research Excellence Fund. The funders did not have any role in the design, collection, analysis, and interpretation of data and in writing this review paper.

REFERENCES

1. Casadevall A, Pirofski L. Host-pathogen interactions: redefining the basic concepts of virulence and pathogenicity. Infect Immun 1999;67(8):3703–13. Available at: http://iai.asm.org/content/67/8/3703.short.
2. Lazzaro BP, Little TJ. Immunity in a variable world. Philos Trans R Soc Lond B Biol Sci 2009;364(1513):15–26.
3. Casadevall A, Pirofski L-A. What is a host? Incorporating the microbiota into the damage-response framework. Infect Immun 2015;83(1):2–7.
4. Villani A-C, Sarkizova S, Hacohen N. Systems immunology: learning the rules of the immune system. Annu Rev Immunol 2018;36(1):813–42.
5. Bishop SC, Woolliams JA. Genomics and disease resistance studies in livestock. Livest Sci 2014;166:190–8.
6. Mallard BA, Emam M, Paibomesai M, et al. Genetic selection of cattle for improved immunity and health. Jpn J Vet Res 2015;63(Suppl 1):S37–44. Available at: http://www.ncbi.nlm.nih.gov/pubmed/25872325.
7. Chaplin DD. Overview of the immune response. J Allergy Clin Immunol 2010; 125(2):S3–23.
8. Toka FN, Kenney MA, Golde WT. Rapid and transient activation of γδ T cells to IFN-γ production, NK cell-like killing, and antigen processing during acute virus infection. J Immunol 2011;186(8):4853–61.
9. Guzman E, Hope J, Taylor G, et al. Bovine γδ T cells are a major regulatory T cell subset. J Immunol 2014;193(1):208–22.
10. Hine BC, Cartwright SL, Mallard BA. Analysis of leukocyte populations in Canadian Holsteins classified as high or low immune responders for antibody- or cell-mediated immune response. Can J Vet Res 2012;76(2):149–56. Available at: http://www.ncbi.nlm.nih.gov/pubmed/23024458.
11. Zerbino DR, Achuthan P, Akanni W, et al. Ensembl 2018. Nucleic Acids Res 2018;46(D1):D754–61.

12. Casey ME, Meade KG, Nalpas NC, et al. Analysis of the bovine monocyte-derived macrophage response to mycobacterium avium subspecies paratuberculosis infection using RNA-seq. Front Immunol 2015;6:23.

13. Greives TJ, Dochtermann NA, Stewart EC. Estimating heritable genetic contributions to innate immune and endocrine phenotypic correlations: a need to explore repeatability. Horm Behav 2017;88:106–11.

14. Minozzi G, Williams JL, Stella A, et al. Meta-analysis of two genome-wide association studies of bovine paratuberculosis. PLoS One 2012;7(3):e32578.

15. Geczy AF, Geczy CL, de Weck AL. Histocompatibility antigens and genetic control of the immune response in guinea pigs. II. Specific inhibition of antigen-induced lymphocyte proliferation by anti-receptor alloantisera. Eur J Immunol 1975;5(10):711–9.

16. Caldwell J. Polymorphism of the BoLA system. Tissue Antigens 1979;13(5):319–26. Available at: http://www.ncbi.nlm.nih.gov/pubmed/91208.

17. Pokorska J, Kulaj D, Dusza M, et al. The influence of BoLA-DRB3 alleles on incidence of clinical mastitis, cystic ovary disease and milk traits in Holstein Friesian cattle. Mol Biol Rep 2018. https://doi.org/10.1007/s11033-018-4238-0.

18. Hayashi T, Mekata H, Sekiguchi S, et al. Cattle with the BoLA class II DRB3*0902 allele have significantly lower bovine leukemia proviral loads. J Vet Med Sci 2017;79(9):1552–5.

19. Duangjinda M, Jindatajak Y, Tipvong W, et al. Association of BoLA-DRB3 alleles with tick-borne disease tolerance in dairy cattle in a tropical environment. Vet Parasitol 2013;196(3–4):314–20.

20. Leach RJ, O'Neill RG, Fitzpatrick JL, et al. Quantitative trait loci associated with the immune response to a bovine respiratory syncytial virus vaccine. PLoS One 2012;7(3):e33526.

21. Maillard J-C, Berthier D, Chantal I, et al. Selection assisted by a BoLA-DR/DQ haplotype against susceptibility to bovine dermatophilosis. Genet Sel Evol 2003;35(Suppl 1):S193–200.

22. Sharif S, Mallard BA, Wilkie BN, et al. Associations of the bovine major histocompatibility complex DRB3 (BoLA-DRB3) alleles with occurrence of disease and milk somatic cell score in Canadian dairy cattle. Anim Genet 1998;29(3):185–93.

23. Rupp R, Hernandez A, Mallard BA. Association of bovine leukocyte antigen (BoLA) DRB3.2 with immune response, mastitis, and production and type traits in Canadian Holsteins. J Dairy Sci 2007;90(2):1029–38.

24. Maillard J-C, Chantal I, Berthier D, et al. Molecular immunogenetics in susceptibility to bovine dermatophilosis: a candidate gene approach and a concrete field application. Ann N Y Acad Sci 2002;969:92–6.

25. Zhang X, Lourenco D, Aguilar I, et al. Weighting strategies for single-step genomic BLUP: an iterative approach for accurate calculation of GEBV and GWAS. Front Genet 2016;7:151.

26. Weigel KA, VanRaden PM, Norman HD, et al. A 100-year review: methods and impact of genetic selection in dairy cattle-From daughter-dam comparisons to deep learning algorithms. J Dairy Sci 2017;100(12):10234–50.

27. Cui H, Dhroso A, Johnson N, et al. The variation game: cracking complex genetic disorders with NGS and omics data. Methods 2015;79-80:18–31.

28. Liu GE, Van Tassell CP, Sonstegard TS, et al. Detection of germline and somatic copy number variations in cattle. In: Pinard M, Gay C, Pastoret P, et al, editors. Animal genomics for animal health, vol. 132. Basel (Switzerland): KARGER; 2008. p. 231–7.

29. Fontanesi L, Martelli PL, Beretti F, et al. An initial comparative map of copy number variations in the goat (Capra hircus) genome. BMC Genomics 2010; 11(1):639.
30. Jenkins GM, Goddard ME, Black MA, et al. Copy number variants in the sheep genome detected using multiple approaches. BMC Genomics 2016;17(1):441.
31. Liu S, Kang X, Catacchio CR, et al. Computational detection and experimental validation of segmental duplications and associated copy number variations in water buffalo (Bubalus bubalis). Funct Integr Genomics 2019. https://doi.org/10. 1007/s10142-019-00657-4.
32. Szyda J, Mielczarek M, Frąszczak M, et al. The genetic background of clinical mastitis in Holstein-Friesian cattle. Animal 2019;1–8. https://doi.org/10.1017/ S1751731119000338.
33. Xu L, Hou Y, Bickhart DM, et al. A genome-wide survey reveals a deletion polymorphism associated with resistance to gastrointestinal nematodes in Angus cattle. Funct Integr Genomics 2014;14(2):333–9.
34. Durán Aguilar M, Román Ponce SI, Ruiz López FJ, et al. Genome-wide association study for milk somatic cell score in holstein cattle using copy number variation as markers. J Anim Breed Genet 2017;134(1):49–59.
35. Viginier B, Dolmazon C, Lantier I, et al. Copy number variation and differential expression of a protective endogenous retrovirus in sheep. PLoS One 2012; 7(7):e41965.
36. Bickhart DM, Liu GE. The challenges and importance of structural variation detection in livestock. Front Genet 2014;5:37.
37. Kemper KE, Littlejohn MD, Lopdell T, et al. Leveraging genetically simple traits to identify small-effect variants for complex phenotypes. BMC Genomics 2016; 17(1):858.
38. Hayes B, Goddard ME. The distribution of the effects of genes affecting quantitative traits in livestock. Genet Sel Evol 2001;33(3):209–29.
39. Bishop SC, Doeschl-Wilson AB, Woolliams JA. Uses and implications of field disease data for livestock genomic and genetics studies. Front Genet 2012; 3:114.
40. Nagahata H. Bovine leukocyte adhesion deficiency (BLAD): a review. J Vet Med Sci 2004;66(12):1475–82.
41. Biffani S, Del Corvo M, Capoferri R, et al. An alternative experimental case–control design for genetic association studies on bovine mastitis. Animal 2017;11(04):574–9.
42. Moose SP, Mumm RH. Molecular plant breeding as the foundation for 21st century crop improvement. Plant Physiol 2008;147(3):969–77.
43. Mahmoud M, Zeng Y, Shirali M, et al. Genome-wide pleiotropy and shared biological pathways for resistance to bovine pathogens. PLoS One 2018;13(4): e0194374.
44. Stear M, Fairlie-Clarke K, Jonsson N, et al. Genetic variation in immunity and disease resistance in dairy cows and other livestock. Cambridge (United Kingdom): Burleigh Dodds; 2017. p. 509–31. https://doi.org/10.19103/AS. 2016.0006.25.
45. Stefan T, Matthews L, Prada JM, et al. Divergent allele advantage provides a quantitative model for maintaining alleles with a wide range of intrinsic merits. Genetics 2019. https://doi.org/10.1534/genetics.119.302022.
46. Ali AOA, Murphy L, Stear A, et al. Association of MHC class II haplotypes with reduced faecal nematode egg count and IgA activity in British Texel sheep. Parasite Immunol 2019;e12626. https://doi.org/10.1111/pim.12626.

47. Stoop CL, Thompson-Crispi KA, Cartwright SL, et al. Short communication: variation in production parameters among Canadian Holstein cows classified as high, average, and low immune responders. J Dairy Sci 2016;99(6):4870–4.

48. Fleming K, Thompson-Crispi KA, Hodgins DC, et al. Short communication: variation of total immunoglobulin G and β-lactoglobulin concentrations in colostrum and milk from Canadian Holsteins classified as high, average, or low immune responders. J Dairy Sci 2016;99(3):2358–63.

49. Aleri JW, Hine BC, Pyman MF, et al. Associations between immune competence, stress responsiveness, and production in Holstein-Friesian and Holstein-Friesian × Jersey heifers reared in a pasture-based production system in Australia. J Dairy Sci 2019;102(4):3282–94.

50. Aleri JW, Hine BC, Pyman MF, et al. Assessing adaptive immune response phenotypes in Australian Holstein-Friesian heifers in a pasture-based production system1. J Anim Sci 2015;93(7):3713–21.

51. Raphaka K, Sánchez-Molano E, Tsairidou S, et al. Impact of genetic selection for increased cattle resistance to bovine tuberculosis on disease transmission dynamics. Front Vet Sci 2018;5:237.

52. Beavers L, Van Doormaal B. Canadian Dairy Network - Pro$ & LPI: enhancements and updates. Available at: https://www.cdn.ca/document.php?id=516.

53. Biozzi G, Stiffel C, Mouton D, et al. Cytodynamics of the immune response in two lines of mice genetically selected for "high" and "low" antibody synthesis. J Exp Med 1972;135(5):1071–94.

54. Amor S, Smith PA, Hart B, et al. Biozzi mice: of mice and human neurological diseases. J Neuroimmunol 2005;165(1–2):1–10.

55. Wagter LC, Mallard BA, Wilkie BN, et al. The relationship between milk production and antibody response to ovalbumin during the peripartum period. J Dairy Sci 2003;86(1):169–73.

56. Larmer S, Mallard B. High immune response sires reduce disease incidence in North American large commercial dairy populations. Cattle Pract 2016;25(2):74–81.

57. Thompson-Crispi KA, Sewalem A, Miglior F, et al. Genetic parameters of adaptive immune response traits in Canadian Holsteins. J Dairy Sci 2012;95(1):401–9.

58. Thompson-Crispi K a, Sargolzaei M, Ventura R, et al. A genome-wide association study of immune response traits in Canadian Holstein cattle. BMC Genomics 2014;15(1):559.

59. Thomas MG, Marwood RM, Parsons AE, et al. The effect of foetal bovine serum supplementation upon the lactate dehydrogenase cytotoxicity assay: important considerations for in vitro toxicity analysis. Toxicol In Vitro 2015;30(1):300–8.

60. Ramakrishnan L. Revisiting the role of the granuloma in tuberculosis. Nat Rev Immunol 2012;12(5):352–66.

61. Wilkie B, Mallard B. Selection for high immune response: an alternative approach to animal health maintenance? Vet Immunol Immunopathol 1999;72(1–2):231–5.

62. Thompson-Crispi KA, Mallard BA. Type 1 and type 2 immune response profiles of commercial dairy cows in 4 regions across Canada. Can J Vet Res 2012;76(2):120–8.

63. Sarker N, Tsudzuki M, Nishibori M, et al. Cell-mediated and humoral immunity and phagocytic ability in chicken Lines divergently selected for serum immunoglobulin M and G levels. Poult Sci 2000;79(12):1705–9.

64. Cheng S, Lamont SJ. Genetic analysis of immunocompetence measures in a white leghorn chicken line. Poult Sci 1988;67(7):989–95.

65. de Klerk B, Emam M, Thompson-Crispi KA, et al. A genome-wide association study for natural antibodies measured in blood of Canadian Holstein cows. BMC Genomics 2018;19(1):694.

66. Rahyab AS, Alam A, Kapoor A, et al. Natural antibody - Biochemistry and functions. Glob J Biochem 2011;2(4):283–8.

67. Thompson-Crispi KA, Miglior F, Mallard BA. Genetic parameters for natural antibodies and associations with specific antibody and mastitis in Canadian Holsteins. J Dairy Sci 2013;96(6):3965–72.

68. Ko DC, Jaslow SL. The marriage of quantitative genetics and cell biology: a novel screening approach reveals people have genetically encoded variation in microtubule stability. Bioarchitecture 2014;4(2):58–61.

69. Ko DC, Shukla KP, Fong C, et al. A genome-wide in vitro bacterial-infection screen reveals human variation in the host response associated with inflammatory disease. Am J Hum Genet 2009;85(2):214–27.

70. Alvarez MI, Glover LC, Luo P, et al. Human genetic variation in VAC14 regulates Salmonella invasion and typhoid fever through modulation of cholesterol. Proc Natl Acad Sci U S A 2017;114(37):E7746–55.

71. Alvarez MI, Ko DC. Reply to Gilchrist et al.: possible roles for VAC14 in multiple infectious diseases. Proc Natl Acad Sci U S A 2018;115(16):E3604–5.

72. Gilchrist JJ, Mentzer AJ, Rautanen A, et al. Genetic variation in VAC14 is associated with bacteremia secondary to diverse pathogens in African children. Proc Natl Acad Sci U S A 2018;115(16):E3601–3.

73. Denholm SJ, McNeilly TN, Banos G, et al. Estimating genetic and phenotypic parameters of cellular immune-associated traits in dairy cows. J Dairy Sci 2017;100(4):2850–62.

74. Emam M, Tabatabaei S, Canovas A, et al. Cellular immuno-genomics: a novel approach to examine genetic regulation of disease resistance in cattle. Proc World Congr Genet Appl Livest Prod. 2018:738. Available at: http://www.wcgalp.org/proceedings/2018/cellular-immuno-genomics-novel-approach-examine-genetic-regulation-disease.

75. Emam M, Tabatabaei S, Sargolzaei M, et al. The effect of host genetics on in vitro performance of bovine monocyte-derived macrophages. J Dairy Sci, in press.

76. Emam M, Tabatabaei S, Sargolzaei M, et al. Identifying the genetic regions associated with bovine monocyte-derived macrophage nitric oxide production: a cellular genome-wide association study. Proceeding of the second Animal genetics and diseases conference. Wellcome Genome Campus, United Kingdom, May 8–10, 2019.

77. Donovan DM, Kerr DE, Wall RJ. Engineering disease resistant cattle. Transgenic Res 2005;14(5):563–7.

78. Wang Z. Genome engineering in cattle: recent technological advancements. Chromosome Res 2015;23(1):17–29.

79. Felsenfeld G. A brief history of epigenetics. Cold Spring Harb Perspect Biol 2014;6(1):a018200.

80. Allis CD, Jenuwein T. The molecular hallmarks of epigenetic control. Nat Rev Genet 2016;17(8):487–500. https://doi.org/10.1038/nrg.2016.59.

81. Carlberg C, Molnár F. Human Epigenomics. Singapore: Springer; 2018. https://doi.org/10.1007/978-981-10-7614-5.

82. Sevane N, Martínez R, Bruford MW. Genome-wide differential DNA methylation in tropically adapted Creole cattle and their Iberian ancestors. Anim Genet 2019;50(1):15–26.

83. Zhang X, Zhang S, Ma L, et al. Reduced representation bisulfite sequencing (RRBS) of dairy goat mammary glands reveals DNA methylation profiles of integrated genome-wide and critical milk-related genes. Oncotarget 2017;8(70): 115326–44.

84. Wang X, Chen Y, Ma S, et al. Whole-genome bisulfite sequencing of goat skins identifies signatures associated with hair cycling. BMC Genomics 2018; 19(1):1–9.

85. O'Doherty AM, Rue-Albrecht KC, Magee DA, et al. The bovine alveolar macrophage DNA methylome is resilient to infection with Mycobacterium bovis. Sci Rep 2019. https://doi.org/10.1038/s41598-018-37618-z.

86. Couldrey C, Brauning R, Bracegirdle J, et al. Genome-wide DNA methylation patterns and transcription analysis in sheep muscle. PLoS One 2014;9(7):1–7.

87. Frattini S, Capra E, Lazzari B, et al. Genome-wide analysis of DNA methylation in hypothalamus and ovary of Capra hircus. BMC Genomics 2017;18(1):1–9.

88. Wang X, Lan X, Radunz AE, et al. Maternal nutrition during pregnancy is associated with differential expression of imprinted genes and DNA methyltranfereases in muscle of beef cattle offspring. J Anim Sci 2015;93(1):35–40.

89. Zhang Y, Wang X, Jiang Q, et al. DNA methylation rather than single nucleotide polymorphisms regulates the production of an aberrant splice variant of IL6R in mastitic cows. Cell Stress Chaperones 2018;23(4):617–28.

90. Osorio JS, Jacometo CB, Zhou Z, et al. Hepatic global DNA and peroxisome proliferator-activated receptor alpha promoter methylation are altered in peripartal dairy cows fed rumen-protected methionine. J Dairy Sci 2015;99(1):234–44.

91. Lan X, Cretney EC, Kropp J, et al. Maternal diet during pregnancy induces gene expression and DNA methylation changes in fetal tissues in sheep. Front Genet 2013;4:1–12.

92. Fang L, Hou Y, An J, et al. Genome-wide transcriptional and post-transcriptional regulation of innate immune and defense responses of bovine mammary gland to Staphylococcus aureus. Front Cell Infect Microbiol 2016;6:193.

93. Paibomesai MA. Epigenetic influences on bovine T-helper 1 and T-helper 2 cytokines (interferon-gamma and Interleukin-4) in high and low immune responders around the peripartum period. [PhD thesis]. Guelph, Ontario: University of Guelph; 2017.

94. Korkmaz FT, Kerr DE. Genome-wide methylation analysis reveals differentially methylated loci that are associated with an age-dependent increase in bovine fibroblast response to LPS. BMC Genomics 2017;18(1):1–18.

95. Chang G, Zhang K, Xu T, et al. Epigenetic mechanisms contribute to the expression of immune related genes in the livers of dairy cows fed a high concentrate diet. PLoS One 2015;10(4):e0123942.

96. Magee DA, Spillane C, Berkowicz EW, et al. Imprinted loci in domestic livestock species as epigenomic targets for artificial selection of complex traits. Anim Genet 2014;45(SUPPL.1):25–39.

97. Dechow CD, Liu WS. DNA methylation patterns in peripheral blood mononuclear cells from Holstein cattle with variable milk yield. BMC Genomics 2018; 19(1):1–12.

98. Doherty R, Whiston R, Cormican P, et al. The CD4+ T cell methylome contributes to a distinct CD4+ T cell transcriptional signature in Mycobacterium bovis-infected cattle. Sci Rep 2016;6(1):1–15.

99. Paibomesai M, Hussey B, Nino-Soto M, et al. Effects of parturition and dexamethasone on DNA methylation patterns of IFN-γ and IL-4 promoters in CD4+ T-lymphocytes of Holstein dairy cows. Can J Vet Res 2013;77(1):54–62.

100. Zhou Y, Connor EE, Bickhart DM, et al. Comparative whole genome DNA methylation profiling of cattle sperm and somatic tissues reveals striking hypomethylated patterns in sperm. Gigascience 2018;7(5):1–13.

101. Shi B, Thomas AJ, Benninghoff AD, et al. Genetic and epigenetic regulation of major histocompatibility complex class I gene expression in bovine trophoblast cells. Am J Reprod Immunol 2018;79(1):e12779.

102. Wiles ET, Selker EU. H3K27 methylation: a promiscuous repressive chromatin mark. Curr Opin Genet Dev 2017;43:31–7.

103. He Y, Yu Y, Zhang Y, et al. Genome-wide bovine H3K27me3 modifications and the regulatory effects on genes expressions in peripheral blood lymphocytes. PLoS One 2012;7(6). https://doi.org/10.1371/journal.pone.0039094.

104. He Y, Song M, Zhang Y, et al. Whole-genome regulation analysis of histone H3 lysin 27 trimethylation in subclinical mastitis cows infected by Staphylococcus aureus. BMC Genomics 2016;17(1):1–12.

105. Izumi H, Tsuda M, Tsuda M, et al. Bovine milk exosomes contain microRNA and mRNA and are taken up by human macrophages. J Dairy Sci 2015;98(5): 2920–33.

106. Izumi H, Kosaka N, Shimizu T, et al. Bovine milk contains microRNA and messenger RNA that are stable under degradative conditions. J Dairy Sci 2012;95(9):4831–41.

107. Chen X, Gao C, Li H, et al. Identification and characterization of microRNAs in raw milk during different periods of lactation, commercial fluid, and powdered milk products. Cell Res 2010;20(10):1128–37.

108. Liang G, Malmuthuge N, Guan LL, et al. Model systems to analyze the role of miRNAs and commensal microflora in bovine mucosal immune system development. Mol Immunol 2015;66(1):57–67.

109. Yáñez-Mó M, Siljander, Pia R-M, et al. Biological properties of extracellular vesicles and their physiological functions. J Extracell Vesicles 2015;4(1):27066.

110. Atalla H, Mallard B, Karrow NA. Characterization of exosomal immune- related micrornas in colostrum and milk from average, low and high immune responder cows. J Anim Sci 2016;94(suppl_4):74–5.

111. Ross M, Atalla H, Mallard B. Bioactivity of colostrum and milk exosomes containing microrna from cows genetically selected as high, average and low immune responders based on their estimated breeding values. J Anim Sci 2016; 94(suppl_4):65–7.

112. Chen T, Xie M-Y, Sun J-J, et al. Porcine milk-derived exosomes promote proliferation of intestinal epithelial cells. Sci Rep 2016;6(1):1–12.

113. van Herwijnen MJC, Driedonks TAP, Snoek BL, et al. Abundantly present miRNAs in milk-derived extracellular vesicles are conserved between mammals. Front Nutr 2018;5:1–6.

114. Chen T, Xi Q-Y, Ye R-S, et al. Exploration of microRNAs in porcine milk exosomes. BMC Genomics 2014;15(1):100.

115. Gu Y, Li M, Wang T, et al. Lactation-related microRNA expression profiles of porcine breast milk exosomes. PLoS One 2012;7(8):pe43691.

116. Intergovernmental Panel on Climate Change. Climate change 2013 – the physical science basis working group I contribution to the fifth assessment report of the intergovernmental panel on climate change. Cambridge (United Kingdom): Cambridge University Press; 2014.

117. Hoffmann I. Adaptation to climate change–exploring the potential of locally adapted breeds. Animal 2013. https://doi.org/10.1017/S1751731113000815.

118. Rojas-Downing MM, Nejadhashemi AP, Harrigan T, et al. Climate change and livestock: impacts, adaptation, and mitigation. Clim Risk Manag 2017;16: 145–63.

119. Collier RJ, Baumgard LH, Zimbelman RB, et al. Heat stress: physiology of acclimation and adaptation. Animal Front 2018;9(1):12–9.

120. Nienaber JA, Hahn GL. Livestock production system management responses to thermal challenges. Int J Biometeorol 2007. https://doi.org/10.1007/s00484-007-0103-x.

121. Williams SE, Shoo LP, Isaac JL, et al. Towards an integrated framework for assessing the vulnerability of species to climate change. PLoS Biol 2008. https://doi.org/10.1371/journal.pbio.0060325.

122. Das R, Sailo L, Verma N, et al. Impact of heat stress on health and performance of dairy animals: a review. Vet World 2016;9(3):260–8.

123. Misztal I. Breeding and genetics symposium: resilience and lessons from studies in genetics of heat stress. J Anim Sci 2017;95(4):1780–7.

124. Colditz IG, Hine BC. Resilience in farm animals: biology, management, breeding and implications for animal welfare. Anim Prod Sci 2016. https://doi.org/10.1071/an15297.

125. Johnson HD. Environmental temperature and lactation (with special reference to cattle). Int J Biometeorol 1965. https://doi.org/10.1007/BF02188466.

126. Correa-Calderon A, Armstrong D, Ray D, et al. Thermoregulatory responses of Holstein and Brown Swiss Heat-Stressed dairy cows to two different cooling systems. Int J Biometeorol 2004. https://doi.org/10.1007/s00484-003-0194-y.

127. Silanikove N, Koluman DN. Impact of climate change on the dairy industry in temperate zones: predications on the overall negative impact and on the positive role of dairy goats in adaptation to earth warming. Small Rumin Res 2015. https://doi.org/10.1016/j.smallrumres.2014.11.005.

128. Gantner V, Bobic T, Gantner R, et al. Differences in response to heat stress due to production level and breed of dairy cows. Int J Biometeorol 2017;61(9): 1675–85.

129. Ingraham RH, Gillette DD, Wagner WD. Relationship of temperature and humidity to conception rate of Holstein cows in subtropical climate. J Dairy Sci 1974. https://doi.org/10.3168/jds.S0022-0302(74)84917-9.

130. Ibrahim MN, Stevens DG, Shanklin MD, et al. Model of broiler performance as affected by temperature and humidity. Trans Am Soc Agric Eng 1975;18:960–2.

131. Gaughan JB, Mader TL, Holt SM, et al. Heat tolerance of Boran and Tuli crossbred steers. J Anim Sci 1999. https://doi.org/10.2527/1999.7792398x.

132. Zimbelman RB, Rhoads RP, Collier RJ, et al. A re-evaluation of the impact of temperature humidity index (THI) and black globe humidity index (BGHI) on milk production in high producing dairy cows. Proc Western Dairy Management Conference. Reno, NV, USA. March 9–11, 2009. p. 158–69.

133. Brügemann K, Gernand E, von Borstel UU, et al. Genetic analyses of protein yield in dairy cows applying random regression models with time-dependent and temperature x humidity-dependent covariates. J Dairy Sci 2011. https://doi.org/10.3168/jds.2010-4063.

134. Dikmen S, Hansen PJ. Is the temperature-humidity index the best indicator of heat stress in lactating dairy cows in a subtropical environment? J Dairy Sci 2009. https://doi.org/10.3168/jds.2008-1370.

135. Curtis AK, Scharf B, Eichen PA, et al. Relationships between ambient conditions, thermal status, and feed intake of cattle during summer heat stress with access to shade. J Therm Biol 2017;63:104–11.

136. Garner JB, Douglas ML, Williams SRO, et al. Genomic selection improves heat tolerance in dairy cattle. Sci Rep 2016;6:1–8.

137. Shikano I, Cory JS. Impact of environmental variation on host performance differs with pathogen identity: implications for host-pathogen interactions in a changing climate. Sci Rep 2015. https://doi.org/10.1038/srep15351.

138. Burton JL, Burnside EB, Kennedy BW, et al. Antibody responses to human erythrocytes and ovalbumin as marker traits of disease resistance in dairy calves. J Dairy Sci 1989;72:1252–65.

139. Pighetti GM, Sordillo LM. Specific immune responses of dairy cattle after primary inoculation with recombinant bovine interferon-?? as an adjuvant when vaccinating against mastitis. Am J Vet Res 1996;57(6):819–24.

140. Diez-Fraile A, Meyer E, Burvenich C. Sympathoadrenal and immune system activation during the periparturient period and their association with bovine coliform mastitis. A review. Vet Q 2003. https://doi.org/10.1080/01652176.2003.9695142.

141. Eskandari F, Sternberg EM. Neural-immune interactions in health and disease. Ann N Y Acad Sci 2002. https://doi.org/10.1111/j.1749-6632.2002.tb04198.x.

142. Veissier I, Van laer E, Palme R, et al. Heat stress in cows at pasture and benefit of shade in a temperate climate region. Int J Biometeorol 2018. https://doi.org/10.1007/s00484-017-1468-0.

143. Bharati J, Dangi SS, Mishra SR, et al. Expression analysis of Toll like receptors and interleukins in Tharparkar cattle during acclimation to heat stress exposure. J Therm Biol 2017. https://doi.org/10.1016/j.jtherbio.2017.02.002.

144. Scheffer M, Bolhuis JE, Borsboom D, et al. Quantifying resilience of humans and other animals. Proc Natl Acad Sci U S A 2018;115(47):11883–90.

145. Sharp AJ, Locke DP, McGrath SD, et al. Segmental duplications and copy-number variation in the human genome. Am J Hum Genet 2005;77(1):78–88.

146. Park E, Pan Z, Zhang Z, et al. The expanding landscape of alternative splicing variation in human populations. Am J Hum Genet 2018;102(1):11–26.

147. Wang XG, Ju ZH, Hou MH, et al. Deciphering transcriptome and complex alternative splicing transcripts in mammary gland tissues from cows naturally infected with Staphylococcus aureus Mastitis. PLoS One 2016;11(7):e0159719.

148. Govignon-Gion A, Dassonneville R, Baloche G, et al. Multiple trait genetic evaluation of clinical mastitis in three dairy cattle breeds. Animal 2016;10(04):558–65.

149. Koeck A, Loker S, Miglior F, et al. Genetic relationships of clinical mastitis, cystic ovaries, and lameness with milk yield and somatic cell score in first-lactation Canadian Holsteins. J Dairy Sci 2014;97(9):5806–13.

150. Narayana SG, Miglior F, Naqvi SA, et al. Genetic analysis of subclinical mastitis in early lactation of heifers using both linear and threshold models. J Dairy Sci 2018;101(12):11120–31.

151. Brito LF, Mallikarjunappa S, Sargolzaei M, et al. The genetic architecture of milk ELISA scores as an indicator of Johne's disease (paratuberculosis) in dairy cattle. J Dairy Sci 2018;101(11):10062–75.

152. Kirkpatrick BW, Lett BM. Short communication: heritability of susceptibility to infection by Mycobacterium avium ssp. paratuberculosis in Holstein cattle. J Dairy Sci 2018;101(12):11165–9.

153. Chapinal N, Koeck A, Sewalem A, et al. Genetic parameters for hoof lesions and their relationship with feet and leg traits in Canadian Holstein cows. J Dairy Sci 2013;96(4):2596–604.
154. Abdalla EA, Rosa GJM, Weigel KA, et al. Genetic analysis of leukosis incidence in United States Holstein and Jersey populations. J Dairy Sci 2013;96(9): 6022–9.
155. Passafaro TL, Carrera JPB, dos Santos LL, et al. Genetic analysis of resistance to ticks, gastrointestinal nematodes and Eimeria spp. in Nellore cattle. Vet Parasitol 2015;210(3–4):224–34.
156. Mallard B, Cartwright S, Nayeri S, et al. Genome-wide association and functional annotation of positional candidate genes for immune response in Canadian Holstein Cattle. Proc World Congr Genet Appl to livest Prod. 2018:711. http://www.wcgalp.org/proceedings/2018/genome-wide-association-and-functional-annotation-positional-candidate-genes-immune.
157. Emam M, Paibomesai MA, Thompson-Crispi KA, et al. The association between sire estimated breeding value for antibody-mediated immune response (AMIR) and offspring AMIR phenotype. Proc World Congr Genet Appl Livest Prod. 2014:522. Available at: http://www.wcgalp.org/proceedings/2014/association-between-sire-estimated-breeding-value-antibody-mediated-immune-response.

Mucosal Immune System of Cattle

All Immune Responses Begin Here

Christopher Chase, DVM, MS, PhD[a],*,
Radhey S. Kaushik, BVSc, MVSc, PhD[b]

KEYWORDS

- Bovine • Mucosal • Immunology • Gastrointestinal • Respiratory • Reproductive
- Microbiome

KEY POINTS

- The largest organ of the immune system is the mucosa making the management of it essential for productivity and health.
- The mucosal barrier consists of mucous, antimicrobial peptides, and IgA and is a "kill zone" to prevent microbial invasion of the epithelium.
- The mucosal epithelial cells are key cells that maintain the "kill zone" and "mucosal firewall" and respond to metabolites and microbial components from the lumen and signals from immune cells to maintain tight junctions and prevent leaky gut.
- The mucosal immune system has a unique circulatory system where immune cells that have activated in mucosal region recirculate to mucosal regions, a system termed the common mucosal system.

INTRODUCTION

In the last decade, there has been an explosion of knowledge on the mucosal immune system with substantial implications for cattle health. The concept of microbiome and its interaction with epithelial cells of the gastrointestinal (GI), reproductive, and mammary systems to influence immune function is discussed in detail by Diego E. Gomez and colleagues' article, "The Cattle Microbiota and the Immune System: An Evolving Field," in this issue. The use of nutraceuticals and their interaction with the microbiome and GI tract (GIT) is discussed in detail by Michael A. Ballou and colleagues' article, "Neutraceuticals: An Alternative Strategy for the Use of Antimicrobials," in this issue. In this article, we review key concepts important for mucosal immunity including epithelial cell immune function in the GI, respiratory, and reproductive tract; the common

[a] Department of Veterinary and Biomedical Sciences, South Dakota State University, PO Box 2175, SAR Room 125, North Campus Drive, Brookings, SD 57007, USA; [b] Department of Biology and Microbiology, South Dakota State University, Brookings, SD 57007, USA
* Corresponding author.
E-mail address: Christopher.Chase@SDSTATE.edu

Vet Clin Food Anim 35 (2019) 431–451
https://doi.org/10.1016/j.cvfa.2019.08.006
0749-0720/19/© 2019 Elsevier Inc. All rights reserved.

vetfood.theclinics.com

mucosal system; and vaccine and disease responses. It is now understood that the maturation of the immune responses begin where microorganisms and/or their products interact with epithelial cells of the mucosa in the neonatal calf (discussed in Diego E. Gomez and colleagues' article, "The Cattle Microbiota and the Immune System: An Evolving Field," elsewhere in this issue) and is necessary for proper development of the immune system and regulation and maintenance of immune homeostasis.

The mucosal immune system provides the first immune defense barrier for more than 90% of potential pathogens and represents the largest immune organ in the body. The mucosal immune system is an integrated system that fortifies the mucosal barrier with immune reinforcements from the innate and adaptive response and at the same time regulates and engages the immune system (**Fig. 1**) and has a greater concentration of antibodies than any other tissue in the body. It must not only protect against harmful pathogens but the mucosal system also tolerizes the immune system to dietary antigens and normal microbial flora. If the barrier is breached the next line of defense is the innate immune response in the lamina propria (LP) with phagocytic cells and production of various cytokines, chemokines, and proteins that not only provide antimicrobial protection but also recruit cells through the proinflammatory process and activate the acquired immune response (see **Fig. 1**). The acquired immune response with its myriad of B cells, T cells, cytokines, and antibodies provides the pathogen-specific memory with continued duration protective for subsequent infections with the same pathogen (see **Fig. 1**).

MUCOSAL FIREWALL: THE MUCOUS BARRIER, MUCOSAL EPITHELIAL CELLS, AND LAMINA PROPRIA

The health of the mucosa depends on three distinct structures: (1) the mucous barrier, (2) the mucosal epithelial cell, and (3) the immune cells of the LP. The mucous barrier

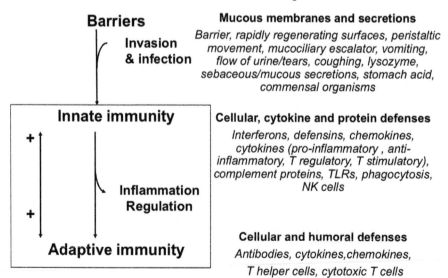

Fig. 1. Mucosal immune responses: the barrier, innate, and adaptive immune components. NK, natural killer cell; TLR, toll-like receptor. (*From* C. Chase, Enteric Immunity Happy Gut, Healthy Animal. *Elsevier.* 2018; 34(1); with permission.)

consists of the mucous and mucins, antimicrobial peptides (AMPs), and IgA. The goblet cells in the mucosa secrete mucous and mucins that constitute the major portion of the barrier (**Fig. 2**).[1–3] Mucins are also produced to a lesser degree by mucosa epithelial cells.[4] The mucous barrier contains AMPs produced by the enterocytes and ciliated epithelial cells (CEC) (see **Fig. 2**; **Figs. 3–9**). Secretory IgA (sIgA) is produced when dimeric IgA is secreted by the plasma cells in the LP and is transported to the mucosal surface of the epithelial cell. The inner mucous layer along with the AMPs and sIgA form a "killing zone" that few pathogens or commensals have evolved strategies to penetrate (see **Fig. 2**). This killing zone along with the tight junctions that knit the enterocytes and CEC form a barrier against pathogens.

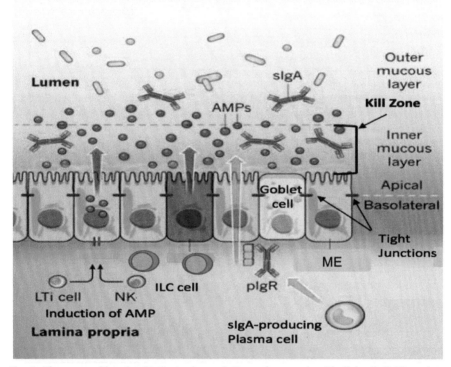

Fig. 2. The mucosal barrier. Distinct subpopulations of mucosal epithelial cells (ME) are integrated into a continuous, single cell layer that is divided into apical and basolateral regions by tight junctions. ME sense the microbiota and their metabolites to induce the production of AMPs. Goblet cells produce mucin and mucous, which is organized into a dense, more highly cross-linked inner proteoglycan gel that forms an adherent inner mucous layer, and a less densely cross-linked outer mucous layer. The outer layer is highly colonized by constituents of the microbiota. The inner mucous layer is largely impervious to bacterial colonization or penetration because of its high concentration of bactericidal AMPs, and commensals specific secretory IgA, which is moved from their basolateral surface, where it is bound by the receptor, to the inner mucous layer. Responding to the microbiotal components, innate lymphoid cells, lymphoid tissue inducer cells, and NK cells produce cytokines, which stimulate AMP production and maintain the epithelial barrier. ILC, innate lymphoid cells; LTi, lymphoid tissue inducer cells; pIgR, polymeric Ig receptor; sIgA, secretory IgA. (*Adapted from* Maynard CL, Elson CO, Hatton RD, Weaver CT. Reciprocal interactions of the intestinal microbiota and immune system. *Nature*. 2012;489(7415):231-241; with permission.)

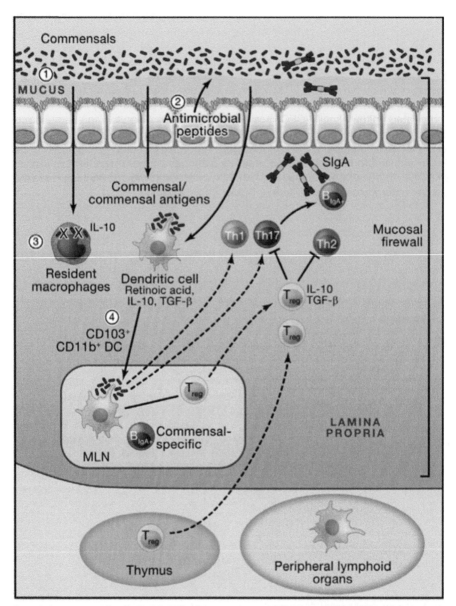

Fig. 3. The mucosal firewall. (1) The mucus represents the primary barrier limiting contact between the microbiota and host tissue preventing microbial translocation. (2) Epithelial cells produce antimicrobial peptides that also play a significant role in limiting exposure to the commensal microbiota. (3) Translocating commensals are rapidly eliminated by tissue-resident macrophages. (4) Commensals or commensal antigens can also be captured by dendritic cells (DCs) that traffic to the mesenteric lymph node from the lamina propria but do not penetrate further. Presentation of commensal antigens by these DCs leads to the differentiation of commensal-specific regulatory cells, Th$_{17}$ cells, and IgA-producing B cells. Commensal-specific lymphocytes traffic to the lamina propria and Peyer patches. In the Peyer patches, regulatory T cells can further promote class switching and IgA generation against commensals. The combination of the epithelial barrier, mucus layer, IgA, and DCs and T cells comprises the mucosal firewall, which limits the passage and exposure of commensals to the gut. IL, interleukin; MLN, mesenteric lymph nodes; TGF, transforming growth factor; T$_{reg}$, regulatory T cells. (*Adapted from* Belkaid Y, Hand TW. Role of the Microbiota in Immunity and Inflammation. *Cell.* 2014;157(1):121-141; with permission.)

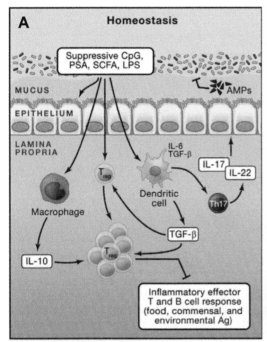
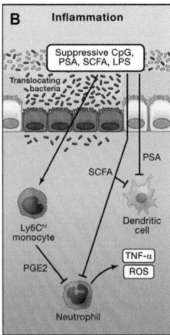

Fig. 4. Mucosal immune regulation during homeostasis and inflammation. (*A*) Commensals promote the induction of regulatory T cells via direct sensing of microbial products or metabolites by T cells or dendritic cells. Further commensals promote the induction of Th17 cells that can regulate the function and homeostasis of epithelial cells. In the context of inflammation, similar mechanisms may account for the regulatory role of the microbiota. (*B*) Commensal-derived metabolites can also have a local and systemic effect on inflammatory cells. For example, short-chain fatty acids can inhibit neutrophil activation. On entrance in the tissue, inflammatory monocytes can also respond to microbial-derived ligands by producing mediators, such as prostaglandin E_2, which limit neutrophil activation and tissue damage. CpG, cytosine-polyguanine nucleotides; LPS, lipopolysaccharide; PGE2, prostaglandin E_2; PSA, polysaccharide A; ROS, reactive oxygen species; SCFA, short-chain fatty acids; TNF, tumor necrosis factor. (*Adapted from* Belkaid Y, Hand TW. Role of the Microbiota in Immunity and Inflammation. *Cell.* 2014;157(1):121-141; with permission.)

The mucosal epithelium (ME) are the cells that line the GIT, uterus, and upper respiratory tract (URT). The ME is important not only for the animal's health and productivity by their normal function (secretion and absorption in the gut, fetal development in the uterus, and oxygen exchange and clearance of particulate and pathogens for proper lung function in the URT), but these epithelial cells (known as enterocytes in the gut and CEC in the URT) are the first responders to microorganisms. The epithelial cells are coated with mucus-glycocalyx layer (see **Fig. 2**) that helps protect cells but are continually in contact with commensal and pathogenic organisms (see **Figs. 2–4**). Because the ME is constantly in contact with microorganisms, their response is quite different.[5] The mucous barrier is first line of defense and ME provide several defensive tools. One of the major defensive tools of the ME are AMP (host defense proteins) that are released into the mucous barrier and their ME production is stimulated by microbial components or products and/or the immune system (see **Figs. 2–5, 8** and **9**). AMPs are cationic molecules produced to defend the host against microbial

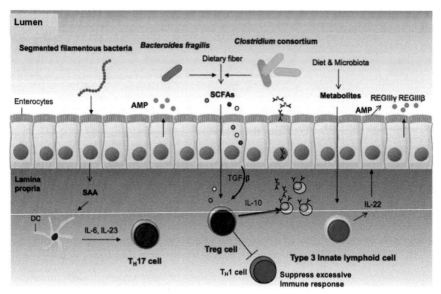

Fig. 5. Contribution of commensals to ME cells and immunity. ME produce serum amyloid A protein after exposure to filamentous bacteria (related to *Clostridium*), which activates DCs to produce IL-6 and IL-23, resulting in the generation of Th17 cells that are important for T-cell development. *Clostridium consortium* and *Bacteroides fragilis* produce SCFAs from dietary carbohydrates that induce directly or indirectly by the production of TGF-β by the ME, the differentiation of Treg cells to enhance IgA production and to help minimize inflammatory response. Diet- or microbiota-derived metabolites upregulate the number of IL-22-secreting type 3 innate lymphoid cells that induce the production of antimicrobial peptides by the ME (AMP/HDP-REGIIIB and REGIIIγ) from epithelial cells. SAA, serum amyloid A. (*Adapted from* Kim D, Yoo S-A, Kim W-U. Gut microbiota in autoimmunity: potential for clinical applications. *Arch Pharm Res.* 2016;39(11):1565-1576; with permission.)

pathogens. AMP act as lytic enzymes that disturb the microbial cell membrane.[6] The AMPs go by different names (ie, defensins, REGIII, lactoferricin) and possess a wide spectrum of antimicrobial activity (at even low micromolar concentrations) against bacteria, fungi, and some enveloped viruses. AMPs attach to the microbial membrane and disrupt it by forming a pore that leads to the efflux of ions and nutrients.[5] ME cells also export IgA and IgG produced by B cells in the LP to the mucous barrier. In addition to providing transport for immunoglobulin through the cell, the polymeric immunoglobulin receptor also adds a secretory component to IgA that lengthens the half-life of IgA (see **Fig. 2**).[1] Secretory IgG (sIgG) in the nasal and URT and the reproductive tract is as or more important than sIgA.[7] A third defensive component to the mucosal barrier that ME contributes are tight junctions (see **Figs. 2** and **6**).[8] These structures consist of several highly regulated structural proteins that have the ability to contract or relax to affect the passage of molecules and ions through the space between cells. When the tight junctions breakdown, this allows the epithelium to become leaky and the inflammatory syndrome associated with it is referred to as "leaky gut"(see **Fig. 6**).[9] This leakiness also occurs in the respiratory and reproductive tract.

ME have important immune regulatory functions that affect the mucous barrier, tight junctions, and the innate and adaptive immune cells in the LP.[10] Like other immune cells, they use pattern-recognition receptors,[11] including the toll-like receptors (TLR) and nucleotide-binding oligomerization domain-like receptors, to monitor

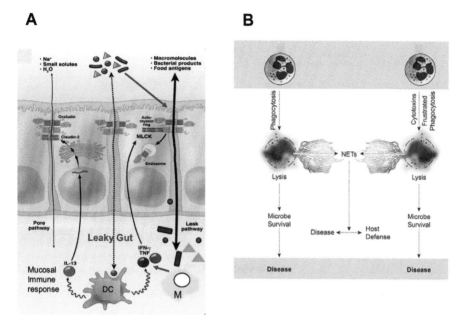

Fig. 6. Innate immunity and the mucosa. (*A*) Pathogenesis of leaky gut. The mucosal barrier normally restricts passage of luminal contents, including microbes and their products, but a small fraction of these materials do cross the tight junction. This diagram shows how DCs and macrophages react to these materials. These innate immune cells release cytokines that exert proinflammatory (TNF and interferon-γ) and anti-inflammatory (IL-13) effects. If proinflammatory signals dominate and signal to the ME, MLCK can be activated to cause barrier dysfunction through the leak pathway, allowing an increase in the amount of luminal material presented to immune cells. In the absence of appropriate immune regulation, immune activation may cause further proinflammatory immune activation, cytokine release, and barrier loss, resulting in a self-amplifying cycle that can result in disease. (*B*) Neutrophil collateral damage from neutrophil extracellular traps (NET) formation. Neutrophil lysis after phagocytosis. Cytolysis is programmed (eg, necroptosis) or caused by direct damage. Neutrophil lysis is caused by cytolytic toxins, pore-forming agents, physical injury, or frustrated phagocytosis. This can result in the formation of NETs during neutrophil lysis. Hydrolytic enzymes–DNA complexes are released in the NETs, enhancing the proinflammatory response and tissue destruction, contributing to collateral damage and disease. IFN, interferon; M, macrophage; MLCK, myosin light chain kinase. (*Adapted from* Odenwald MA, Turner JR. Intestinal permeability defects: is it time to treat? Clin Gastroenterol Hepatol 2013;11(9):1078, with permission; and Kobayashi SD, Malachowa N, DeLeo FR. Influence of microbes on neutrophil life and death. Front Cell Infect Microbiol 2017;7(4):159, with permission.)

pathogen-associated molecular patterns to recognize danger from microbes and induce different signaling pathways to activate the immune system against infection (discussed in Diego E. Gomez and colleagues' article, "The Cattle Microbiota and the Immune System: An Evolving Field," elsewhere in this issue). They do this by detecting microbial components, such as lipopolysaccharide (gram-negative bacteria) and cytosine-polyguanine nucleotides (found in bacteria and viruses) (see **Fig. 4**). However, ME express TLR not on their surface but rather inside the cell, and are only upregulated when the cell is infected.[11] They also respond to microbial metabolites including short-chain fatty acids (ie, butyrate) and many normal commensal microbial components, such as *Bacteroides fragilis* capsular polysaccharide A (see

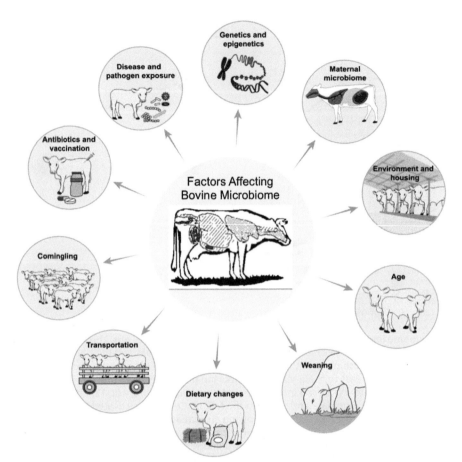

Fig. 7. Factors affecting the development of the bovine microbiota. Microbiota developments are highly dynamic and are shaped by various host and environmental factors, including host genetics, mode of delivery, diet and the microbiota of the mother, environmental housing, weaning, feeding type, transportation, comingling, antibiotic treatment, vaccination, and pathogen exposure. (*Adapted from* Zeineldin M, Lowe J, Aldridge B. Contribution of the Mucosal Microbiota to Bovine Respiratory Health. *Trends Microbiol.* May 2019; with permission.)

Fig. 4).[12,13] Unlike innate immune cells (ie, macrophages and neutrophils), which are proinflammatory and also first responders, ME respond with predominately an anti-inflammatory response. The normal response to TLR and nucleotide-binding oligomerization domain-like receptors like signaling is proinflammatory response through the nuclear factor-κB pathway. Metabolites, such as butyrate, and normal commensal components affect the mucous barrier by enhanced production of mucus by goblet cells. Their effect on ME results in increased production of AMPs, inhibition of nuclear factor-κB, and the production of the anti-inflammatory transforming growth factor-β (TGF-β) by the ME.[12,13] The ME also express chemokines that are chemotactic and bind the chemokine receptor on mucosal system T cells. The production of chemokines by epithelial cells recruits these lymphocytes to the LP and into ME. These metabolites and normal commensal components also affect the immune response in the LP by increased production of sIgA by B cells; reduced expression of T cell–activating

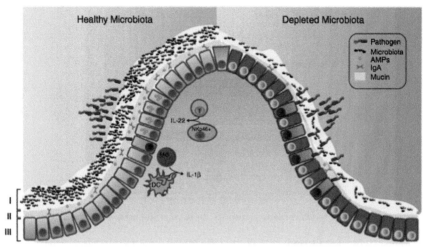

Current Opinion in Microbiology

Fig. 8. Healthy mucosal defenses and mucosal dysbiosis. The intestinal microbiota promotes three levels of protection against enteric infection. (I) Saturation of colonization sites and competition for nutrients by the microbiota limit pathogen association with host tissue. (II) Kill zone. Commensal microbes prime barrier immunity by driving expression of mucin, IgA, and AMPs that further prevents pathogen contact with host mucosa. (III) Finally, the microbiota enhances immune responses to invading pathogens. This is achieved by promoting IL-22 expression by T cells and NK cells, which increases epithelial resistance against infection, and priming secretion of IL-1b by intestinal monocytes (MΦ) and DCs, which promotes recruitment of inflammatory cells into the site of infection. In conditions where the microbiota is absent there is reduced competition, barrier resistance, and immune defense against pathogen invasion. (*From* Khosravi A, Mazmanian SK. Disruption of the gut microbiome as a risk factor for microbial infections. *Curr Opin Microbiol.* 2013;16(2):221-227; with permission.)

molecules on antigen-presenting cells (APC), such as dendritic cells (DCs); and increased number and function of regulatory T (T_{reg}) cells and their production of anti-inflammatory cytokines (TGF-β) and interleukin (IL)-10 (see **Figs. 3–5**).[12,13] The mucous barrier plus the immune regulatory function maintain tight junctions, blocking a major proinflammatory response while maintaining an anti-inflammatory environment that results in T_{reg} cells (T cells that do not cause an inflammatory response), the production of IgA by the mucosal firewall results in homeostasis, the steady-state process where the function and integrity of the mucosa is maintained. Homeostasis is imperative for host survival. This process relies on a complex and coordinated set of barriers, innate and adaptive responses that selects and calibrates responses against self, food, commensals, and pathogens in the most appropriate manner. The interactions with commensals is key and is discussed later. ME have to integrate local cues, such as defined metabolites, cytokines, or hormones, allowing the induction of responses in a way that preserves the physiologic and functional requirements of each tissue (see **Fig. 5**). The regulatory pathways that are involved in the maintenance of a homeostatic relationship with the microbiota are tissue specific (see **Fig. 4**A).[13] These same homeostatic processes also aid in repairing and limiting the damage in the face of inflammation (see **Fig. 4**B).[13]

A local increase of the anti-inflammatory cytokine IL-10 results in inhibition of the local proinflammatory response and increases eosinophils in the tissue. With only a proinflammatory response there is little resolution of disease and enhanced

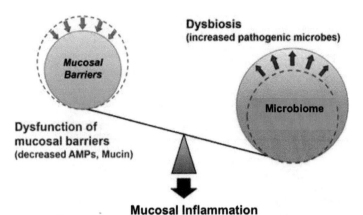

Fig. 9. Microbial dysbiosis promotes susceptibility to mucosal inflammation. Dysfunction of mucosal barriers because of decreased production of AMPs and mucin allows intestinal bacteria to gain access to gut immune cells, thereby contributing to the development of intestinal inflammation. Dysbiosis induced by environmental factors, such as a high-fat diet and various antimicrobials and stressors, accelerates intestinal inflammation in situations where the mucosal barrier is disrupted. (*Adapted from* Okumura R, Takeda K. Roles of intestinal epithelial cells in the maintenance of gut homeostasis. *Exp Mol Med.* 2017;49(5):e338. https://doi.org/10.1038/emm.2017.20 with permission.)

collateral damage and immunopathology.[14] The proinflammatory/anti-inflammatory mucosal response increases with age and results in less disease. Neutrophils (eg, polymorphonuclear cells) die after a short time at sites of inflammation. Hydrolytic enzymes are released and contribute to the inflammatory response and tissue destruction contributing to collateral damage and enhanced disease. Neutrophil granule proteins induce adhesion and emigration of inflammatory monocytes to the site of inflammation. Neutrophils also create extracellular defenses by the formation of neutrophil extracellular traps (see **Fig. 6**B).[15–17] This neutrophil extracellular trap formation is induced by such agents as bacterial aggregates and biofilms, fungal hyphae, and protozoan parasites (cryptosporidia, *Neospora*, and coccidiosis) that cannot be phagocytized.[18–21] Neutrophils use the potent oxidative metabolism system to kill bacteria. This reaction is one of the most potent bactericidal mechanisms and is potentially fungicidal, parasiticidal, and viricidal. The eosinophil is capable of the same phagocytic and metabolic functions as the neutrophils but focuses the host's defense against the tissue phase of parasitic infections. Basophils and mast cells have been associated primarily with allergic reactions because of their binding of IgE. They release inflammatory mediators necessary for the activation of the acquired immune response.[22,23] Alpha- and beta-interferon, the last component of this innate response, sets up an immediate wall against virus infections and also provides anti-inflammatory response. The second wave occurs a day or two later, when natural killer cells enhance AMP production,[1,5] kill parasites[18,19] and virally infected cells,[24] but also produce cytokines to help the adaptive immune response.[24]

The adaptive phase occurs in the organized mucosa-associated lymphoid tissues (MALT) (discussed later).[25] MALT is the initial induction site for mucosal immunity for antigens that are sampled from mucosal surfaces. The DC are important because they are APC that help in discriminating between dietary antigens, commensal microflora, and pathogens, and interacting with T cells. Another T cell, Gamma delta T cells, are found in high levels in the mucosa and the LP in cattle have a unique role in ruminant immunology (discussed in Mariana Guerra-Maupome and colleagues' article, "Gamma Delta T Cell Function in Ruminants," elsewhere in this issue).

MICROBIOME AND ENTERIC IMMUNITY

The microbiome is essential for immune development in the neonatal calf and maintenance of health in the older animals. The microbiome-gut-immune-brain axis maintains the health of all animals.[13,26–32] As the calf develops there is a succession of microbes that finally culminates in what is called a "climax" community that occurs as the GIT transitions to an anaerobic environment.[29,33] This succession is influenced by nutrition, stress, and environment. This microbial community of commensals and their metabolites control the health of the mucosa and the underlying immune cells in the LP (see **Figs. 4** and **5**).[32,34,35] These commensal metabolites stimulate ME to produce TGF-β, which is essential for the development of T_{reg} lymphocytes that produce anti-inflammatory IL-10 (see **Figs. 4** and **5**). The microbial components in the microbiome also stimulate ME to produce serum amyloid A, which stimulates DCs to activate another important mucosa T_{reg} cell, T_H17 cells (see **Fig. 4**).[36] These microbial metabolites also directly stimulate a natural killer–like cell type 3 innate lymphoid cells to produce IL-22 to induce the enterocytes to produce more defensins (eg, REGIIIγ and REGIIIβ) (see **Fig. 5**). The composition of the microbiome varies by location with the numbers and diversity of populations being high in the rumen and increasing dramatically from the abomasum to the colon, with the ileum being a key organ for microbial-immune development. In URT, there are dramatic differences between the nasopharyngeal region and lung in numbers and diversity of populations.[31,37] These microbiome communities have evolved to help protect the animal by improving barrier and immune function; understanding the complexity of the microbial ecosystem is essential.[38,39]

The stress of weaning, comingling, transportation, dietary changes, antimicrobial therapy, and abrupt diet changes results in major microbial population shifts in the luminal microbial ecosystem, the microbiome (see **Fig. 7**).[26] This lowers the defenses against pathogen entry, leading to increased risk of disease. This leads to dysbiosis, the loss of good bacteria with an overgrowth of harmful organisms (see **Fig. 8**).[35,40] However, dysbiosis is not just the loss of microbiome, it results in depletion of the kill zone (see **Fig. 2**); the mucous layer becomes thinner and the amount of sIgA and AMP declines weakening the barrier, allowing pathogens to interact with the mucosa and cause disease. Commensal organisms that help stimulate the mucosa to be anti-inflammatory are no longer available so tight junctions become weakened, leaky gut occurs, and proinflammatory responses occur that further weaken the gut epithelium (see **Figs. 6** and **9**).[30] One major factor leading to the dysbiosis and diarrhea that one can learn from pigs is low feed and water intake.[41] Dysbiosis is also associated with susceptibility to Johne disease.[40]

ORGANIZED AND DIFFUSE MUCOSAL LYMPHOCYTES

Organized MALT is widely distributed in mucosal surfaces throughout the body. MALT is the initial induction site for mucosal immunity for antigens that are sampled from mucosal surfaces and where the mucosal adaptive immune response develops. These mucosal aggregates or follicles (also known as lymphoid follicles [LF]) of B cells, T cells, and DCs and macrophages APCs are covered by epithelium that contains specialized epithelial cells called dome or M cells that are found in the bronchus-associated lymphoid tissues (BALT) (**Fig. 10**),[42] gut-associated lymphoid

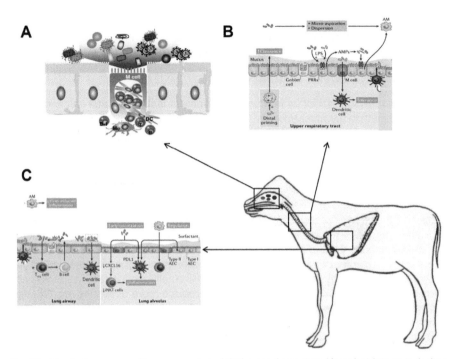

Fig. 10. Respiratory mucosal immune system. (*A*) The nasal associated lymphoid tissue including the tonsils is an important site for immune responses and microbiome interactions and respiratory pathogen carriage. Microfold cells (M cells) specialize in antigen uptake and are present throughout the respiratory and GI mucosal immune system. The cilia of M cells are shorter than those of conventional epithelium cells. These cells are like a window to the immune system and allow interaction with viruses, bacteria, and other components of the microbiome. On its basal side, the M cell develops a pocket-like structure that can hold immunocompetent cells. M cells, such as macrophages (MΦ), function in active antigen uptake. Because lysosome development in M cells is poor, in most cases the incorporated antigens are just passed through the M cells unmodified and then taken up by DCs, which then interact with T cells, which in turn interact with B cells. (*B*) URT and (*C*) lower respiratory tract (LRT). The URT mucous is thicker than the LRT and the ME are taller and decrease in size as one descends into the LRT and the alveoli. Resident microorganisms prime immune cells include ME, neutrophils, and dendritic cells, which all contribute to the clearance of pathogens. Moreover, microbial signaling is necessary for the recruitment and activation of regulatory cells, such as anti-inflammatory alveolar macrophages and T_{reg} cells. The host responds to microbial colonization through the release of AMPs and sIgA. Sensing of the microbiota involves microfold (M) cells that activate tolerogenic dendritic cells. In addition, alveolar dendritic cells can directly sample luminal microorganisms. These pathways lead to the regulation of inflammation and the induction of tolerance in the respiratory tract. It is also likely that early bacterial colonization is key to long-term immune regulation, which is illustrated by the microbiota-induced decrease in CXC-16 (*Cxcl16*) gene, which prevents the accumulation of inducible natural killer T cells, and by the programmed death ligand 1–mediated induction of tolerogenic dendritic cells. This tolerant milieu, in turn, contributes to the normal development and maintenance of resident bacterial communities, which are also influenced by host and environmental factors. AEC, alveolar epithelial cell; AM, alveolar macrophages; iNKT, inducible natural killer T cells; PDL1, programmed death ligand 1; PRR, pattern recognition receptor; URT, upper respiratory tract. (*Adapted from* Sato S, Kiyono H. The mucosal immune system of the respiratory tract. *Curr Opin Virol.* 2012;2(3):225-232 and Man WH, de Steenhuijsen Piters WAA, Bogaert D. The microbiota of the respiratory tract: gatekeeper to respiratory health. *Nat Rev Microbiol.* 2017;15(5):259-270; with permission.)

tissues (GALT) (**Fig. 11**),[43] and in the uterus (**Fig. 12**).[44] These dome cells pinocytose antigen and transport it across the ME (see **Fig. 10A**).[45] The antigen may then be processed by APCs and presented to T and B lymphocytes; indeed, APCs play a central role in the induction and maintenance of mucosal immunity.[46] The lymphocytes that emigrate from these LF into the surrounding LP are referred to as diffuse lymphocytes.[47] The hallmark of this system is that local stimulation results in memory T and B cells in the nearby mucosal tissue but also in other mucosal tissues (**Fig. 13**).

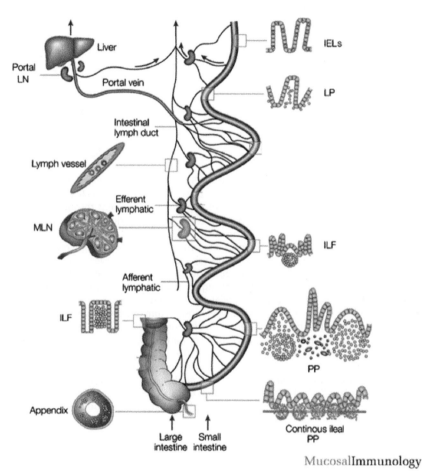

MucosalImmunology

Fig. 11. Gastrointestinal mucosal immune system. Lymphocytes can leave the surface epithelium (intraepithelial lymphocytes) or LP via draining afferent lymphatics to mesenteric lymph nodes, or via portal blood reaching the liver where induction of tolerance occurs. The M cells in the follicle-associated epithelium of Peyers patches (PPs) transport antigen to prime B cells in the isolated lymphoid follicles of the PPs of the jejunum, ileum, and the large intestine. The continuous ileal PP (IPP) are a primary lymphoid organ responsible for B-cell development. The IPP are up to 2 m long and constitute 80% to 90% of the intestinal lymphoid tissue. IEL, intraepithelial lymphocytes; ILF, isolated lymphoid follicles; LN, lymph node; MLN, mesenteric lymph nodes. (*Adapted from* Brandtzaeg P, Kiyono H, Pabst R, Russell MW. Terminology: nomenclature of mucosa-associated lymphoid tissue. *Mucosal Immunol.* 2008;1(1):31-37; with permission.)

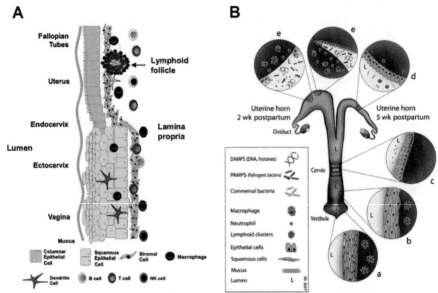

Fig. 12. Reproductive mucosal immune system. (*A*) Schematic of the mucosal immune system throughout the nongravid female reproductive tract. The vagina and ectocervix are lined with squamous epithelial cells. Columnar mucosa epithelium is present throughout the upper female reproductive tract including the endocervix, uterine endometrium, and fallopian tubes. (*B*) Schematic of the mucosal immune system of postpartum female bovine reproductive tract. The vulvar opening acts as the portal for entry and clearance of microbial contaminants. Multiple epithelial layers in the vestibule (a) and vagina (b) prevent bacterial entry at these anatomic sites unless they have been breached because of laceration during delivery. The cervix (c), although still dilated after calving, provides another barrier to the entry of microbes into the uterus because of epithelial folding and secretion of mucus that flows outward to the vagina. Around the second week postpartum (e), the simple columnar uterine epithelial barrier is breached at the caruncles because of death of epithelial cells. For the next 3 weeks, the uterus responds to microbial contamination and colonization while reestablishing the integrity of the epithelial barrier (d). (*Adapted from* Wira CR, Fahey JV, Rodriguez-Garcia M, et al. Regulation of mucosal immunity in the female reproductive tract: the role of sex hormones in immune protection against sexually transmitted pathogens. *Am J Reprod Immunol.* 2014;72(2):236-258 and *from* Dadarwal D, Palmer C, Griebel P. Mucosal immunity of the postpartum bovine genital tract. *Theriogenology.* 2017;104:62-71; with permission.)

RESPIRATORY MUCOSAL IMMUNE SYSTEM

The respiratory mucosal immune system contains a large number of lymphocytes. Unlike the GI mucosal immune system, sIgG is an important mucosal defense mechanism of the nasopharyngeal associated lymphoid tissue (NALT). The NALT ME varies from squamous to more columnar ME in the tonsillar regions.[28] NALT contains organized LF making it an optimal target for mucosal vaccines (**Fig. 14**).[28,42] The NALT microbiome contains commensals along with several possible pathogens including *Mycoplasma bovis*, *Mannheimia haemolytica*, *Histophilus somni*, and *Pasteurella multicida*.[28,37] The NALT, like the GALT and BALT, contains M cells (see **Fig. 10**A) that provide easy access for antigens to the immune system and induction of adaptive immune responses.[45] The URT is lined by ciliated ME cells and has a major role in

3rd Line of Defense | Mucosal Immune System

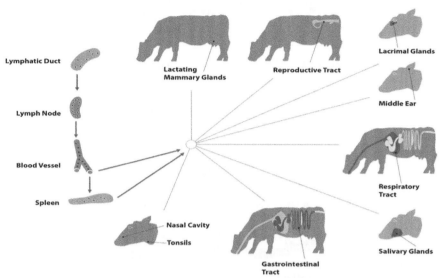

Fig. 13. Lymphocyte circulation and common mucosal immune system of the bovine. As illustrated on the left side of the figure, lymphocyte circulation with lymphocytes entering the lymph nodes by afferent lymphatics and exiting by efferent lymphatics. The common mucosal system involves the circulation of B and T cells between lymphoid tissues on mucosal surfaces.

clearance of particulates via the mucociliary escalator (see **Fig. 10**B).[48] The URT ME maintains the kill zone (see **Fig. 10**B).[48] The URT ME also regulate the anti-inflammatory response in the LP. The URT also contains BALT that are active in the production of IgA and in tolerance against normal respiratory microbiome. The microbiome is less complex in the URT and contains fewer organisms than the NALT.[28,31,48] The lower respiratory tract (LRT) contains the larger bronchial airways and the alveoli. ME in LRT are shorter and have the same functions as the ME of the URT (see **Fig. 10**C). In the alveoli, the mucous has been replaced by surfactant and the primary function of ME and the alveolar macrophages is to minimize inflammation (see **Fig. 10**C). The microbiome in the LRT is less complex than URT and contains fewer organisms. In healthy animals, there should be no microorganisms in the alveoli (see **Fig. 10**C).[48]

GASTROINTESTINAL TRACT MUCOSAL IMMUNE SYSTEM

The GI mucosal immune system alone contains more than a trillion (10^{12}) lymphocytes and has a greater concentration of antibodies than other tissue in the body. Mucous varies in depth and character throughout the length of the GIT with less viscous mucous being present in the upper GIT and a more viscous mucous in the lower GIT. The GI mucosal lymphoid organ system begins developing at 100 days of gestation when the mesenteric lymph nodes are present (see **Fig. 11**).[25,43] The jejunum contains the discrete Peyer patches and the continuous ileal Peyer patches (IPP) (see **Fig. 11**). There are also discrete LF distributed throughout the GIT; these are less developed than the Peyer patches and are often temporary as the result of a local immune response. IPP play a continual role in immune development particularly of

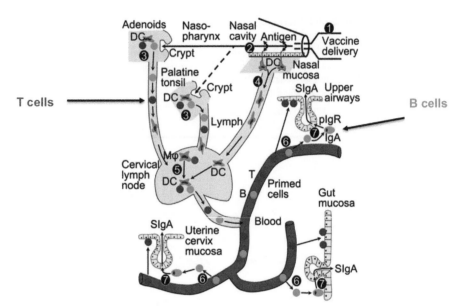

Fig. 14. Induction immunity after nasal vaccine administration. (1) Delivery of nasal vaccine. (2) Uptake of vaccine antigen through nasal mucosa. (3) Immune induction in nasal-associated lymphoid tissue including tonsils. (4) Antigen targeting and migration of mucosal DCs to regional lymph node. (5) Immune induction and amplification in regional (cervical) lymph nodes by antigen-loaded DCs and macrophages (MΦ). (6) Compartmentalized homing and exit of nasal-associated lymphoid tissue–induced T and B cells to secretory effector sites in airways, gut, and uterine cervix. (7) Local production and pIgR-mediated external transport of dimeric IgA to generate sIgA. (*Adapted from* Brandtzaeg P. Potential of nasopharynx-associated lymphoid tissue for vaccine responses in the airways. *Am J Respir Crit Care Med.* 2011;183(12):1595-1604; with permission.)

B lymphocytes. The B lymphocytes present are almost exclusively IgM$^+$ cells and if the IPP are removed, the animals remain deficient in B cells for at least 1 year because the IPP is the major source of the peripheral B-cell pool. Because the IPP is the site of proliferation and negative selection, IPP follicles are inferred as the major site[49] for generation of the preimmune B-cell repertoire in ruminants,[50] whereas the discreet Peyer patches, distributed throughout the jejunum, function as induction sites for the generation of IgA plasma cells (see **Fig. 11**).[50] Unfortunately, the role of the rumen in mucosal immunity is unclear.

FEMALE REPRODUCTIVE MUCOSAL IMMUNE SYSTEM

The female reproductive tract (FRT) is a dynamic immune system because of the cyclicity of hormonal regulation and pregnancy (see **Fig. 12**). The thickness and character of mucous varies by the anatomic location in the reproductive tract and time of the reproductive cycle. There are elevated levels of IgG and IgA in cervicovaginal mucus, and IgA, IgE, and IgG in the uterus. sIgG is an important mucosal defense mechanism for the FRT.[7] Only the endocervix and uterus has the columnar ME and these cells are sloughed and repopulated during normal estrus cycle (see **Fig. 12A**).[44] Following delivery of a calf, the FRT undergoes an active inflammatory process to clear cellular debris from the placenta and respond to bacterial contamination. The ME cells of the uterus completely slough. In healthy cows, uterine inflammation subsides by the fourth to fifth week postpartum. However, FRT (mainly of the uterus) repair is not complete until the sixth to eighth week postpartum (see **Fig. 12B**).[27] The normal uterine ME are leakier than the GIT and URT. The LP of a healthy reproductive tract normally has fewer innate and adaptive cells with a few LF (see **Fig. 12A**). Following calving, activation of the innate immune system is essential for placental separation. During the first week postpartum, there is increased influx of neutrophils recruitment following normal parturition and this neutrophil recruitment is closely associated with increased cytokine secretion seen in clinically normal cows until 24 days in milk.[51] Neutrophil levels decline by the fourth week postpartum when uterine involution is almost complete. Macrophages also provide a crucial component in phagocytosis, antigen presentation, and regulation of uterine inflammation. Once bacteria have been cleared, anti-inflammatory macrophages are present to aid in uterine involution. Isolated LF are found throughout the bovine genital tract (see **Fig. 12**). The LF located in the LP are believed to be immune induction sites because they have been observed following infection with bovine genital tract pathogens. T cells and B cells are also present in the lumen. Microflora of the FRT depend on fertility and parturition status of the animal. In the healthy FRT, the microbial flora are a combination of aerobic, facultatively anaerobic, and obligately anaerobic microorganisms.[52] Following parturition, bacterial contamination of the uterus occurs for 2 to 3 weeks postpartum because of calving-associated relaxation of physical barriers, including an open cervix. Negative pressure events created by repeated uterine contraction and relaxation enhances bacterial contamination by a vacuum effect. Gram-negative bacteria predominate in bovine uteri during the first week after calving and are gradually replaced by gram-positive bacteria during the second and third week postpartum. Bacterial contamination is cleared in most cows by the end of the fourth week postpartum.[27]

COMMON MUCOSAL SYSTEM

Lymphocytes are divided into two populations: those that circulate between the bloodstream and the systemic lymphoid tissues, and those that circulate between the bloodstream and lymphoid tissues associated with mucosal surfaces. In the MALT, mature T cells and B cells that have been stimulated by antigen and induced to switch to produce IgA leave the submucosal lymphoid tissue and reenter the bloodstream (see **Fig. 13**).[42,43] These lymphocytes exit the bloodstream through high endothelial venule and locate in the LP (see **Figs. 10–12**). B cells differentiate into plasma cells that secrete dimeric IgA. Many of these cells return to the same mucosal surface from which they originated but others are found at different mucosal surfaces throughout the body. This homing of lymphocytes to other MALT sites throughout the body is referred to as the "common immune system" (see **Fig. 13**). For example, oral immunization can result in the migration of IgA precursor cells to the bronchi and subsequent secretion of IgA onto the bronchial mucosa. There is a special affinity for lymphocytes, which have been sensitized in the gut to migrate to the mammary gland to become plasma cells and secrete IgA into the milk.

MUCOSAL VACCINE RESPONSES

Protecting the animal from infection at mucosal surfaces, such as the GIT, respiratory tract, mammary glands, and FRT, is especially difficult for the systemic immune system. The antibodies responsible for humoral immunity and lymphocytes responsible for cell-mediated immunity are predominantly in the bloodstream and tissues; they are typically not found on the mucosal surfaces. Therefore, although lymphocytes assist in preventing systemic invasion through the mucosal surface, they are often not effective at controlling infection on the mucosal surface. Even in the lungs and the mammary gland, where IgG and lymphocytes are found in relative abundance, they are not able to function as effectively in mucosal tissues. Adaptive immune protection on mucosal surfaces is caused in large part by sIgA, cytotoxic T cells, and γδ T cells. The route of vaccine administration is important when attempting to induce mucosal immunity. To induce sIgA production at mucosal surfaces, it is best for the vaccine to enter the body via a mucosal surface. This is accomplished by administering the vaccine to mucosal surfaces by aerosolizing the vaccine so the animal inhales it (intranasal vaccination) or by feeding the vaccine to the animal (oral vaccination). Parenteral vaccines can generate mucosal responses that produce mucosal sIgA.[53] Work in our laboratory has demonstrated mucosal immunity following parenteral vaccination in the face of maternal immunity, which generated bovine respiratory syncytial virus–specific mucosal IgA that protected against bovine respiratory syncytial virus disease.[54]

Intranasal vaccines have been used because of the high concentration of lymphoid tissue in the NALT,[42] the induction of a rapid interferon response,[55] the induction of immunity against bovine respiratory disease pathogens,[28] and the lack of interference from maternal antibodies.[56] Induction of the NALT also has implications for induction of other mucosal sites as a result of the common mucosal response (see **Figs. 13** and **14**).[28,42]

The main portal of entry for oral vaccines is the lymphoid tissue in the NALT. Timing seems to be critical for immunization of GALT, like Peyers patches in the GIT. Administration of modified live virus vaccine within the first 24 hours after birth would be at risk of neutralization and inactivation by the colostral maternal antibody. Numerous studies have shown that rotavirus-coronavirus modified live virus vaccines studies fail to protect in the presence of maternal antibodies (Geoff Smith, personal communication, 2018). Once animals are 1 to 2 days of age or older, the harsh pH and proteolytic environment of GIT affect antigenicity of vaccines intended to induce GALT.

SUMMARY

The mucosal immune system provides the first immune defense barrier. The health of the ME, is important not only for the growth and development of cattle, through secretion and absorption in the GIT, oxygen exchange and particulate removal in the respiratory tract, and fetal development in the FRT, but also provides the first immune response to microorganisms. The ME maintain a kill zone barrier to keep out pathogens in concert with the commensal microorganisms (microbiome) and other cells of the immune system. The microbiome functions best when it is in a stable condition resulting in immune homeostasis. Immunoregulation by the ME and microbiome results in the establishment of a mucosal firewall. Disruptions in the microbiome results in dysbiosis, which decreases the kill zone, allows leaky gut, and increases inflammation. This increased inflammation is seen as an important part of pathogenesis of infectious diseases of the GIT, respiratory, and reproductive tract. Delivery of vaccines to enhance mucosal immunity is a key strategy to protect animal health particularly with the decreased use of antibiotics. Maintaining the mucosal firewall and inducing mucosal immunity through vaccination are keys to maintaining animal health, increasing animal productivity, and reducing antimicrobial usage.

REFERENCES

1. Maynard CL, Elson CO, Hatton RD, et al. Reciprocal interactions of the intestinal microbiota and immune system. Nature 2012;489:231–41.
2. Pelaseyed T, Bergström JH, Gustafsson JK, et al. The mucus and mucins of the goblet cells and enterocytes provide the first defense line of the gastrointestinal tract and interact with the immune system. Immunol Rev 2014;260:8–20.
3. Zanin M, Baviskar P, Webster R, et al. The interaction between respiratory pathogens and mucus. Cell Host Microbe 2016;19:159–68.
4. Johansson MEV, Hansson GC. Is the intestinal goblet cell a major immune cell? Cell Host Microbe 2014;15:251–2.
5. Maldonado-Contreras AL, McCormick BA. Intestinal epithelial cells and their role in innate mucosal immunity. Cell Tissue Res 2011;343:5–12.
6. Zhang L-J, Gallo RL. Antimicrobial peptides. Curr Biol 2016;26:R14–9.
7. Horton RE, Vidarsson G. Antibodies and their receptors: different potential roles in mucosal defense. Front Immunol 2013;4:200.
8. Marchiando AM, Graham WV, Turner JR. Epithelial barriers in homeostasis and disease. Annu Rev Pathol 2010;5:119–44.
9. Kvidera SK, Dickson MJ, Abuajamieh M, et al. Intentionally induced intestinal barrier dysfunction causes inflammation, affects metabolism, and reduces productivity in lactating Holstein cows. J Dairy Sci 2017;100:4113–27.
10. Villena J J, Aso H, Rutten VPMG, et al. Immunobiotics for the bovine host: their interaction with intestinal epithelial cells and their effect on antiviral immunity. Front Immunol 2018;9:326.
11. Katwal P, Thomas M, Uprety T, et al. Development and biochemical and immunological characterization of early passage and immortalized bovine intestinal epithelial cell lines from the ileum of a young calf. Cytotechnology 2019;71: 127–48.
12. Troy EB, Kasper DL. Beneficial effects of *Bacteroides fragilis* polysaccharides on the immune system. Front Biosci (Landmark Ed) 2010;15:25–34.
13. Belkaid Y, Hand TW. Role of the microbiota in immunity and inflammation. Cell 2014;157:121–41.
14. Angus KW, Tzipori S, Gray EW. Intestinal lesions in specific-pathogen-free lambs associated with a cryptosporidium from calves with diarrhea. Vet Pathol 1982;19: 67–78.
15. Kobayashi SD, Malachowa N, Deleo FR. Influence of microbes on neutrophil life and death. Front Cell Infect Microbiol 2017;7:159.
16. de Buhr N, Reuner F, Neumann A, et al. Neutrophil extracellular trap formation in the Streptococcus suis-infected cerebrospinal fluid compartment. Cellular Microbiology 2017;19(2):e12649.
17. Branzk N, Lubojemska A, Hardison SE, et al. Neutrophils sense microbe size and selectively release neutrophil extracellular traps in response to large pathogens. Nat Immunol 2014;15:1017–25.
18. McDonald V, Korbel DS, Barakat FM, et al. Innate immune responses against *Cryptosporidium parvum* infection. Parasite Immunol 2013;35:55–64.
19. Leitch GJ, He Q. Cryptosporidiosis: an overview. J Biomed Res 2012;25:1–16.
20. Bruns S, Kniemeyer O, Hasenberg M, et al. Production of extracellular traps against *Aspergillus fumigatus* in vitro and in infected lung tissue is dependent on invading neutrophils and influenced by hydrophobin RodA. PLoS Pathog 2010;6:e1000873.

21. Behrendt JH, Ruiz A, Zahner H, et al. Neutrophil extracellular trap formation as innate immune reactions against the apicomplexan parasite *Eimeria bovis*. Vet Immunol Immunopathol 2010;133:1–8.

22. Abraham SN, St John AL. Mast cell-orchestrated immunity to pathogens. Nat Rev Immunol 2010;10:440–52.

23. Galli SJ, Tsai M. Mast cells in allergy and infection: versatile effector and regulatory cells in innate and adaptive immunity. Eur J Immunol 2010;40:1843–51.

24. Shekhar S, Yang X. Natural killer cells in host defense against veterinary pathogens. Vet Immunol Immunopathol 2015;168:30–4.

25. Liebler-Tenorio EM, Pabst R. MALT structure and function in farm animals. Vet Res 2006;37:257–80.

26. Zeineldin M, Lowe J, Aldridge B. Contribution of the mucosal microbiota to bovine respiratory health. Trends Microbiol 2019. https://doi.org/10.1016/j.tim.2019.04.005.

27. Dadarwal D, Palmer C, Griebel P. Mucosal immunity of the postpartum bovine genital tract. Theriogenology 2017;104:62–71.

28. Osman R, Malmuthuge N, González-Cano P, et al. Development and function of the mucosal immune system in the upper respiratory tract of neonatal calves. Annu Rev Anim Biosci 2018;6:141–55.

29. Malmuthuge N, Guan LL. Understanding the gut microbiome of dairy calves: opportunities to improve early-life gut health. J Dairy Sci 2017;100:1–10.

30. Okumura R, Takeda K. Roles of intestinal epithelial cells in the maintenance of gut homeostasis. Exp Mol Med 2017;49:e338.

31. Timsit E, Workentine M, van der Meer F, et al. Distinct bacterial metacommunities inhabit the upper and lower respiratory tracts of healthy feedlot cattle and those diagnosed with bronchopneumonia. Vet Microbiol 2018;221:105–13.

32. Taschuk R, Griebel PJ. Commensal microbiome effects on mucosal immune system development in the ruminant gastrointestinal tract. Anim Health Res Rev 2012;13:129–41.

33. Malmuthuge N, Guan LL. Gut microbiome and omics: a new definition to ruminant production and health. Animal Frontiers 2016;6(2):8–12.

34. Kim YH, Nagata R, Ohtani N, et al. Effects of dietary forage and calf starter diet on Ruminal pH and bacteria in Holstein calves during weaning transition. Front Microbiol 2016;7:1575.

35. Khosravi A, Mazmanian SK. Disruption of the gut microbiome as a risk factor for microbial infections. Curr Opin Microbiol 2013;16:221–7.

36. Kim D, Yoo S-A, Kim W-U. Gut microbiota in autoimmunity: potential for clinical applications. Arch Pharm Res 2016;39:1565–76.

37. Timsit E, Holman DB, Hallewell J, et al. The nasopharyngeal microbiota in feedlot cattle and its role in respiratory health. Anim Front 2016;6:44–50.

38. Mayer EA, Tillisch K, Gupta A. Gut/brain axis and the microbiota. J Clin Invest 2015;125:926–38.

39. Gomez DE, Arroyo LG, Costa MC, et al. Characterization of the fecal bacterial microbiota of healthy and diarrheic dairy calves. J Vet Intern Med 2017;31:928–39.

40. Derakhshani H, De Buck J, Mortier R, et al. The features of fecal and ileal mucosa-associated microbiota in dairy calves during early infection with *Mycobacterium avium* subspecies paratuberculosis. Front Microbiol 2016;7:426.

41. Fouhse JM, Zijlstra RT, Willing BP. The role of gut microbiota in the health and disease of pigs. Animal Frontiers 2016;6(3):30–6.

42. Brandtzaeg P. Potential of nasopharynx-associated lymphoid tissue for vaccine responses in the airways. Am J Respir Crit Care Med 2011;183:1595–604.

43. Brandtzaeg P, Kiyono H, Pabst R, et al. Terminology: nomenclature of mucosa-associated lymphoid tissue. Mucosal Immunol 2008;1:31–7.
44. Wira CR, Fahey JV, Rodriguez-Garcia M, et al. Regulation of mucosal immunity in the female reproductive tract: the role of sex hormones in immune protection against sexually transmitted pathogens. Am J Reprod Immunol 2014;72:236–58.
45. Sato S, Kiyono H. The mucosal immune system of the respiratory tract. Curr Opin Virol 2012;2:225–32.
46. Inman CF, Haverson K, Konstantinov SR, et al. Rearing environment affects development of the immune system in neonates. Clin Exp Immunol 2010;160: 431–9.
47. Brandtzaeg P. 'ABC' of mucosal immunology. Nestle Nutr Workshop Ser Pediatr Program 2009;64:23–38 [discussion: 38–43, 251–7].
48. Man WH, de Steenhuijsen Piters WAA, Bogaert D. The microbiota of the respiratory tract: gatekeeper to respiratory health. Nat Rev Microbiol 2017;15:259–70.
49. Butler JE. Immunoglobulin diversity, B-cell and antibody repertoire development in large farm animals. Rev Off Int Epizoot 1998;17:43–70.
50. Liang G, Malmuthuge N, Bao H, et al. Transcriptome analysis reveals regional and temporal differences in mucosal immune system development in the small intestine of neonatal calves. BMC Genomics 2016;17:602.
51. Gabler C, Fischer C, Drillich M, et al. Time-dependent mRNA expression of selected pro-inflammatory factors in the endometrium of primiparous cows postpartum. Reprod Biol Endocrinol 2010;8:152.
52. Wang Y, Ametaj BN, Ambrose DJ, et al. Characterisation of the bacterial microbiota of the vagina of dairy cows and isolation of pediocin-producing *Pediococcus acidilactici*. BMC Microbiol 2013;13:19.
53. Su F, Patel GB, Hu S, et al. Induction of mucosal immunity through systemic immunization: phantom or reality? Hum Vaccin Immunother 2016;12:1070–9.
54. Kolb et al. Protection against bovine respiratory syncytial virus in calves vaccinated with adjuvanted modified live vaccine administered in the face of maternal antibody. Vaccine, in press.
55. Todd JD, Volenec FJ, Paton IM. Interferon in nasal secretions and sera of calves after intranasal administration of avirulent infectious bovine rhinotracheitis virus: association of interferon in nasal secretions with early resistance to challenge with virulent virus. Infect Immun 1972;5:699–706.
56. Vangeel I, Antonis AF, Fluess M, et al. Efficacy of a modified live intranasal bovine respiratory syncytial virus vaccine in 3-week-old calves experimentally challenged with BRSV. Vet J 2007;174:627–35.

Gamma Delta T Cell Function in Ruminants

Mariana Guerra-Maupome, DVM, PhD, Jamison R. Slate, BS, MSc,
Jodi L. McGill, MSc, PhD*

KEYWORDS

- Veterinary immunology • Bovine • Ruminant • Gamma delta T cells
- Nonconventional T cells • Workshop cluster 1
- Immune response to intracellular pathogens

KEY POINTS

- Gamma delta ($\gamma\delta$) T cells are prominent in the immune system of ruminant and other domestic animal species.
- $\gamma\delta$ T cells are nonconventional T cells that bridge the innate and adaptive immune response.
- $\gamma\delta$ T cells influence the outcome of some infectious diseases by rapidly homing to sites of infection.
- $\gamma\delta$ T cells respond directly and specifically to a broad range of antigens but are not major histocompatibility complex restricted.
- $\gamma\delta$ T cells protect against intracellular pathogens directly, by cytolytic activity against infected cells, and indirectly through the activation of other immune populations.

INTRODUCTION

Gamma delta ($\gamma\delta$) T cells have been identified in all vertebrate species examined thus far.[1] Since they were first identified, a considerable effort has been made to understand their function and importance in human and animal health. In ruminants, $\gamma\delta$ T cells constitute a major lymphocyte population in peripheral blood, epithelial tissues, and sites of inflammation.[2] The high frequency of $\gamma\delta$ T cells in the peripheral blood of ruminants (constituting 15%–60% of peripheral blood mononuclear cells), particularly in young animals, suggests an important role in host defense.[2,3]

A large proportion of ruminant $\gamma\delta$ T cells express workshop cluster 1 (WC1), a transmembrane glycoprotein and member of the scavenger receptor cysteine rich (SRCR). WC1 is thought to act as pattern recognition receptor (PRR) and/or costimulatory

Disclosure Statement: National Institutes of Health: Kansas INBRE P20 GM103418 and COBRE P20 GM103638 to JLM.
Department of Veterinary Microbiology and Preventive Medicine, Iowa State University, 1907 Christensen Drive, VMRI Building 5, Ames, IA 50010, USA
* Corresponding author.
E-mail address: jlmcgill@iastate.edu

molecule[4,5] and has historically been used as a surface marker to define $\gamma\delta$ T cell populations in sheep and cattle. $\gamma\delta$ T cells share functions of the innate and the adaptive response and have been proposed to bridge the 2 arms of the immune system. Contrary to $\alpha\beta$ T cells, they can recognize a broad range of antigens (Ags) without restriction by major histocompatibility complex (MHC) molecules. On Ag recognition, $\gamma\delta$ T cells are primed for rapid effector function that correlates with their defined tissue distribution, T cell receptor (TCR) gene expression and WC1 pheno-type. Identified $\gamma\delta$ T cell functional responses include chemokine and cytokine pro-duction,[6–10] cytotoxicity,[7,11–13] Ag presentation,[8,14] and a regulation of inflammatory processes.[11,15,16] However, $\gamma\delta$ T cell functions, particularly in tissue sites such as the mucosa, are still not well understood; thus, a better understanding of their func-tions, and development of improved strategies for engaging these functions in protec-tive immune responses, will be beneficial to both human and animal health. This review describes the main roles of ruminant $\gamma\delta$ T cell subsets in various bovine disease models and discusses the identified mechanisms by which they influence the immune response.

$\gamma\delta$ T CELLS COMPRISE HETEROGENEOUS SUBSETS

Bovine $\gamma\delta$ T cells are typically characterized by the expression or lack thereof, of the receptor WC1.[17,18] WC1 is a transmembrane molecule member of the SRCR family, thought to act as pathogen recognition receptor and/or costimulatory molecule.[4,5] In cattle, the WC1 molecule is encoded by at least 13 genes.[16] Although genes have been identified in humans and mice that share some homology with WC1, the receptor is not expressed in species other than ruminants and pigs.[19] Bovine WC1$^+$ $\gamma\delta$ T cells are CD2$^-$, CD4$^-$, and CD8$^-$ and are a predominant subset in periph-eral blood of cattle. In contrast, the WC1^{neg} $\gamma\delta$ T cell population is most numerous in the spleen, uterus, intestinal mucosa, and mesenteric lymph nodes (LNs), and the ma-jority express CD2 and CD8.[18,20] WC1$^+$ $\gamma\delta$ T cells in cattle can be further divided into 3 defined populations, differentiated by the WC1 genes they express and the pathogens to which they respond: WC1.1$^+$, WC1.2$^+$, and WC1.3$^+$.[21,22]

Like cattle, a large frequency of $\gamma\delta$ T cells in sheep also expresses the WC1 receptor (also known as T19). The ovine WC1 gene family is predicted to contain at least 50 genes.[23,24] $\gamma\delta$ T cells in bison also express the WC1 receptor.[25] A population of WC1^{neg}, CD8$^{low/+}$ has been identified in both sheep[26–28] and bison.[25] Consistent with reports in cattle, WC1^{neg} $\gamma\delta$ T cells from sheep seem to preferentially home to tissue sites such as the uterus.[26–28]

$\gamma\delta$ T CELLS RECOGNIZE ANTIGENS THROUGH WC1, THE T CELL RECEPTOR, AND PATTERN RECOGNITION RECEPTORS

$\gamma\delta$ T cells are able to recognize a variety of protein and nonprotein ligands [reviewed in[29]]. This capacity can be mediated by the TCR, similar to $\alpha\beta$ T cells; however, other receptors also play important roles in $\gamma\delta$ T cell activation, including PRR and WC1 (**Fig. 1**).

Unlike primates, ruminant $\gamma\delta$ T cells do not respond to phosphoantigens but do recognize soluble fractions from many pathogens. Bovine $\gamma\delta$ T cells proliferate and produce interferon gamma (IFNγ) specifically and directly to complex, protein, and nonprotein mycobacterial Ags that cannot be recognized by $\alpha\beta$ T cells; for example, mycolylarabinogalactan peptidoglycan, a component of the *Mycobacterial* cell wall, is differentially recognized by $\gamma\delta$ T cells but not $\alpha\beta$ T cells.[16,30–32] Bovine $\gamma\delta$ T cells respond to both the protein and nonprotein Ags,[33] and TCR Ag binding is required

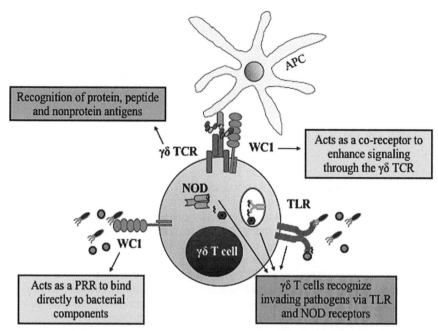

Fig. 1. Ruminant γδ T cells have the capacity to respond to antigens and pathogen-associated molecules via multiple receptors. γδ T cells have the capacity to bind to both protein and nonprotein antigens via their TCR. This type of activation requires antigen presentation by an antigen-presenting cell (APC). γδ T cells also express an array of PRR such as TLR and nucleotide oligomerization domain (NOD) receptors to directly recognize invading pathogens. WC1 is expressed on most of the peripheral blood γδ T cells and likely plays a role as both a PRR and a coreceptor to enhance antigen-specific responses induced via the TCR. It is not well understood how activation through the TCR, WC1, and PRR receptors is coordinated.

for activation.[12,34] Interestingly, bovine γδ T cells respond to certain peptide Ags, such as those from *Mycobacterium bovis* and from *Anaplasma marginale*.[31,34] Unlike αβ T cells, which recognize peptides bound to MHC molecules, bovine γδ T cells are not MHC restricted. They recognize peptides via a mechanism that requires direct cell-cell contact with an antigen-presenting cell and signaling through the γδ TCR, but this recognition is independent of MHC class I or class II complexes that CD8 cytotoxic and CD4 helper T cells require.[31,34]

As an important bridge between the innate and adaptive immune systems, γδ T cells also respond directly to pathogen-associated molecular patterns (PAMPs) through ligation of PRRs such as toll-like receptors (TLRs) and nucleotide oligomerization domain—like receptors—all of which are capable of activating bovine γδ T cells independent of additional TCR signals—as well as WC1 and the TCR itself.[35] For example, purified γδ T cells from bovine peripheral blood secrete the chemokines CCL3 and CCL5 (see **Table 2**) in direct response to both TLR2 and TLR4 ligands, lipopolysaccharide (LPS) and peptidoglycan, which results in recruiting leukocytes into inflammatory sites.[35] The activation of γδ T cells by TLR3 ligand (poly(I:C)) and TLR9 ligand (CpG) enhances in vitro type I IFN production, an important innate immune cytokine. At the gene expression level, bovine γδ T cells express TLR3 and TLR7, receptors that are key for the recognition of virus such as bovine respiratory syncytial virus (BRSV).[10,36]

WC1 molecules play a particularly important role in activation of ruminant γδ T cells. WC1 has the capacity to act as a coreceptor on γδ T cells, similar to CD4 and CD8 on αβ T cells. Some researchers have suggested that WC1 has additional functionality in Ag recognition; it is thought WC1 can act as a hybrid PRR by binding directly to the surface of certain pathogenic bacteria.[3] Ultimately, understanding how signaling through the γδ TCR, PRR, and the various forms of WC1 contribute to Ag-specific responses will be essential to our understanding of overall γδ T cell biology in ruminants.

γδ T CELLS ARE CRITICAL IN YOUNG ANIMALS

γδ T cells constitute up to 60% of the T-lymphocyte population in peripheral blood of young animals, but the relative proportion of circulating γδ T cells decreases to 10% to 20% as the animal ages.[2] The high frequency of γδ T cells in ruminants suggests an important role in the host defense against pathogens, perhaps more so in young animals. Newborn calves are born immunologically naïve. Although all essential immune components are present at birth, many of their functions are "suboptimal" until calves are at least 2 to 4 weeks of age, making newborns more vulnerable to infections (reviewed[37]). Thus, a large pool of preactivated γδ T cells may be critical to immune function in young ruminants, by providing early non–MHC-restricted cellular immunity until CD8 and CD4 T cells become fully established[2] (**Fig. 2**, adapted from[38]). Supporting this, a proportion of γδ T cells in young ruminants express perforin directly ex vivo, simulating a "natural killer" (NK) phenotype that disappears over time.[6,39]

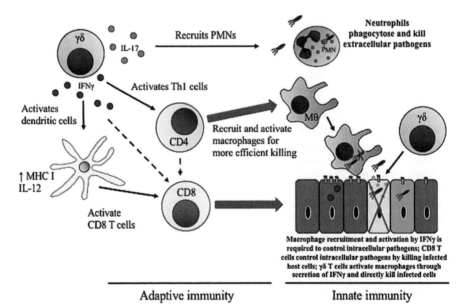

Adaptive immunity Innate immunity

Fig. 2. γδ T cells bridge the innate and adaptive immune system. γδ T cells share features of both the innate and adaptive immune systems. Given their location in the mucosa, a common site of pathogen invasion, γδ T cells are thought to be important in protecting the host in the early stages of disease and to assist with the induction of a robust adaptive immune response. (*Modified from* Baldwin CL, Hsu H, Chen C, et al. The role of bovine γδ T cells and their WC1 co-receptor in response to bacterial pathogens and promoting vaccine efficacy: a model for cattle and humans. *Vet Immunol Immunopathol* 2014;159:144-155; with permission.)

γδ T CELL ANATOMIC DISTRIBUTION

γδ T cells express the same TCRs in a given tissue site, reflecting distinct capabilities for recognition of tissue-specific Ags.[36,40] For example, γδ T cells distributed throughout epithelial surfaces might lack TCR diversity, but exist in a "preactivated" or primed state, which would favor their role as "frontline defenders." Consistent with this concept, sheep γδ T cells patrol the dermal and epidermal areas of the skin.[41,42] Isolation of skin-recirculating γδ T cells from the afferent lymph has the capacity for immediate interleukin 17 (IL-17) and IFNγ secretion, regardless of the state of inflammation in the skin.[41]

Most of the WC1[neg] γδ T cells in cattle are enriched in the intestinal epithelium and lamina propria, red pulp of the spleen, and mesenteric LNs.[2,18,43] Compatible with the role of sentinel mucosal cells, analysis of resting WC1[neg] γδ T cells shows expression of genes promoting tissue quiescence and apoptosis.[36] WC1[+] γδ T cells are well represented in peripheral blood, peripheral LNs, and the skin[18,44]; furthermore, these T cells are more transcriptionally active and primed for rapid effector function including proinflammatory cytokine secretion and cytotoxicity.[36,45,46]

γδ T CELLS RAPIDLY HOME TO SITES OF INFECTION

The tissue distribution and accumulation of γδ T cells is important, as the presence or absence of defined subsets influences the outcome of some infectious diseases. In vivo, following experimental BRSV infection, WC1[+] γδ T cells migrate to the nose, trachea, and lungs of calves 10 days postinfection, and this migration suggests their involvement in the early stages of the antiviral immune response.[47] With *Mycobacterium avium* subspecies paratuberculosis (Map; Johne's disease) experimental infection, highly organized granulomas containing increased numbers of WC1[+] γδ T cells occur early after infection.[48] Similarly, during ovine Map infection, overall frequencies of γδ T cells increased in the ileal tissue with highest densities localized at the periphery of tuberculoid Map lesions.[49] Interestingly, in a bison model of sheep-associated malignant catarrhal fever, CD8[+] WC1[neg] γδ T cells, rather than WC1[+] or CD8 αβ T cells, are the predominant population infiltrating the vascular lesions.[25]

WC1[+] γδ T cells are the first cells to infiltrate the site of delayed-type hypersensitivity reactions following injection with purified protein derivative from *M bovis* (PPD-B), and they accumulate in the periphery of developing tuberculous lesions in the lung and LNs early after infection with virulent or attenuated *M bovis*.[31,50–52] Some studies have attempted to establish a function for γδ T cells in granuloma formation. In a mouse model using fetal bovine tissue (SCID-bo) to reconstitute a functional bovine immune system, depletion of WC1[+] γδ T cells before *M bovis* infection was associated with lack of granuloma organization and increased neutrophil infiltration.[53] In contrast to SCID-bo mouse model, depletion of WC1[+] γδ T cells from calves before *M bovis* challenge had no significant effects on the development or organization of granulomatous lesions.[54]

UNIQUE FUNCTIONAL PROPERTIES OF RUMINANT γδ T CELLS SUBSETS

Since γδ T cells were first identified, a great effort has been made to understand their function and importance in human and animal health. γδ T cells have distinct functions that vary between WC1 subsets, including inflammatory chemokine and cytokine production, cytotoxic activity, Ag presentation, and immunomodulation (**Fig. 3**). The authors further discuss γδ T cell effector functions and define their unique contributions to the immune response in ruminants.

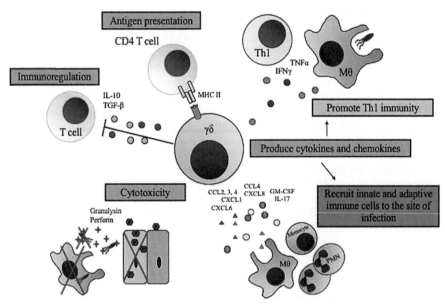

Fig. 3. γδ T cell functions in host defense and immunity. γδ T cells have been shown to play important roles in homeostasis and during disease. They have the capacity to regulate the inflammatory response and promote tissue repair through secretion of antiinflammatory cytokines such as IL-10 and TGF-β; to shape the inflammatory milieu through secretion of innate chemokines; to shape the adaptive immune system by presenting antigens via MHC II and through production of Th1 cytokines such as IFNγ and TNFα; and to control pathogen invasion through direct cytotoxicity against bacterial pathogens and virally infected cells.

Cytokine Production

Although γδ T cells are able to generate a variety of immunomodulatory cytokines (**Table 1**), their differential WC1 gene expression correlates with distinct capacity for cytokine secretion. Ruminant γδ T cells are a significant source of IFNγ (see **Table 1**), but this capacity varies based on WC1 phenotype.[22,34] Depending on environmental stimuli, WC1$^+$ γδ T cells have the capability to secrete inflammatory cytokines, such as IFNγ and tumor necrosis factor alpha (see **Table 1**); immunoregulatory/antiinflammatory cytokines such as IL-4, IL-10, and transforming growth factor beta (TGF-β); and cytokines that support adaptive T cell responses, such as IL-2.[8,16,31,55–57] Bovine and ovine γδ T cells are also major producers of IL-17, another proinflammatory cytokine.[31,41,57–59]

The propensity of γδ T cells to accumulate at lesion sites early in the immune response implicates γδ T cells in initial chemokine production and immune cell recruitment (**Table 2**). In this regard, analysis of chemokine receptor expression profiles indicated that bovine WC1$^+$ γδ T cells express CCR5, CCR7, CXCR3, and CXCR5 transcripts (see **Table 2**) and high levels of L-selectin compared with αβ T cells, suggesting that they are more capable of migration toward inflammatory signals.[50] Directly stimulating circulating bovine γδ T cells with the bacterial cell wall components LPS and peptidoglycan induces expression of chemokines CCL3 and CCL5, two potent chemoattractants for phagocytes of the innate immune system.[35] Other in vitro studies have reported bovine γδ T cell expression of several innate chemokines and receptors, including CCL2, CCL8, CXCL1,

Table 1
Common cytokines and their functions

Cytokine	Function
Proinflammatory Cytokines	
GM-CSF	Key growth factor granulocytes and monocytes. Induces proliferation and differentiation of inflammatory cytokine-secreting cells in inflamed tissues
IFNα/β (Type I IFN)	Induces antiviral states in nearby cells, induces upregulation of MHC I expression, critically important to the innate antiviral immune response
IFNγ (Type II IFN)	Induces a protective antiviral state in cells, increases MHC I and II expression, activates macrophage phagocytosis and iNOS production, promotes Th1 differentiation
IL-17	Master regulator of neutrophil maturation and recruitment, induces expression of downstream proinflammatory chemoattractant such as CXCL8
TNF-α	Potent systemic pyrogen, stimulates apoptosis in various cell types, major chemoattractant for phagocytic neutrophils in localized tissues, important in the Th1 response
Anti-inflammatory/Noninflammatory Cytokines	
IL-2	Potent T cell growth factor, also stimulates proliferation and differentiation of B cells and NK cells
IL-4	Anti-inflammatory cytokine, supports Th2 differentiation and antibody production
IL-10	Anti-inflammatory cytokine, inhibits Th1 differentiation
TGF-β	Anti-inflammatory cytokine, inhibits B and T cell proliferation, promotes tissue repair and resolution

Abbreviations: GM-CSF, granulocyte-macrophage colony-stimulating factor; NK, natural killer; TGF, transforming growth factor; TNF, tumor necrosis factor.

Table 2
Common chemokines and their receptors

Chemokines/Chemotaxis		
Ligands	Receptors	Function
CCL2	CCR2	Monocyte chemoattractant
CCL3	CCR1	Neutrophil chemoattractant, has pyrogenic (fever inducing) effects similar to TNF-α
CCL4	CCR1, CCR5	Chemoattractant for monocytes and natural killer cells
CCL5	CCR5	Strong chemoattractant for granulocytes and leukocytes. Promotes the chemotaxis and proliferation of immune cells into an inflamed tissue
CCL8	CCR1, CCR2B, CCR5	Predominantly a monocyte chemoattractant
CXCL1	CXCR2	Involved in neutrophil chemotaxis and activation
CXCL2	CXCR2	Primarily a neutrophil chemoattractant, has roles in angiogenesis and wound healing
CXCL6	CXCR1, CXCR2	Neutrophil chemoattractant. In addition, it has been reported to have direct bactericidal effects.
CXCL8	CXCR1, CXCR2	Commonly known as IL-8. Potent neutrophil chemoattractant and some other granulocytes, mainly basophils
CXCL13	CXCR5	Regulates B cell homing within the lymph nodes

CXCL2, and CXCL6, which are typically associated with recruitment and activation of myeloid-derived cell types (see **Table 2**).[36] The authors' studies have demonstrated that neonatal bovine $\gamma\delta$ T cell produces CCL2, CCL3, and GM-CSF in response to viral TLR agonists and in vivo during BRSV infection.[10] PAMPs induce "priming" of $\gamma\delta$ T cells, resulting in robust downstream production of chemotactic factors, including CCL3, CCL4, CCL5, CXCL8, and GM-CSF, to presumably promote the influx of lymphocytes and monocytes into the site of infection to control bacterial spread.[9,35] Chemokine expression by $\gamma\delta$ T cells may influence local cellular traffic, promoting the influx of lymphocytes and monocytes and limiting the access of inflammatory cells that may cause tissue damage.[13,16]

Cytotoxicity

$\gamma\delta$ cells are potently cytotoxic and may contribute to the immune response against intracellular pathogens by direct lysis of infected cells or by inhibiting bacterial growth.[7,12,60] Bovine $WC1^+$ $\gamma\delta$ T cells display cytolytic effector functions toward cells infected with a wide-range of pathogens.[7,11,12] This function has been correlated with the expression of granulysin, granzyme B and perforin, all of which are known to affect the viability of intracellular and extracellular pathogens.[6,13,14,45,61] Bovine $\gamma\delta$ T cell cytotoxicity is not MHC restricted, as $\gamma\delta$ T cells from bovine leukemia virus (BLV)-infected animals lysed autologous and xenogenic targets expressing BLV envelope proteins, thus functioning similar to NK cells.[62] Non–MHC-restricted NK-like cytotoxicity has also been observed by $WC1^+$ $\gamma\delta$ T cell lines responding to Babesia bovis[7] and by $\gamma\delta$ T cells isolated from animals with foot-and-mouth disease (FMD) virus.[14] In contrast, lysis of Theileria parva–infected autologous targets by $WC1^+$ $\gamma\delta$ T cell lines was reported to depend on the TCR, but independent of MHC-I and MHC-II.[12]

Antigen Presentation

As an important bridge between the innate and adaptive immune systems, $\gamma\delta$ T cells can be induced to present Ags via MHC class II. Bovine $\gamma\delta$ T cells take up Ag and present it to CD4 T cells, inducing CD4 T cell activation and proliferation.[63] Peripheral blood $WC1^+$ $\gamma\delta$ T cell upregulates MHC II, CD80, and CD86, which are necessary for Ag presentation but also T cell activation, and directly induces CD4 T cell proliferation following FMD infection.[14] In vitro stimulation with M bovis Bacillus Calmette-Guerin (BCG) (the strain used as a vaccine against human tuberculosis) induced upregulation of MHC class II and various costimulatory molecules (CD80, CD86) by $\gamma\delta$ T cells from peripheral blood.[64] Human and murine $\gamma\delta$ T cells have subsequently also been shown to present Ags via MHC class II.

Immunoregulation

$\gamma\delta$ T cells not only play a direct role in pathogen immunity but are also involved in regulating the inflammatory response induced by infection. Depletion of $\gamma\delta$ T cells was shown to increase Ag-specific proliferation of $\alpha\beta$ T cells in cultures from M bovis–infected cattle.[16] It was subsequently shown that[15] bovine $WC1.2^+$ $\gamma\delta$ T cells regulate CD4 T cell responses through secretion of the antiinflammatory cytokines TGF-β and IL-10. Both $WC1^+$ and $WC1^{neg}$ $\gamma\delta$ T cells are able to suppress proliferation and IFN-γ production by CD4 and CD8 T cells through their production of regulatory cytokine IL-10.[56] Thus, $\gamma\delta$ T cells have the capacity to both induce and limit inflammatory responses as a result of infection.

RUMINANT γδ T CELL RESPONSES TO INFECTIOUS DISEASES

γδ T cells are most well characterized for their ability to respond to mycobacterial infections. However, they have been shown to participate in the immune response to a wide variety of viral, bacterial, and parasitic infections (**Table 3**).

Bacterial Pathogens

Bovine γδ T cells proliferate and secrete significant amounts of IFNγ in response to protein and nonprotein Ags from *Mycobacterium*.[16,30,31,33,55] In vivo, the frequency of activated γδ cells increases in the peripheral blood and lungs following experimental *M bovis* infection.[50,54,65,66] BCG vaccination and virulent *M bovis* infection also induce an increase in circulating WC1[+] γδ T cells with the capacity to lyse autologous *M bovis*–infected monocytes.[13,67] γδ T cells are among the first T cells to infiltrate early *M bovis* granuloma lesions, arriving before CD4 T cells.[68] WC1.1[+], WC1.2[+], and WC1[neg] γδ T cells accumulate in the lymphoid mantle surrounding *M bovis* granulomas in the lungs; however, WC1.2[+] γδ T cells seem to dominate during the chronic stage of disease.[31] Depletion of γδ T cells before virulent *M bovis* infection does not significantly alter disease pathology but does result in increased production of Ag-specific IL-4 and impaired lymphocyte proliferative responses, suggesting alterations in the Th1 bias of the immune response following infection.[54]

In both sheep and cattle, γδ T cells accumulate in the ileum during Map (Johne's disease) infection.[49,69] WC1[+] γδ T cells increase significantly in the peripheral blood and milk of Map-infected cattle compared with uninfected cattle.[48] Granuloma organization is associated with differential recruitment of γδ subsets. WC1[+] γδ T cells migrate rapidly to Map lesions, whereas WC1[neg] γδ T cells infiltrate more slowly.[48] In this model, WC1[neg] γδ T cells generate significant quantities of IFNγ during initial infection,[48] perhaps contributing to early local control of the pathogen.

Leptospira borgpetersenii serovar Hardjo is a particularly virulent strain of *Leptospira,* causing kidney damage, infertility, mastitis, abortions, and stillbirths in cattle. Vaccination against *L borgpetersenii* serovar Hardjo stimulates a strong WC1[+] γδ T cell response.[46] Although other vaccines are protective against other serovars of *Leptospira*, only those vaccines that activate WC1[+] γδ T cells are able to protect cows and their fetuses from *L borgpetersenii* serovar Hardjo.[70] Subsequent work using the bovine model of leptospirosis has shown that WC1.1[+] γδ T cells are the subpopulation responsible for vaccine-mediated recognition of *Leptospira* and that WC1 is the PRR responsible for mediating γδ T cell recognition of the bacterium.[4,5,71]

WC1[+] γδ T cells from *A marginale* vaccinated cattle proliferate and secrete IFNγ in specific response to complex *A marginale* Ag and to the immunodominant Ag, major surface protein 2.[34,72] Young calves are more resistant to *A marginale* infection compared with adult animals, a feature that has been attributed to the high circulating frequencies of γδ T cells in young animals.[73] At late stages following *A marginale* infection, the frequency of circulating γδ T cells declines significantly,[74] suggesting that the population is exiting circulation to home to sites of infection in the tissues.

Viral Pathogens

Accumulating evidence suggests that ruminant γδ T cells have the capacity to respond to viral infection. Increased numbers of activated γδ T cells have been reported in peripheral blood of cattle early after exposure to bovine leukemia virus,

Table 3
Main features of bovine γδ T cell subsets in infectious diseases

Pathogen	γδ T Cell Immune Function
Bacterial	
Leptospira spp.	• WC1$^+$ γδ T cells produce robust IFNγ in response to in vitro stimulation with *Leptospira* Ag in vaccinated cattle[70,83] • WC1.1$^+$ γδ T cells mediate protection by proliferating and producing IFNγ in response to *Leptospira* stimulation[22] • WC1 mediates recognition to the bacterium[4,5,71]
M. bovis	• γδ cells undergo dynamic changes in frequency and activation status in the peripheral blood and lungs following experimental *M. bovis* infection[50,54,65,66] • WC1.1$^+$ and WC1.2$^+$ γδ T cells proliferate to in vitro stimulation with complex, protein and nonprotein mycobacterial antigens[31,84] • γδ T cells increase expression of CD25 and CD26 in response to in vitro stimulation with ESTAT6/CFP10 or PPD-b[16] • γδ T cells produce and secrete IL-17 in response to stimulation with *M. bovis* Ag[31] • WC1$^+$ γδ T cells accumulate in early lung and LN following BCG vaccination and in developing granuloma lesions following early after *M. bovis* infection[50,52,66] • WC1.1$^+$, WC1.2$^+$, and WC1^{neg} γδ T cells are found in the lymphoid mantle surrounding *M. bovis* granulomas in the lungs; however, WC1.2$^+$ γδ T cells seem to dominate during the chronic stage of disease[31] • γδ T cells are the first cells to infiltrate the site of intradermal PPD injection in cattle[51] • Depletion of γδ T cells in SCID-bo mice results in impaired granuloma formation[13] • Depletion in vivo of WC1$^+$ γδ T cells from calves before *M. bovis* infection, results in decreased levels of IgG2 and IFNγ and increased IL-4 production[54] • Depletion of γδ T cell from PBMC from *M. bovis*–infected animals results in increased Ag-specific proliferation mediated by TGF-β[16] • BCG vaccination and virulent *M. bovis* infection also induce WC1$^+$ γδ T cell with the capacity to lyse macrophages infected with *M. bovis*[13,67]
M. avium	• In both sheep and cattle, γδ T cells accumulate in the ileum during Map infection[49,65,69] • Highly organized granulomas are characterized by early recruitment of WC1$^+$ γδ T cells, whereas WC1^{neg} γδ T cells infiltrate more slowly[48] • 70% of the γδ T cells in PBMC cultures from Map-infected calves were of WC1$^+$ with increased expression of CD25[65] • WC1^{neg} γδ T cell subset produces IFNγ after experimental Map infection both in vivo and in vitro[68] • Map-specific γδ T cells have immunoregulatory function and exhibit cytotoxic activity against antigen-primed CD4 T cells[11] • γδ T cells suppress CD4 T cell proliferation and produce IL-10 and TGF-β[11]
A. marginale	• WC1.2$^+$ γδ T cells recognize *A. marginale* MSP2 through the TCR, proliferate and produce IFNγ[34]
Viral	
FMD	• FMD vaccine induces increased numbers of γδ T cells with an NK-like phenotype capable of lysing virus-infected target cells[60] • WC1$^+$ γδ T cells increase CD25 and downregulate CD45RO, express IFNγ and perforin, lyse FMD-infected cells, and induce CD4 T cell proliferation[14]

(continued on next page)

Table 3 *(continued)*	
Pathogen	**γδ T Cell Immune Function**
	• γδ T cells from FMD-vaccinated calves localize to the site of FMD infection in the palate mucosa
	• In vivo depletion of WC1$^+$ γδ T cells in cattle after FMD virus infection results in a shorter period of viremia (5 d) compared with depletion of CD4 (6 d) or CD8 T cells (7 d)[77]
BVDV	• γδ T cells increased >100-fold in bronchoalveolar lavage fluid early after infection. Circulating γδ T cells displayed decreased CD45RO expression compared with noninfected animals[75]
	• PI cattle with high frequencies of circulating γδ T cells are resistant to fatal mucosal disease[78]
BRSV	• WC1.1 γδ T cells from BRSV-infected calves' express chemokines[10]
	• In vitro, γδ T cells are a significant source of IL-17 during BRSV/*Mannheimia haemolytica* coinfection[58]
	• Depletion of WC1$^+$ cells have no effect on the kinetics of infection or clinical signs in BRSV-infected calves[79,80]
	• Depletion of WC1$^+$ γδ T cells results in increased IgM and IgA responses in the lung washings[80]
Parasitic	
Theileria spp.	• WC1$^+$ γδ T cells proliferate in response to *Theileria annulata*–infected cells (APC and IL-2 dependent)[8]
	• γδ T cells are activated by and lyse *T parva*–infected cells by recognizing parasite Ag in an MHC-unrestricted fashion and cells acquire the ability to lyse *T. parva*–infected targets[12]
Trypanosoma congolense	• In vitro stimulation with *Trypanosoma* Ag induced proliferation of WC1$^+$ γδ T cells from *Bos taurus* but not *Bos indicus* cattle

Abbreviations: Ig, immunoglobulin; PBMC, peripheral blood mononuclear cell.

bovine herpesvirus 1 (BHV-1), FMD virus, and bovine viral diarrhea virus (BVDV).[14,60,75,76] γδ T cells from FMD-infected animals produced IFN and developed the ability to nonspecifically kill virally infected target cells, including BHV-1 and parainfluenza virus type 3 (PI-3)-infected cells.[14] Furthermore, γδ T cells from FMD-vaccinated cattle localized to the site of FMD infection in the palate mucosa.[60] In vivo depletion of WC1$^+$ γδ T cells in cattle after FMD virus infection results in a shorter period of viremia (5 days) compared with depletion of CD4 (6 days) or CD8 T cells (7 days), suggesting a possible immunosuppressive role for γδ T cell subsets during acute viral infection.[77] Following intrabronchial BVDV infection, early γδ T cell number increased greater than 100-fold higher than background levels in the bronchoalveolar lavage fluid, suggesting that γδ T cells were recruited to the lungs in response to infection.[75] Calves persistently infected (PI) with noncytopathic BVDV are at risk for the development of fatal mucosal disease (MD). However, PI calves with higher frequencies of circulating γδ T cells seem to be more resistant to the development of MD, suggesting a possible role for γδ in mediating innate or nonspecific protection against BVDV superinfection.[78]

The authors' laboratory has demonstrated a correlation between WC1.1 expression and increased chemokine production in γδ T cells from BRSV-infected calves.[10] In vitro, γδ T cells are a significant source of IL-17 during BRSV/*Mannheimia haemolytica* coinfection,[58] and thus they may contribute to disease pathology in this context. Depletion of WC1$^+$ cells has no effect on the kinetics of infection or clinical signs in BRSV-infected calves[79,80]but enhance local and systemic BRSV–specific immunoglobulin (Ig) responses in WC1$^+$-depleted calves.[80] Interestingly, this result was also seen following WC1$^+$ depletion before *M bovis* infection,[54] suggesting the role for γδ T cells in shaping early immunity may extend to responses against viral, as well as intracellular bacterial pathogens.

Parasitic Pathogens

Bovine WC1$^+$ γδ T cells recognize Ags from multiple pathogenic parasites, including *B bovis*,[7] *Theileria annulate*,[8] *T parva*,[12] and *Trypanosoma congolense*.[81] In vitro stimulation with *T parva* Ag induces MHC-independent activation and proliferation of γδ T cells, and cells acquire the ability to lyse *T parva*–infected targets.[12] During early *Neospora caninum* infection, γδ T cells infiltrate the placental tissue and produce IFNγ in response to parasite Ag.[82] Although it seems that a Th1 response eliminates the parasite in this infection, the immune-mediated destruction of placental tissues is likely fatal to the fetus. In vitro, stimulation with *N. caninum*–infected fibroblasts polarizes γδ T cells to differentiate into IL-17–producing cells with the capacity to preferentially kill parasite-infected targets.[59]

SUMMARY

γδ T cells have an important role in many infectious diseases that are of economic importance to domestic species. Thus, engaging them in productive immune responses through vaccination or immunomodulatory strategies may prove highly beneficial to domestic animal health. The understanding of γδ T cell biology, especially in the bovine, has made impressive advancements, particularly in the context of mycobacterial infections. However, several opportunities for study remain regarding the role of individual subsets, γδ T cell participation in immunity to infectious diseases, importance for tissue homeostasis, and development of efficient approaches for engaging particularly subsets in protective, vaccine-induced immune responses. The tools and reagents for addressing these in-depth questions continue to improve, and the field holds great promise for elucidating and engaging this important population for improvement of ruminant and domestic animal health.

REFERENCES

1. Hayday AC. [gamma][delta] cells: a right time and a right place for a conserved third way of protection. Annu Rev Immunol 2000;18:975–1026.
2. Hein WR, Mackay CR. Prominence of gamma delta T cells in the ruminant immune system. Immunol Today 1991;12:30–4.
3. Davis WC, Brown WC, Hamilton MJ, et al. Analysis of monoclonal antibodies specific for the gamma delta TcR. Vet Immunol Immunopathol 1996;52:275–83.
4. Hsu H, Chen C, Nenninger A, et al. WC1 is a hybrid gammadelta TCR coreceptor and pattern recognition receptor for pathogenic bacteria. J Immunol 2015;194:2280–8.
5. Wang F, Herzig CT, Chen C, et al. Scavenger receptor WC1 contributes to the gammadelta T cell response to Leptospira. Mol Immunol 2011;48:801–9.
6. Bonneville M, O'Brien RL, Born WK. Gammadelta T cell effector functions: a blend of innate programming and acquired plasticity. Nat Rev Immunol 2010;10:467–78.
7. Brown WC, Davis WC, Choi SH, et al. Functional and phenotypic characterization of WC1+ gamma/delta T cells isolated from Babesia bovis-stimulated T cell lines. Cell Immunol 1994;153:9–27.

8. Collins RA, Sopp P, Gelder KI, et al. Bovine gamma/delta TcR+ T lymphocytes are stimulated to proliferate by autologous Theileria annulata-infected cells in the presence of interleukin-2. Scand J Immunol 1996;44:444–52.

9. Jutila MA, Holderness J, Graff JC, et al. Antigen-independent priming: a transitional response of bovine gammadelta T-cells to infection. Anim Health Res Rev 2008;9:47–57.

10. McGill JL, Nonnecke BJ, Lippolis JD, et al. Differential chemokine and cytokine production by neonatal bovine gammadelta T-cell subsets in response to viral toll-like receptor agonists and in vivo respiratory syncytial virus infection. Immunology 2013;139:227–44.

11. Chiodini RJ, Davis WC. The cellular immunology of bovine paratuberculosis: the predominant response is mediated by cytotoxic gamma/delta T lymphocytes which prevent CD4+ activity. Microb Pathog 1992;13:447–63.

12. Daubenberger CA, Taracha EL, Gaidulis L, et al. Bovine gammadelta T-cell responses to the intracellular protozoan parasite Theileria parva. Infect Immun 1999;67:2241–9.

13. Skinner MA, Parlane N, McCarthy A, et al. Cytotoxic T-cell responses to Mycobacterium bovis during experimental infection of cattle with bovine tuberculosis. Immunology 2003;110:234–41.

14. Toka FN, Kenney MA, Golde WT. Rapid and transient activation of gammadelta T cells to IFN-gamma production, NK cell-like killing, and antigen processing during acute virus infection. J Immunol 2011;186:4853–61.

15. Hoek A, Rutten VP, Kool J, et al. Subpopulations of bovine WC1(+) gammadelta T cells rather than CD4(+)CD25(high) Foxp3(+) T cells act as immune regulatory cells ex vivo. Vet Res 2009;40:6.

16. Rhodes SG, Hewinson RG, Vordermeier HM. Antigen recognition and immunomodulation by gamma delta T cells in bovine tuberculosis. J Immunol 2001; 166:5604–10.

17. Telfer JC, Baldwin CL. Bovine gamma delta T cells and the function of gamma delta T cell specific WC1 co-receptors. Cell Immunol 2015;296:76–86.

18. Machugh ND, Mburu JK, Carol MJ, et al. Identification of two distinct subsets of bovine gamma delta T cells with unique cell surface phenotype and tissue distribution. Immunology 1997;92:340–5.

19. Crocker G, Sopp P, Parsons K, et al. Analysis of the gamma/delta T cell restricted antigen WC1. Vet Immunol Immunopathol 1993;39:137–44.

20. Baldwin CL, Sathiyaseelan T, Rocchi M, et al. Rapid changes occur in the percentage of circulating bovine WC1(+)gamma delta Th1 cells. Res Vet Sci 2000;69:175–80.

21. Chen C, Herzig CT, Telfer JC, et al. Antigenic basis of diversity in the gammadelta T cell co-receptor WC1 family. Mol Immunol 2009;46:2565–75.

22. Rogers AN, VanBuren DG, Hedblom E, et al. Function of ruminant gammadelta T cells is defined by WC1.1 or WC1.2 isoform expression. Vet Immunol Immunopathol 2005;108:211–7.

23. O'Keeffe MA, Metcalfe SA, Glew MD, et al. Lymph node homing cells biologically enriched for gamma delta T cells express multiple genes from the T19 repertoire. Int Immunol 1994;6:1687–97.

24. Walker ID, Glew MD, O'Keeffe MA, et al. A novel multi-gene family of sheep gamma delta T cells. Immunology 1994;83:517–23.

25. Nelson DD, Davis WC, Brown WC, et al. CD8(+)/perforin(+)/WC1(-) gammadelta T cells, not CD8(+) alphabeta T cells, infiltrate vasculitis lesions of American

bison (Bison bison) with experimental sheep-associated malignant catarrhal fever. Vet Immunol Immunopathol 2010;136:284–91.

26. Fox A, Maddox JF, de Veer MJ, et al. GammadeltaTCR+ cells of the pregnant ovine uterus express variable T cell receptors and contain granulysin. J Reprod Immunol 2010;84:52–6.

27. Fox A, Lee CS, Brandon MR, et al. Effects of pregnancy on lymphocytes within sheep uterine interplacentomal epithelium. Am J Reprod Immunol 1998;40: 295–302.

28. Meeusen E, Fox A, Brandon M, et al. Activation of uterine intraepithelial gamma delta T cell receptor-positive lymphocytes during pregnancy. Eur J Immunol 1993; 23:1112–7.

29. Born WK, Kemal Aydintug M, O'Brien RL. Diversity of gammadelta T-cell antigens. Cell Mol Immunol 2013;10:13–20.

30. Maue AC, Waters WR, Davis WC, et al. Analysis of immune responses directed toward a recombinant early secretory antigenic target six-kilodalton protein-culture filtrate protein 10 fusion protein in Mycobacterium bovis-infected cattle. Infect Immun 2005;73:6659–67.

31. McGill JL, Sacco RE, Baldwin CL, et al. Specific recognition of mycobacterial protein and peptide antigens by gammadelta T cell subsets following infection with virulent Mycobacterium bovis. J Immunol 2014;192:2756–69.

32. Vesosky B, Turner OC, Turner J, et al. Gamma interferon production by bovine gamma delta T cells following stimulation with mycobacterial mycolylarabinogalactan peptidoglycan. Infect Immun 2004;72:4612–8.

33. Welsh MD, Kennedy HE, Smyth AJ, et al. Responses of bovine WC1(+) gammadelta T cells to protein and nonprotein antigens of Mycobacterium bovis. Infect Immun 2002;70:6114–20.

34. Lahmers KK, Norimine J, Abrahamsen MS, et al. The CD4+ T cell immunodominant Anaplasma marginale major surface protein 2 stimulates gammadelta T cell clones that express unique T cell receptors. J Leukoc Biol 2005;77:199–208.

35. Hedges JF, Lubick KJ, Jutila MA. Gamma delta T cells respond directly to pathogen-associated molecular patterns. J Immunol 2005;174:6045–53.

36. Hedges JF, Cockrell D, Jackiw L, et al. Differential mRNA expression in circulating gammadelta T lymphocyte subsets defines unique tissue-specific functions. J Leukoc Biol 2003;73:306–14.

37. Chase CC, Hurley DJ, Reber AJ. Neonatal immune development in the calf and its impact on vaccine response. Vet Clin North Am Food Anim Pract 2008;24: 87–104.

38. Baldwin CL, Hsu H, Chen C, et al. The role of bovine γδ T cells and their WC1 coreceptor in response to bacterial pathogens and promoting vaccine efficacy: a model for cattle and humans. Vet Immunol Immunopathol 2014;159:144–55.

39. De Rosa SC, Andrus JP, Perfetto SP, et al. Ontogeny of gamma delta T cells in humans. J Immunol 2004;172:1637–45.

40. Wilson E, Hedges JF, Butcher EC, et al. Bovine gamma delta T cell subsets express distinct patterns of chemokine responsiveness and adhesion molecules: a mechanism for tissue-specific gamma delta T cell subset accumulation. J Immunol 2002;169:4970–5.

41. Geherin SA, Lee MH, Wilson RP, et al. Ovine skin-recirculating γδ T cells express IFN-γ and IL-17 and exit tissue independently of CCR7. Vet Immunol Immunopathol 2013;155:87–97.

42. Gorrell MD, Townsend WL, Ladds PW. The distribution of lymphocyte subpopulations in normal and acanthotic ovine skin. Vet Immunol Immunopathol 1995;44: 151–67.

43. Itohara S, Farr AG, Lafaille JJ, et al. Homing of a gamma delta thymocyte subset with homogeneous T-cell receptors to mucosal epithelia. Nature 1990;343:754–7.

44. Wilson E, Aydintug MK, Jutila MA. A circulating bovine gamma delta T cell subset, which is found in large numbers in the spleen, accumulates inefficiently in an artificial site of inflammation: correlation with lack of expression of E-selectin ligands and L-selectin. J Immunol 1999;162:4914–9.

45. Blumerman SL, Herzig CT, Wang F, et al. Comparison of gene expression by co-cultured WC1+ gammadelta and CD4+ alphabeta T cells exhibiting a recall response to bacterial antigen. Mol Immunol 2007;44:2023–35.

46. Blumerman SL, Herzig CT, Baldwin CL. WC1+ gammadelta T cell memory population is induced by killed bacterial vaccine. Eur J Immunol 2007;37:1204–16.

47. Thomas LH, Cook RS, Howard CJ, et al. Influence of selective T-lymphocyte depletion on the lung pathology of gnotobiotic calves and the distribution of different T-lymphocyte subsets following challenge with bovine respiratory syncytial virus. Res Vet Sci 1996;61:38–44.

48. Plattner BL, Doyle RT, Hostetter JM. Gamma-delta T cell subsets are differentially associated with granuloma development and organization in a bovine model of mycobacterial disease. Int J Exp Pathol 2009;90:587–97.

49. Little D, Alzuherri HM, Clarke CJ. Phenotypic characterisation of intestinal lymphocytes in ovine paratuberculosis by immunohistochemistry. Vet Immunol Immunopathol 1996;55:175–87.

50. Price S, Davies M, Villarreal-Ramos B, et al. Differential distribution of WC1(+) gammadelta TCR(+) T lymphocyte subsets within lymphoid tissues of the head and respiratory tract and effects of intranasal M. bovis BCG vaccination. Vet Immunol Immunopathol 2010;136:133–7.

51. Doherty ML, Bassett HF, Quinn PJ, et al. A sequential study of the bovine tuberculin reaction. Immunology 1996;87:9–14.

52. Cassidy JP, Bryson DG, Pollock JM, et al. Early lesion formation in cattle experimentally infected with Mycobacterium bovis. J Comp Pathol 1998;119:27–44.

53. Smith RA, Kreeger JM, Alvarez AJ, et al. Role of CD8+ and WC-1+ gamma/delta T cells in resistance to Mycobacterium bovis infection in the SCID-bo mouse. J Leukoc Biol 1999;65:28–34.

54. Kennedy HE, Welsh MD, Bryson DG, et al. Modulation of immune responses to Mycobacterium bovis in cattle depleted of WC1(+) gamma delta T cells. Infect Immun 2002;70:1488–500.

55. Smyth AJ, Welsh MD, Girvin RM, et al. In vitro responsiveness of gammadelta T cells from Mycobacterium bovis-infected cattle to mycobacterial antigens: predominant involvement of WC1(+) cells. Infect Immun 2001;69:89–96.

56. Guzman E, Hope J, Taylor G, et al. Bovine gammadelta T cells are a major regulatory T cell subset. J Immunol 2014;193:208–22.

57. Steinbach S, Vordermeier HM, Jones GJ. CD4+ and gammadelta T Cells are the main Producers of IL-22 and IL-17A in Lymphocytes from Mycobacterium bovis-infected Cattle. Sci Rep 2016;6:29990.

58. McGill JL, Rusk RA, Guerra-Maupome M, et al. Bovine Gamma Delta T Cells Contribute to Exacerbated IL-17 Production in Response to Co-Infection with Bovine RSV and Mannheimia haemolytica. PLoS One 2016;11:e0151083.

59. Peckham RK, Brill R, Foster DS, et al. Two distinct populations of bovine IL-17(+) T-cells can be induced and WC1(+)IL-17(+)gammadelta T-cells are effective killers of protozoan parasites. Sci Rep 2014;4:5431.

60. Amadori M, Archetti IL, Verardi R, et al. Role of a distinct population of bovine gamma delta T cells in the immune response to viral agents. Viral Immunol 1995;8:81–91.

61. Alvarez AJ, Endsley JJ, Werling D, et al. WC1(+) gammadelta T cells indirectly regulate chemokine production during mycobacterium bovis infection in SCID-bo mice. Transbound Emerg Dis 2009;56:275–84.

62. Bukowski JF, Morita CT, Brenner MB. Recognition and destruction of virus-infected cells by human gamma delta CTL. J Immunol 1994;153:5133–40.

63. Collins RA, Werling D, Duggan SE, et al. Gammadelta T cells present antigen to CD4+ alphabeta T cells. J Leukoc Biol 1998;63:707–14.

64. Price SJ, Hope JC. Enhanced secretion of interferon-gamma by bovine gamma-delta T cells induced by coculture with Mycobacterium bovis-infected dendritic cells: evidence for reciprocal activating signals. Immunology 2009;126:201–8.

65. Koets A, Rutten V, Hoek A, et al. Progressive bovine paratuberculosis is associated with local loss of CD4(+) T cells, increased frequency of gamma delta T cells, and related changes in T-cell function. Infect Immun 2002;70:3856–64.

66. Pollock JM, Pollock DA, Campbell DG, et al. Dynamic changes in circulating and antigen-responsive T-cell subpopulations post-Mycobacterium bovis infection in cattle. Immunology 1996;87:236–41.

67. Olin MR, Hwa Choi K, Lee J, et al. Gammadelta T-lymphocyte cytotoxic activity against Mycobacterium bovis analyzed by flow cytometry. J Immunol Methods 2005;297:1–11.

68. Plattner BL, Huffman EL, Hostetter JM. Gamma-delta T-cell responses during subcutaneous Mycobacterium avium subspecies paratuberculosis challenge in sensitized or naive calves using matrix biopolymers. Vet Pathol 2013;50:630–7.

69. Charavaryamath C, Gonzalez-Cano P, Fries P, et al. Host responses to persistent Mycobacterium avium subspecies paratuberculosis infection in surgically isolated bovine ileal segments. Clin Vaccine Immunol 2013;20:156–65.

70. Brown RA, Blumerman S, Gay C, et al. Comparison of three different leptospiral vaccines for induction of a type 1 immune response to Leptospira borgpetersenii serovar Hardjo. Vaccine 2003;21:4448–58.

71. Damani-Yokota P, Telfer JC, Baldwin CL. Variegated transcription of the WC1 hybrid PRR/co-receptor genes by individual γδ T cells and correlation with pathogen responsiveness. Front Immunol 2018;9:717.

72. Tuo W, Bazer FW, Davis WC, et al. Differential effects of type I IFNs on the growth of WC1- CD8+ gamma delta T cells and WC1+ CD8- gamma delta T cells in vitro. J Immunol 1999;162:245–53.

73. Jones WE, Kliewer IO, Norman BB, et al. Anaplasma marginale infection in young and aged cattle. Am J Vet Res 1968;29:535–44.

74. Wyatt CR, Davis WC, Knowles DP, et al. Effect on intraerythrocytic Anaplasma marginale of soluble factors from infected calf blood mononuclear cells. Infect Immun 1996;64:4846–9.

75. Silflow RM, Degel PM, Harmsen AG. Bronchoalveolar immune defense in cattle exposed to primary and secondary challenge with bovine viral diarrhea virus. Vet Immunol Immunopathol 2005;103:129–39.

76. Endsley JJ, Quade MJ, Terhaar B, et al. BHV-1-specific CD4+, CD8+, and gammadelta T cells in calves vaccinated with one dose of a modified live BHV-1 vaccine. Viral Immunol 2002;15:385–93.

77. Juleff N, Windsor M, Lefevre EA, et al. Foot-and-mouth disease virus can induce a specific and rapid CD4+ T-cell-independent neutralizing and isotype class-switched antibody response in naïve cattle. J Virol 2009;83:3626–36.

78. Bruschke CJ, Haghparast A, Hoek A, et al. The immune response of cattle, persistently infected with noncytopathic BVDV, after superinfection with antigenically semi-homologous cytopathic BVDV. Vet Immunol Immunopathol 1998;62: 37–50.

79. Mcinnes E, Sopp P, Howard CJ, et al. Phenotypic analysis of local cellular responses in calves infected with bovine respiratory syncytial virus. Immunology 1999;96:396–403.

80. Taylor G, Thomas LH, Wyld SG, et al. Role of T-lymphocyte subsets in recovery from respiratory syncytial virus infection in calves. J Virol 1995;69:6658–64.

81. Flynn JN, Sileghem M. Involvement of gamma delta T cells in immunity to trypanosomiasis. Immunology 1994;83:86–92.

82. Maley SW, Buxton D, Macaldowie CN, et al. Characterization of the immune response in the placenta of cattle experimentally infected with Neospora caninum in early gestation. J Comp Pathol 2006;135:130–41.

83. Naiman BM, Alt D, Bolin CA, et al. Protective killed Leptospira borgpetersenii vaccine induces potent Th1 immunity comprising responses by CD4 and gamma-delta T lymphocytes. Infect Immun 2001;69:7550–8.

84. Vesosky B, Turner OC, Turner J, et al. Activation marker expression on bovine peripheral blood gammadelta T cells during post-natal development and following vaccination with a commercial polyvalent viral vaccine. Dev Comp Immunol 2003;27:439–47.

Mycoplasma bovis

Interactions with the Immune System and Failure to Generate an Effective Immune Response

Fiona P. Maunsell, BVSc, PhD[a],*, Christopher Chase, DVM, MS, PhD[b]

KEYWORDS

- *Mycoplasma bovis* • Pathogenesis • Immune response

KEY POINTS

- Host responses are often ineffective at clearing *Mycoplasma bovis* infection and may contribute to the pathogenesis of disease. The optimal immune response for the control of *M bovis* infection is unknown.
- For such a small and structurally simple pathogen, *M bovis* possesses a surprisingly large repertoire of strategies to disrupt, evade, and modulate almost every aspect of the host immune response.
- Immune modulation occurs through direct effects on neutrophils, macrophages, and lymphocytes as well as indirect effects via the induction of cytokine secretion. *M bovis* can also evade immune responses through surface antigen variation, and possibly by intracellular invasion and biofilm production.

INTRODUCTION

Over the last half century *Mycoplasma bovis* has emerged as a globally important pathogen of cattle. A variety of clinical syndromes are associated with *M bovis* infection, particularly bovine respiratory disease (BRD) and mastitis but also otitis media, conjunctivitis, arthritis, genital tract infections, and decubital abscesses.[1] *M bovis* is primarily an inhabitant of respiratory mucosal surfaces, and, like the other opportunistic pathogens of the BRD complex, it is often found in the upper respiratory tract of healthy cattle. *M bovis* is able to persist at sites of colonization for long periods in some cattle, with or without intermittent shedding.[1–3]

Disclosure: The author has nothing to disclose.
[a] Department of Large Animal Clinical Sciences, College of Veterinary Medicine, University of Florida, PO Box 100136, Gainesville, FL 32610, USA; [b] Department of Veterinary and Biomedical Sciences, South Dakota State University, PO Box 2175, SAR Room 125 North Campus Drive, Brookings, SD 57007, USA
* Corresponding author.
E-mail address: maunsellf@ufl.edu

Both intramammary[4–6] and respiratory[7–9] infection elicit active humoral and cell-mediated immune responses. Some animals effectively control infection, although how they do so is poorly understood. Consistent with an effective immune response in some animals, infection often remains subclinical.[1–3,10,11] In addition, prior intra-mammary infection with *M bovis* provides at least short-term protection from future cases of clinical mycoplasmal mastitis,[4] and outbreaks of severe mastitis are unusual in endemically infected herds. Also consistent with the potential for an effective immune response against *M bovis*, there are some examples of successful vaccination of calves against experimental respiratory challenge.[12–14] However, vaccines that have seemed promising in experimental challenge models have often failed to provide protection in the field.[12,15,16] Overall, the body of research suggests that host responses can control *M bovis* infection under poorly defined circumstances, but that this pathogen is often successful in evading these responses.

M bovis–associated disease occurs when host and/or pathogen factors result in rapid replication in the upper respiratory tract and subsequent dissemination to the lung and/or middle ear, or invasion and hematogenous spread to other tissues. Mastitis occurs after hematogenous spread of *M bovis* or after intramammary inoculation. Once clinical disease has occurred, host responses are often ineffective at resolving *M bovis* infection, with chronic, debilitating disease being a frequent outcome.

Mycoplasmas are pathogens of many species, and are known to use multiple strategies that disrupt host responses to promote chronic infection. However, despite the importance of *M bovis* as a bovine pathogen, there is limited understanding of the factors that allow the establishment, persistence, and dissemination of infection, and why host defenses frequently fail to resolve disease. There are also limited data on mycoplasmal pathogens of other species from which to draw parallels; for example, despite *Mycoplasma pneumoniae* being a leading cause of community-acquired pneumonia in humans, the host-pathogen interactions that allow it to establish chronic infection of the respiratory tract are poorly understood.[17] Many factors have been identified in vitro that may contribute to the modulation and evasion of the immune response by *M bovis*, but there is a need for data evaluating their role in vivo. This article focuses on current knowledge of the host-pathogen interactions that allow *M bovis* to be such a successful pathogen of cattle.

MICROBIAL CHARACTERISTICS IMPORTANT IN *MYCOPLASMA BOVIS* PATHOGENESIS

Mycoplasmas lack a cell wall and interact with their environment through a large number of proteins in, or anchored to, the cytoplasmic membrane. These proteins play vital roles in nutrient acquisition, adhesion, and modulation of host immune responses. Characteristics of *M bovis* imparted by membrane proteins include the ability to adhere to a wide variety of cell types, surface antigen variation, and biofilm production.

Adhesins

Adhesion to host epithelial cells is an essential first step for the establishment of respiratory tract infection. *M bovis* adheres to a wide variety of respiratory and nonrespiratory epithelial cell types in vitro.[18–21] The ability of different strains of *M bovis* to adhere to epithelial cells is related to virulence, with less pathogenic or nonpathogenic strains having lower adherence rates than more virulent strains.[21]

Several adhesins have been identified in *M bovis*. The variable surface lipoprotein (Vsp) family is discussed later, but, in addition to acting as major immunogens, some members are important adhesins.[21,22] Other adhesins include 3 enzymes that adhere to fibronectin and/or plasminogen in addition to their metabolic functions.[23–25] Many *M bovis* membrane proteins predicted from genome sequencing remain hypothetical,[26] and it is likely that additional adhesins remain to be identified. Little is known of the host environments under which specific adhesins are important. However, it is clear that *M bovis* has a complex adhesion strategy that likely enhances its ability to infect multiple tissue types and cause a wide variety of clinical manifestations.

Surface Antigens and Antigenic Variation

One of the best-studied features of *M bovis* is a large family of highly immunodominant variable surface lipoproteins (Vsps).[27–30] The 13 members of the Vsp family undergo high-frequency phase and size variation, providing a vast and complex capacity for antigenic variation.[28–31] Some Vsps contain adhesive domains[22] and others are thought to play a role in biofilm formation.[32] Perhaps most importantly, variation in these immunodominant surface lipoproteins likely plays a key role in evading host immune defenses.[22,33] Exposure to antibodies directed against specific Vsps results in selection for new dominant Vsp variants.[33] The Vsp family therefore provides *M bovis* with a highly dynamic surface structure that allows populations of this pathogen to adapt to varying conditions both within the host and in the external environment, including immune evasion. Outside of the Vsp family, other variable surface proteins have been identified in *M bovis*, further enhancing capacity for antigenic variation.[34]

In addition to variable surface proteins, several conserved surface proteins are expressed by *M bovis*.[18,24,35,36] Theoretically these should provide good targets for an adaptive immune response, but many animals remain chronically infected despite producing antibodies against these immunogens.

Biofilm Formation

Biofilms provide protection from host defenses, such as opsonization and complement-mediated lysis, as well as from environmental stressors and antimicrobial penetration. They are an important feature of many chronic bacterial infections. Most strains of *M bovis* form biofilms in vitro and *M bovis* is a prolific biofilm former compared with many other mycoplasmal species.[32] Using an immunoproteomics approach, Chen and colleagues[37] (2018) found that 6 proteins uniquely expressed by *M bovis* in biofilms, but not by planktonic cells, were immunoreactive with bovine convalescent serum. This finding supports the hypothesis that *M bovis* forms biofilms in vivo, where they may be important in chronic colonization of the upper respiratory tract.

Hydrogen Peroxide Production

Hydrogen peroxide (H_2O_2) production is an important virulence factor of several *Mycoplasma* pathogens.[38,39] H_2O_2 is produced by *M bovis* in vitro[40] and may be important in causing oxidative injury to lung tissue.[41] The importance of H_2O_2 production in the pathogenesis of *M bovis*–associated disease still needs to be elucidated, but H_2O_2 production by other *Mycoplasma* pathogens contributes to cytotoxity.[38]

ANTIBODY AND T-CELL RESPONSES TO *MYCOPLASMA BOVIS* INFECTION

Experimental *M bovis* respiratory infection elicits a humoral response, with a median time to seroconversion of 21 days.[42] Antibody titers to *M bovis* increase for several weeks after challenge.[9] In calves, adaptive immune responses to *M bovis* seem to have a T-helper (Th) 2 bias, with immunoglobulin (Ig) G_1 predominating in serum,[7,9] and little IgG_2 produced.[9] Consistent with these findings, IgG_1-producing plasma cells predominate in the lungs of calves with experimentally induced *M bovis* pneumonia.[43]

M bovis infection also results in IgA production in the upper and lower respiratory tract.[8,10] Natural infection of calves elicits a more variable intensity of antibody responses than experimental infection, with some calves failing to produce a detectable systemic antibody response.[44] In summary, local and systemic antibody responses occur in response to *M bovis* colonization of the respiratory tract in some, but not all, cattle. When these responses occur they are often ineffective in controlling *M bovis* infection. Intramammary inoculation of *M bovis* in adult cows stimulates both systemic IgG_1 and IgG_2 responses.[5] Concentrations and total production of IgA and IgG also increase in the mammary gland after inoculation[4–6] and may be important in protection from subsequent infection because their concentrations are higher in glands resistant to reinfection than in susceptible glands.[4] More work is needed to better define the humoral responses that are most efficient at *M bovis* clearance from the respiratory tract and mammary gland, as well as responses that protect from new infections.

In nonbovine species, mycoplasma infections of the respiratory tract are characterized by production of both proinflammatory and antiinflammatory cytokines.[45] The intensity of lung inflammation during mycoplasma infection is thought to be driven by the balance of cytokines produced.[45,46] Peripheral blood mononuclear cells (PBMCs) from calves infected with *M bovis* secrete both interferon (IFN)-γ and interleukin (IL)-4, suggesting a mixed Th1-Th2 systemic cytokine response, although a lack of IgG_2 production is more consistent with a Th2-biased response.[9] After *M bovis* respiratory infection of 12-week-old calves, cluster of differentiation (CD) 4+, CD8+, and $\gamma\delta$ T cells showed higher in vitro activation in response to *M bovis* antigens than did cells from uninfected calves.[9] Strong major histocompatibility complex (MHC) class II expression is observed in bronchus-associated lymphoid tissue in calves experimentally infected with *M bovis*, consistent with the stimulation of local T-cell responses by antigen-presenting cells.[43]

In addition to the microbial characteristics, such as surface antigen variation, that may contribute to evasion of immune responses, *M bovis* exerts a broad range of immunomodulatory effects on host cells that may promote ineffective responses. Ongoing, ineffective immune responses contribute to the chronic inflammation that is commonly associated with mycoplasmal diseases.

HOST-PATHOGEN INTERACTIONS, IMMUNE EVASION, AND DYSREGULATION
Strategies to Avoid Opsonization

Effective phagocytosis of *M bovis* by bovine neutrophils and macrophages depends on opsonization.[47] The humoral immune response to *M bovis* tends to be skewed toward IgG_1 production, which is a less effective opsonin for neutrophil phagocytosis and killing than IgG_2.[43,48] *M bovis* has several additional strategies that may help it to evade opsonization (**Fig. 1**). First, variation in surface antigens is driven at least partly by antibody-mediated selection pressure,[33] an important strategy by which antigenic variants could evade opsonization. Second, the formation of biofilms may provide *M bovis* with physical protection from opsonization and phagocytosis.[32] Third, some species of *Mycoplasma* have been found to express 2 proteins that damage host immunoglobulins, one that binds IgG (Mycoplasma Ig binding protein) and another that cleaves IgG heavy chains (Mycoplasma Ig protease).[49] Although this system has not been studied in *M bovis*, there are several copies of the *mip* and *mib* genes in all the *M bovis* genomes that have been fully sequenced.[50] This system may provide *M bovis* with an additional strategy for avoiding antibody-mediated phagocytosis (see **Fig. 1**).

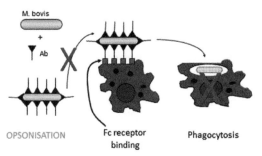

OPSONISATION   Fc receptor   Phagocytosis
                binding

Fig. 1. Mycoplasma bovis Interferes with Opsonization. Opsonization with antibody or complement greatly increases the chances that a bacteria will be phagocytized and then killed by phagocytic cells (neutrophils and macrophages). M bovis has several mechanisms it uses to prevent opsonization thus escaping phagocytosis and killing.

Neutrophil Interactions with Mycoplasma bovis

Neutrophils use a variety of strategies to remove invaders, including degranulation, phagocytosis, killing by release of reactive oxygen species, antibody-derived cell cytotoxicity, and the release of neutrophil extracellular traps (NETs). Neutrophils are the most abundant immune cell type in the lungs, middle ear, and joints of cattle with *M bovis*–associated disease.[51–54] The extent of neutrophil recruitment to sites of *M bovis* infection seems directly correlated with the severity of disease, and ongoing recruitment while failing to clear infection is likely a contributor to the severe inflammatory lung lesions observed in many cattle with chronic *M bovis* disease.

Neutrophils show impaired function in vitro after exposure to *M bovis*.[47,55,56] Unopsonized *M bovis* exerts a wide variety of effects on bovine neutrophils, adhering to the cell surface without being phagocytosed, inhibiting respiratory burst activity and nitric oxide production, inducing the production of the proinflammatory cytokines IL-12 and TNF-α, and enhancing neutrophil apoptosis.[55,56]

Many pathogens induce neutrophils to form NETs. NETs are webs of extracellular DNA and antimicrobial neutrophil granule proteins that trap and kill pathogens. Several *Mycoplasma* species, including *M pneumoniae*, secrete extracellular nucleases, allowing escape from NET-mediated killing.[57] Mycoplasmas have been shown to use host nucleotides from degraded NETs for DNA synthesis.[58] Recent research has shown that bovine neutrophils produce NETs in response to *M bovis*, but those NETs are rapidly degraded by a membrane nuclease.[59] This membrane nuclease likely plays an important role in virulence. Given that several of the other bacterial pathogens of the BRD complex are potent stimulators of NET production,[60,61] the ability to degrade such NETs may be especially important in allowing *M bovis* to persist in the mixed bacterial infections common in BRD.

In summary, *M bovis* has a surprisingly diverse array of strategies to evade opsonization as well as phagocytosis and killing by neutrophils, perhaps indicating the importance of neutrophils in combatting mycoplasma infections.

Macrophage Interactions with Mycoplasma bovis

Macrophages play a crucial role in the early control of bacterial infections, with effective recognition, clearance of bacteria, cytokine production, and antigen presentation all being important to a successful immune response. Opsonization is critical for bovine alveolar macrophages to phagocytose and kill mycoplasmas in vitro.[47] Strategies *M bovis* uses to evade opsonization are discussed earlier.

The local cytokine environment drives the inflammatory response in bacterial pneumonia. Although many cell types can contribute to cytokine production, alveolar macrophages are especially important in driving downstream immune responses in BRD. *M bovis* stimulates cytokine production by alveolar macrophages and by blood monocytes. The expression of the proinflammatory cytokines TNF-α and IFN-γ was induced in vivo in alveolar macrophages in the lung and local lymphoid tissue of cattle in experimentally induced *M bovis* pneumonia.[62] TNF-α production by alveolar macrophages was similarly stimulated by in vitro incubation with *M bovis*.[63] However, in natural *M bovis* infection, increased alveolar macrophage expression of the antiinflammatory cytokine IL-10, as well as TNF-α and IFN-γ, is reported, indicating a more mixed cytokine response.[64] Cytokine production by blood monocytes exposed to *M bovis* differs from that reported for tissue macrophages. Bovine blood monocytes did not produce TNF-α or IFN-γ but did produce IL-10 when incubated with *M bovis*.[65] PBMCs from calves with clinical *M bovis*–associated disease have reduced IFN-γ production on stimulation with *M bovis* compared with those from clinically healthy cattle.[66] Therefore, the response to *M bovis* infection seems to vary between body compartments, and further work is needed to understand the major effects of *M bovis* on activation of circulating monocytes and tissue macrophages and cytokine production in vivo.

Oxidative injury induced by alveolar macrophages may contribute to the caseonecrotic lesions that are typical of pneumonia and arthritis caused by *M bovis*, with large numbers of inducible nitric oxide (iNOS)–expressing macrophages identified in or adjacent to necrotic lung and joint lesions.[67,68] Both *M bovis* antigen and macrophages that strongly express iNOS colocalize to the margins of caseonecrotic lesions,[67] and alveolar macrophages produce nitric oxide when incubated with *M bovis*.[63]

Tissue macrophages play a key role in antigen presentation. MHC class II expression is increased in local lymphoid tissues during experimental infection with *M bovis* but is downregulated in macrophages at the margins of chronic *M bovis* lung[43,69] and joint[68] lesions. The mechanism of MHC class II downregulation on activated macrophages is yet to be determined, but it has been hypothesized that it may be caused by iNOS expression and nitric oxide production.[43] MHC class II expression by dendritic cells in airway mucosa is increased in *M bovis* pneumonia, but is downregulated at the margins of lung lesions.[43] Downregulation of MHC class II expression by the major antigen-presenting cells at the site of *M bovis* infection may contribute to ongoing, ineffective local responses.

Another mechanism by which *M bovis* modulates host immune responses is through effects on programmed cell death. *M bovis* delays apoptosis in monocytes[65,70] and alveolar macrophages (**Fig. 2**).[71] Delayed monocyte/macrophage apoptosis could be expected to reduce the effector functions of these important phagocytic and antigen-presenting cells, and alter the orchestration of the immune response.

Immunomodulatory Effects of Mycoplasma bovis on Lymphocytes

Several research teams have shown the immunomodulatory effects of *M bovis* on bovine lymphocytes in vitro. At least some strains of *M bovis* inhibit the proliferation of lymphocytes[70–72]; the mechanism is currently unknown. In addition, live *M bovis* induces apoptosis of bovine lymphocytes in vitro,[73] which may be another mechanism by which it modulates the host response.

Recent work suggests that T-cell exhaustion is an important mechanism whereby *M bovis* alters lymphocyte function (see **Fig. 2**).[66,74] T-cell exhaustion is a state of reduced responsiveness of antigen-specific CD8+ and CD4+ T cells induced by

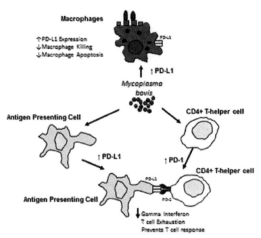

Fig. 2. Mycoplasma bovis Immune Suppression by the Induction of PD-1 and/or PD-L1. Programmed death 1 (PD-1) receptor is expressed normally at low levels on activated T cells. M. bovis increases PD-1 levels on T helper and cytotoxic T cells. M. bovis also increases the expression of Programmed death ligand 1 (PD-L1) on activated antigen-presenting cells and macrophages. The expression of PD-L1 on macrophages decreases macrophage killing of bacteria and also prevents the cells from undergoing apoptosis. The co-expression of PD-1 on the T cells and PD-L1 on the antigen presenting cells inhibits the ability of T cells to both replicate and also to kill, resulting in T cell exhaustion.

chronic, continuous antigen presentation and T-cell receptor stimulation. It contributes to ineffective ongoing immune responses in chronic infections,[75] including some chronic diseases of cattle.[76–78] T-cell exhaustion is characterized by reversible progressive loss of effector functions such as antigen-specific proliferative responses, cytokine production, and cytotoxic activity, as well as failure of normal memory T-cell responses. Exhausted T cells have upregulation of multiple inhibitory receptors, the best characterized of which is the programmed death 1 (PD-1) receptor, which is normally expressed at low to moderate levels on activated T cells.[75] When PD-1 binds to its ligand, PD ligand 1 (PD-L1) on activated antigen-presenting cells, T-cell effector functions are inhibited.[75] Substantial upregulation of PD-1 and PD1-1 expression results in T-cell exhaustion.[75] PBMCs from cattle with *M bovis*–associated disease have upregulation of PD-1 on CD4+ and CD8+ T cells, reduced IFN-γ production, and increased PD-L1 expression on macrophages; and blocking PD-1 and PD-L1 restores antigen-specific IFN-γ production.[66] The expression of PD-L1 is substantially upregulated in tracheal epithelial cells, lung epithelial cells, and lung lavage macrophages after in vitro incubation with *M bovis* (see **Fig. 2**).[74] In addition, the PD-1/PD-L1 axis is upregulated in immune cells in the lungs of cattle experimentally infected with *M bovis*.[74] Together these data support an important role for T cell exhaustion in maintaining the host-pathogen stalemate that occurs during chronic *M bovis*–associated disease.

Cell Invasion and Intracellular Survival of Mycoplasma bovis

Although most *M bovis* organisms reside on mucosal surfaces or extracellularly within lesions, *M bovis* can invade and survive in a variety of host cell types.[31,70,71] *M bovis* survives inside bovine alveolar macrophages in vitro and in vivo.[71] *M bovis* also invades and survives in a variety of circulating cells, including some lymphocyte populations in PBMCs and in erythrocytes.[70] In addition, invasion and intracellular survival of *M bovis* occurs in a diverse array of epithelial cell types, including bovine embryonic tracheal or lung epithelial cells,[71] primary embryonic calf turbinate cells,[19] and primary bovine mammary epithelial cells.[20] It can be hypothesized that intracellular survival is another strategy that *M bovis* uses to evade host immune responses and enhance dissemination, although its importance in the pathogenesis of *M bovis* infection is currently unknown.

OTHER FACTORS THAT INFLUENCE *MYCOPLASMA BOVIS*–HOST INTERACTIONS

Coinfection with other pathogens of the BRD complex is common in *M bovis*–associated respiratory disease. Synergy between *M bovis* and other respiratory pathogens has been proposed and readers are referred to Burki and colleagues[19] (2015) for a review of these relationships.

Interaction of *M bovis* with the microbiota of the upper respiratory tract may prove to be important in disease progression. Recent studies of the nasopharyngeal microbiota of cattle suggests that the composition and stability of the microbiota play important roles in susceptibility to respiratory disease.[79] A reduction in bacterial diversity accompanied by a large increase in the relative abundance of *M bovis* in the nasopharynx within a few days of transport to a feedlot has been reported.[80] Other investigators have reported a large increase in the proportion of cattle shedding *M bovis* in respiratory secretions after transport to a feedlot.[11] *M bovis* is more frequently present in the nasopharyngeal microbiota of feedlot cattle that develop BRD than in healthy cattle.[81] Therefore, under certain conditions, *M bovis* is able to undergo rapid replication in the upper respiratory tract, and this is associated with reduced diversity of the nasal microbiota and increased risk of BRD. As with other pathogens of the BRD complex, conditions that damage the physical defenses of the respiratory tract (eg, poor air quality, viral infections) or that suppress innate immunity (eg, stressors that cause glucocorticoid release, such as transportation, heat or cold stress, weaning, nutritional stress, or overcrowding) are likely to predispose to such replication events. However, the host, pathogen, and local microbiota dynamics that allow *M bovis* to be especially adept at taking advantage of these situations remain to be elucidated. Understanding the factors that control the replication and expansion of *M bovis* in the upper respiratory tract will be essential to advancing the understanding of *M bovis*–associated disease.

SUMMARY

M bovis can induce a broad range of immunomodulatory events through direct effects on neutrophils, macrophages, and lymphocytes, and indirectly through the induction of cytokine secretion. *M bovis* can also evade immune responses through surface antigen variation, and possibly by intracellular invasion and biofilm production. However, further investigation of the host and microbial factors that control *M bovis* infection dynamics in the upper respiratory tract, and that lead to the development of disease or to the production of an effective immune response, is needed in order to formulate improved control and preventive strategies for this pathogen.

REFERENCES

1. Maunsell FP, Woolums AR, Francoz D, et al. *Mycoplasma bovis* infections in cattle. J Vet Intern Med 2011;25:772–83.

2. Punyapornwithaya V, Fox LK, Hancock DD, et al. Association between an outbreak strain causing *Mycoplasma bovis* mastitis and its asymptomatic carriage in the herd: a case study from Idaho, USA. Prev Vet Med 2010;93:66–70.
3. Biddle MK, Fox LK, Hancock DD. Patterns of mycoplasma shedding in the milk of dairy cows with intramammary mycoplasma infection. J Am Vet Med Assoc 2003; 223:1163–6.
4. Bennett RH, Jasper DE. Factors associated with differentiation between cattle resistant and susceptible to intramammary challenge exposure with *Mycoplasma bovis*. Am J Vet Res 1978;39:407–16.
5. Bennett RH, Jasper DE. Bovine mycoplasmal mastitis from intramammary inoculations of small numbers of *Mycoplasma bovis*: local and systemic antibody response. Am J Vet Res 1980;41:889–92.
6. Boothby JT, Jasper DE, Thomas CB. Experimental intramammary inoculation with *Mycoplasma bovis* in vaccinated and unvaccinated cows: effect on local and systemic antibody response. Can J Vet Res 1987;51:121–5.
7. Howard CJ, Gourlay RN. Immune response of calves following the inoculation of *Mycoplasma dispar* and *Mycoplasma bovis*. Vet Microbiol 1983;8:45–56.
8. Howard CJ, Thomas LH, Parsons KR. Immune response of cattle to respiratory mycoplasmas. Vet Immunol Immunopathol 1987;17:401–12.
9. Vanden Bush TJ, Rosenbusch RF. Characterization of the immune response to *Mycoplasma bovis* lung infection. Vet Immunol Immunopathol 2003;94:23–33.
10. Maunsell FP, Brown MB, Powe J, et al. Oral inoculation of young dairy calves with *Mycoplasma bovis* results in colonization of tonsils, development of otitis media and local immunity. PLoS One 2012;7:E44523.
11. Castillo-Alcala F, Bateman KG, Cai HY, et al. Prevalence and genotype of *Mycoplasma bovis* in beef cattle after arrival at a feedlot. Am J Vet Res 2012;73: 1932–43.
12. Nicholas RA, Ayling RD, Stipkovits LP. An experimental vaccine for calf pneumonia caused by *Mycoplasma bovis*: clinical, cultural, serological and pathological findings. Vaccine 2002;20:3569–75.
13. Zhang R, Han X, Chen Y, et al. Attenuated *Mycoplasma bovis* strains provide protection against virulent infection in calves. Vaccine 2014;32:3107–14.
14. Dudek K, Bednarek D, Ayling RD, et al. An experimental vaccine composed of two adjuvants gives protection against *Mycoplasma bovis* in calves. Vaccine 2016;34:3051–8.
15. Boothby JT, Jasper DE, Thomas CB. Experimental intramammary inoculation with *Mycoplasma bovis* in vaccinated and unvaccinated cows: effect on the mycoplasmal infection and cellular inflammatory response. Cornell Vet 1986;76: 188–97.
16. Soehnlen MK, Aydin A, Lengerich EJ, et al. Blinded, controlled field trial of two commercially available *Mycoplasma bovis* bacterin vaccines in veal calves. Vaccine 2011;29:5347–54.
17. Waites KB, Xiao L, Liu Y, et al. *Mycoplasma pneumoniae* from the respiratory tract and beyond. Clin Microbiol Rev 2017;30:747–809.
18. Sachse K, Pfutzner H, Heller M, et al. Inhibition of *Mycoplasma bovis* cytadherence by a monoclonal antibody and various carbohydrate substances. Vet Microbiol 1993;36:307–16.
19. Burki S, Gaschen V, Stoffel MH, et al. Invasion and persistence of *Mycoplasma bovis* in embryonic calf turbinate cells. Vet Res 2015;46:53.
20. Josi C, Burki S, Stojiljkovic A, et al. Bovine epithelial *in vitro* infection models for *Mycoplasma bovis*. Front Cell Infect Microbiol 2018;8:329.

21. Thomas A, Sachse K, Dizier I, et al. Adherence to various host cell lines of *Mycoplasma bovis* strains differing in pathogenic and cultural features. Vet Microbiol 2003;91:101–13.
22. Sachse K, Helbig JH, Lysnyansky I, et al. Epitope mapping of immunogenic and adhesive structures in repetitive domains of *Mycoplasma bovis* variable surface lipoproteins. Infect Immun 2000;68:680–7.
23. Zhao G, Zhang H, Chen X, et al. *Mycoplasma bovis* NADH oxidase functions as both a NADH oxidizing and O_2 reducing enzyme and an adhesin. Sci Rep 2017; 7:44.
24. Song Z, Li Y, Liu Y, et al. alpha-Enolase, an adhesion-related factor of *Mycoplasma bovis*. PLoS One 2012;7:E38836.
25. Guo Y, Zhu H, Wang J, et al. TrmFO, a fibronectin-binding adhesin of *Mycoplasma bovis*. Int J Mol Sci 2017;18:E1732.
26. Adamu JY, Wawegama NK, Browning GF, et al. Membrane proteins of *Mycoplasma bovis* and their role in pathogenesis. Res Vet Sci 2013;95:321–5.
27. Behrens A, Heller M, Kirchhoff H, et al. A family of phase- and size-variant membrane surface lipoprotein antigens (Vsps) of *Mycoplasma bovis*. Infect Immun 1994;62:5075–84.
28. Lysnyansky I, Sachse K, Rosenbusch R, et al. The vsp locus of *Mycoplasma bovis*: gene organization and structural features. J Bacteriol 1999;181:5734–41.
29. Lysnyansky I, Ron Y, Yogev D. Juxtaposition of an active promoter to vsp genes via site-specific DNA inversions generates antigenic variation in *Mycoplasma bovis*. J Bacteriol 2001;183:5698–708.
30. Nussbaum S, Lysnyansky I, Sachse K, et al. Extended repertoire of genes encoding variable surface lipoproteins in *Mycoplasma bovis* strains. Infect Immun 2002;70:2220–5.
31. Burki S, Frey J, Pilo P. Virulence, persistence and dissemination of *Mycoplasma bovis*. Vet Microbiol 2015;179:15–22.
32. McAuliffe L, Ellis RJ, Miles K, et al. Biofilm formation by mycoplasma species and its role in environmental persistence and survival. Microbiology 2006;152:913–22.
33. Le Grand D, Solsona M, Rosengarten R, et al. Adaptive surface antigen variation in *Mycoplasma bovis* to the host immune response. FEMS Microbiol Lett 1996; 144:267–75.
34. Behrens A, Poumarat F, Le Grand D, et al. A newly identified immunodominant membrane protein (pMB67) involved in *Mycoplasma bovis* surface antigenic variation. Microbiology 1996;142:2463–70.
35. Robino P, Alberti A, Pittau M, et al. Genetic and antigenic characterization of the surface lipoprotein P48 of *Mycoplasma bovis*. Vet Microbiol 2005;109:201–9.
36. Wawegama NK, Browning GF, Kanci A, et al. Development of a recombinant protein-based enzyme-linked immunosorbent assay for diagnosis of *Mycoplasma bovis* infection in cattle. Clin Vaccine Immunol 2014;21:196–202.
37. Chen S, Hao H, Zhao P, et al. Differential immunoreactivity to bovine convalescent serum between *Mycoplasma bovis* biofilms and planktonic cells revealed by comparative immunoproteomic analysis. Front Microbiol 2018;9:379.
38. Pilo P, Vilei EM, Peterhans E, et al. A metabolic enzyme as a primary virulence factor of *Mycoplasma mycoides* subsp. *mycoides* small colony. J Bacteriol 2005;187:6824–31.
39. Ferrarini GM, Mucha SG, Parrot D, et al. Hydrogen peroxide production and myo-inositol metabolism as important traits for virulence of *Mycoplasma hyopneumoniae*. Mol Microbiol 2018;108:683–96.

40. Khan LA, Miles RJ, Nicholas RA. Hydrogen peroxide production by *Mycoplasma bovis* and *Mycoplasma agalactiae* and effect of *in vitro* passage on a *Mycoplasma bovis* strain producing high levels of H_2O_2. Vet Res Commun 2005;29: 181–8.

41. Schott C, Cai H, Parker L, et al. Hydrogen peroxide production and free radical-mediated cell stress in *Mycoplasma bovis* pneumonia. J Comp Pathol 2014;150: 127–37.

42. Grissett GP, White BJ, Larson RL. Structured literature review of responses of cattle to viral and bacterial pathogens causing bovine respiratory disease complex. J Vet Intern Med 2015;29:770–80.

43. Hermeyer K, Buchenau I, Thomasmeyer A, et al. Chronic pneumonia in calves after experimental infection with *Mycoplasma bovis* strain 1067: characterization of lung pathology, persistence of variable surface protein antigens and local immune response. Acta Vet Scand 2012;54:9.

44. Virtala AM, Mechor GD, Grohn YT, et al. Epidemiologic and pathologic characteristics of respiratory tract disease in dairy heifers during the first three months of life. J Am Vet Med Assoc 1996;208:2035–42.

45. Razin S, Yogev D, Naot Y. Molecular biology and pathogenicity of mycoplasmas. Microbiol Mol Biol Rev 1998;62:1094–156.

46. Yang J, Hooper WC, Phillips DJ, et al. Cytokines in *Mycoplasma pneumoniae* infections. Cytokine Growth Factor Rev 2004;15:157–68.

47. Howard CJ, Taylor G. Interaction of mycoplasmas and phagocytes. Yale J Biol Med 1983;56:643–8.

48. Howard CJ. Comparison of bovine IgG1, IgG2 and IgM for ability to promote killing of *Mycoplasma bovis* by bovine alveolar macrophages and neutrophils. Vet Immunol Immunopathol 1984;6:321–6.

49. Arfi Y, Minder L, Di Primo C, et al. MIB-MIP is a mycoplasma system that captures and cleaves immunoglobulin G. Proc Natl Acad Sci U S A 2016;113:5406–11.

50. Calcutt MJ, Lysnyansky I, Saschse K, et al. Gap analysis of *Mycoplasma bovis* disease, diagnosis and control: An aid to identify future development requirements. Transbound Emerg Dis 2018;65(Suppl 1):91–109.

51. Adegboye DS, Hallbur PG, Cavanaugh DL, et al. Immunohistochemical and pathological study of *Mycoplasma bovis*-associated lung abscesses in calves. J Vet Diagn Invest 1995;7:333–7.

52. Rodriguez F, Bryson DG, Ball HJ, et al. Pathological and immunohistochemical studies of natural and experimental *Mycoplasma bovis* pneumonia in calves. J Comp Pathol 1996;115:151–62.

53. Maeda T, Shibahara T, Kimura K, et al. *Mycoplasma bovis*-associated suppurative otitis media and pneumonia in bull calves. J Comp Pathol 2003;129:100–10.

54. Gagea MI, Bateman KG, Shanahan RA, et al. Naturally occurring *Mycoplasma bovis*-associated pneumonia and polyarthritis in feedlot beef calves. J Vet Diagn Invest 2006;18:29–40.

55. Jimbo S, Suleman M, Maina T, et al. Effect of *Mycoplasma bovis* on bovine neutrophils. Vet Immunol Immunopathol 2017;188:27–33.

56. Thomas CB, Van Ess P, Wolfram LJ, et al. Adherence to bovine neutrophils and suppression of neutrophil chemiluminescence by *Mycoplasma bovis*. Vet Immunol Immunopathol 1991;27:365–81.

57. Yamamoto T, Kida Y, Sakamoto Y, et al. Mpn491, a secreted nuclease of *Mycoplasma pneumoniae*, plays a critical role in evading killing by neutrophil extracellular traps. Cell Microbiol 2017;19:E12666.

58. Henthorn CR, Minion F, Sahin O. Utilization of macrophage extracellular trap nucleotides by *Mycoplasma hyopneumoniae*. Microbiology 2018;164:1394–404.

59. Mitiku F, Hartley CA, Sansom FM, et al. The major membrane nuclease MnuA degrades neutrophil extracellular traps induced by *Mycoplasma bovis*. Vet Microbiol 2018;218:13–9.

60. Aulik NA, Hellenbrand KM, Czuprynski CJ. Mannheimia haemolytica and its leukotoxin cause macrophage extracellular trap formation by bovine macrophages. Infect Immun 2012;80:1923–33.

61. Hellenbrand KM, Forsythe KM, Rivera-Rivas JJ, et al. Histophilus somni causes extracellular trap formation by bovine neutrophils and macrophages. Microb Pathog 2013;54:67–75.

62. Rodríguez F, Castro P, Poveda JB, et al. Immunohistochemical labelling of cytokines in calves infected experimentally with *Mycoplasma bovis*. J Comp Pathol 2015;152:243–7.

63. Jungi TW, Krampe M, Sileghem M, et al. Differential and strain-specific triggering of bovine alveolar macrophage effector functions by mycoplasmas. Microb Pathog 1996;21:487–98.

64. Rodríguez F, González JF, Arbelo M, et al. Cytokine expression in lungs of calves spontaneously infected with *Mycoplasma bovis*. Vet Res Commun 2015;39:69–72.

65. Mulongo M, Prysliak T, Scruten E, et al. *In vitro* infection of bovine monocytes with *Mycoplasma bovis* delays apoptosis and suppresses production of gamma interferon and tumor necrosis factor alpha but not interleukin-10. Infect Immun 2014;82:62–71.

66. Goto S, Konnai S, Okagawa T, et al. Increase of cells expressing PD-1 and PD-L1 and enhancement of IFN-γ production via PD-1/PD-L1 blockade in bovine mycoplasmosis. Immun Inflamm Dis 2017;5:355–63.

67. Hermeyer K, Jacobsen B, Spergser J, et al. Detection of *Mycoplasma bovis* by *in-situ* hybridization and expression of inducible nitric oxide synthase, nitrotyrosine and manganese superoxide dismutase in the lungs of experimentally-infected calves. J Comp Pathol 2011;145:240–50.

68. Devi VR, Poumarat F, Le Grand D, et al. Histopathological findings, phenotyping of inflammatory cells, and expression of markers of nitritive injury in joint tissue samples from calves after vaccination and intraarticular challenge with *M. bovis* strain 1067. Acta Vet Scand 2014;56:45.

69. Radaelli E, Luini M, Domeneghini C, et al. Expression of class II major histocompatibility complex molecules in chronic pulmonary Mycoplasma bovis infection in cattle. J Comp Pathol 2009;140:198–202.

70. van der Merwe J, Prysliak T, Perez-Casal J. Invasion of bovine peripheral blood mononuclear cells and erythrocytes by *Mycoplasma bovis*. Infect Immun 2010;78:4570–8.

71. Suleman M, Prysliak T, Clarke K, et al. *Mycoplasma bovis* isolates recovered from cattle and bison (*Bison bison*) show differential *in vitro* effects on PBMC proliferation, alveolar macrophage apoptosis and invasion of epithelial and immune cells. Vet Microbiol 2016;186:28–36.

72. Thomas CB, Mettler J, Sharp P, et al. *Mycoplasma bovis* suppression of bovine lymphocyte response to phytohemagglutinin. Vet Immunol Immunopathol 1990;26:143–55.

73. Vanden Bush TJ, Rosenbusch RF. *Mycoplasma bovis* induces apoptosis of bovine lymphocytes. FEMS Immunol Med Microbiol 2002;32:97–103.

74. Suleman M, Cyprian FS, Jimbo S, et al. *Mycoplasma bovis*-Induced Inhibition of Bovine Peripheral Blood Mononuclear Cell Proliferation Is Ameliorated after Blocking the Immune-Inhibitory Programmed Death 1 Receptor. Infect Immun 2018;86 [pii:e00921-17].

75. Wherry EJ, Kurachi M. Molecular and cellular insights into T cell exhaustion. Nat Rev Immunol 2015;15:486–99.

76. Brown WC, Barbet AF. Persistent infections and immunity in ruminants to arthropod-borne bacteria in the family anaplasmataceae. Annu Rev Anim Biosci 2016;4:177–97.

77. Ikebuchi R, Konnai S, Shirai T, et al. Increase of cells expressing PD-L1 in bovine leukemia virus infection and enhancement of anti-viral immune responses *in vitro* via PD-L1 blockade. Vet Res 2011;42:103.

78. Okagawa T, Konnai S, Nishimori A, et al. Bovine immunoinhibitory receptors contribute to suppression of *Mycobacterium avium* subsp. *paratuberculosis*-specific T-cell responses. Infect Immun 2015;84:77–89.

79. Holman DB, Timsit E, Alexander TW. The nasopharyngeal microbiota of feedlot cattle. Sci Rep 2015;5:15557.

80. Stroebel C, Alexander T, Workentine ML, et al. Effects of transportation to and co-mingling at an auction market on nasopharyngeal and tracheal bacterial communities of recently weaned beef cattle. Vet Microbiol 2018;223:126–33.

81. McMullen C, Orsel K, Alexander TW, et al. Comparison of the nasopharyngeal bacterial microbiota of beef calves raised without the use of antimicrobials between healthy calves and those diagnosed with bovine respiratory disease. Vet Microbiol 2019;231:56–62.

The Cattle Microbiota and the Immune System

An Evolving Field

Diego E. Gomez, DVM, MSc, MVSc, PhD[a],*,
Klibs N. Galvão, DVM, MVPM, PhD[a],
Juan C. Rodriguez-Lecompte, DVM, MSc, PhD[b],
Marcio C. Costa, DVM, DVSc, PhD[c]

KEYWORDS

- Cattle • Mammary gland • Metritis • Mastitis • Calf diarrhea

KEY POINTS

- The advent and refinement of sequencing technologies in the last decade has made possible the opportunity to better assess microbial communities inhabiting various body systems, leading to a surge of unexpected associations between the microbiota and the host.
- The bacteria present on mucosal surfaces throughout the body stimulate the development of both the innate and adaptive immune systems.
- The interaction between the microbiota and the host mucosal immunity plays an important role in the maintenance of the host's homeostasis and prevention against disease caused by pathogenic microorganisms.

INTRODUCTION

The symbiotic interaction between mammals and their diverse microorganisms are of importance because mutualism provides nutritional, developmental, physiologic, and immunologic benefits to the host.[1,2] The host-microbiota interaction occurs principally at the mucosal surfaces, which creates an ecological niche facilitating bacterial colonization and establishment, while developing mechanisms to recognize and respond

Disclosure: The authors have nothing to disclose.
[a] Department of Large Animal Clinical Sciences, College of Veterinary Medicine, University of Florida, 2015 Southwest 16th Avenue, Gainesville, FL 32608, USA; [b] Department of Pathology and Microbiology, Atlantic Veterinary College, University of Prince Edward Island, 550 University Avenue, Charlottetown, Prince Edward Island C1A 4P3, Canada; [c] Department of Veterinary Biomedicine, University of Montreal, 3200 Rue Sicotte, Saint-Hyacinthe, Quebec J2S 2M2, Canada
* Corresponding author.
E-mail address: diegogomeznieto@ufl.edu

to pathogenic microorganisms.[3] The beneficial effects of these commensal bacteria are related to barrier enhancement, immune response modulation, stimulation of the establishment of a healthy microbiota, and inhibition of intestinal colonization by pathogens.[4–7] In addition, the presence of commensal bacteria on the mucosal surface stimulates the development of the innate immune system, including factors such as tight junctions (TJs) and the secretion of mucus, immunoglobulin (Ig) A, and antimicrobial peptides.[8–10] Similarly, bacteria influence adaptive immune system factors such as activation of antigen-presenting cells (APCs; dendritic cells and macrophages), B and T cells, and regulatory T cells (Tregs).[11] Alterations to such factors could lead to increased gut permeability, bacterial translocation, chronic or exacerbated inflammatory response, and the onset of local or systemic disease.[12,13] As such, a clear understanding of the interaction between bacteria and the immune response of various body systems is paramount to advancing understanding of the development of disease.

New insights into the host-microbiota interaction have recently emerged with the advance of new molecular technologies such as next-generation sequencing (NGS). Although the microbiota in its entirety (bacteria, viruses, fungi, archaea, protozoa, and small parasites) play an important role in the development and regulation of local and systemic immunity, most studies have focused on bacterial communities. This article presents the current knowledge and controversies regarding the important role of the microbiota on the immune system at the mucosa surface of the gut and uterus, and the mucin-rich surface of the mammary gland of the cattle.

GUT MICROBIOTA AND THE IMMUNE SYSTEM
How Do Bacteria Colonize the Calf Gut?

Culture-dependent and sequencing-based studies have shown that the development and establishment of the gut microbiota is a dynamic process during the preweaning period and can be influenced by several internal and external factors (**Fig. 1**). Internal factors (ie, those characteristics that are inherent to the host) include the nutritional state, the functional immaturity of the gut and immune system,[1,3,14] intestinal pH, gut motility, biliary secretions, bacterial mucosal receptors, and microbial composition.[14] These factors seem to be responsible for the type of bacteria colonizing the different regions of the gut, as well as the between the mucosa-associated and digesta-associated microbiota of the calf gut[15–17] The list of external factors is broad and includes anything with the potential to influence the calf's environment, such as the composition of the vaginal microbiota of the dam,[18–20] diet,[21–23] and use of antibiotics at the individual[24,25] and at the farm levels[26,27] (see **Fig. 1**).

Internal and external factors can modify the normal composition of the microbiota. For example, antimicrobial administration can result in changes of the structure of the bacteria inhabiting the calf gut.[24,25] In general, the term dysbiosis refers to imbalances present in the microbiota of diseased individuals, but it has also been used to refer to any deviation from the normal composition of the microbiota. Note that there is no consensus about the definition of a normal microbiota. It is logical to assume that the normal microbiota should be the one selected in each species during the evolutionary process, and therefore, the one present in feral individuals. However, modern production systems have changed this normal microbiota and the consequences of these modifications remain unknown in calves. In general, it is accepted that loss of beneficial bacteria, proliferation of pathogens, and reduction of diversity are biomarkers associated with dysbiosis in calves and other species.[1,2,28,29]

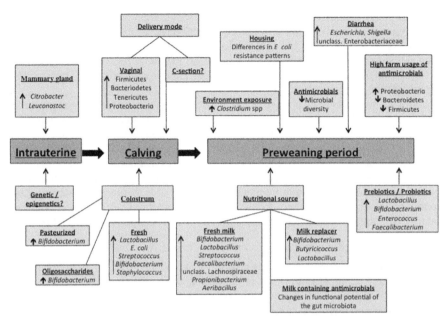

Fig. 1. Factors affecting gut microbiome development and establishment of dairy calves from birth to the weaning period. The model depicted also includes a combination of hypothetical effects (question mark indicates not experimentally supported) or extrapolated data from studies in other species. C-section, cesarean section.

In general, during parturition the calf is exposed to several different bacterial communities, including those acquired during birth through the vagina, perineum, and skin. During the calving process, the calf is exposed to a variety of bacteria that predominate the vaginal canal, including *Truperella pyogenes*, *Staphylococcus* spp, *Clostridium* spp, *Bacteroides* spp, *Ureaplasma* spp, and *Mannheimia* spp.[18–20] After calving, transference of oral and cutaneous microorganisms from the dam to the calf occurs by processes such as licking and suckling.[30] For example, *Citrobacter* spp and *Leuconostoc* spp, which are normally inhabitants of the cow's udder skin, can be detected in meconium and fecal samples within the first 6 hours after calving.[31]

During the first hours of life, colostrum is offered to the calf as an important source of nutrients and to provide factors for development of the gastrointestinal tract and, in particular, the immune system. In general, fresh bovine colostrum contains *Lactobacillus* spp, *Bifidobacterium* spp, *Staphylococcus* spp, *Escherichia coli*, and *Streptococcus uberis*,[32] with *E coli*, *Lactobacillus* spp, and *Bifidobacterium* spp dominating the fecal microbiota of the calf during the first days after calving.[21,33–38] The source and/or processing of colostrum (either fresh or heat treated) seem to influence the prevalence of early gut colonizers.[22] For example, colostrum-deprived calves had a higher relative abundance of *Lactobacillus* and *E coli* in the small intestine,[22] but calves fed heat-treated colostrum had a higher prevalence of *Bifidobacterium* spp.[22,23,39] These neonatal calf studies suggest that bacteria "contaminating" colostrum and colostrum components (ie, oligosaccharides)[39] are essential for bacterial acquisition and promote the colonization of the early calf gut microbiota.

Studies using fingerprinting techniques showed pronounced instability of the fecal bacterial community throughout the first 30 days after birth.[40] The earliest colonizers included *E coli* (days 1–7), *Bifidobacterium* spp (first identified on day 1), and

Clostridium spp (detected during days 1–3). *Faecalibacterium* spp were first identified on day 3 and remained present for the following 30 days. Studies using NGS to characterize the fecal microbiota of healthy calves had similar results. The phyla Bacteroidetes, Firmicutes, and Proteobacteria dominated the fecal bacteria during the first 4 weeks of life of calves, with *Bifidobacterium* spp, *Bacteroides* spp, and *Lactobacillus* spp the dominant genera.[41–44]

Altogether, these findings show that the calf fits the classic pattern of bacterial colonization of neonates in other species.[45,46] First there is rapid colonization by facultative anaerobes, including *Lactobacillus*, *E coli*, and other genera of the Enterobacteriaceae family,[40–47] followed by the colonization of strictly anaerobic bacteria, including *Clostridium* spp, *Bifidobacterium* spp, *Eubacterium* spp, and *Bacteroides* spp, a few days after birth (once oxygen supplies are exhausted), transitioning the gut into an anaerobic milieu.[40–47] An increase in richness (a measure of how many different species are present in a community) and diversity (a measure of the number different species and their abundance) of the microbiota accompany the changes in bacterial taxa.[40–44]

The Calf Gastrointestinal Immune System

During in utero fetal development, several immune defense mechanisms begin their development (**Fig. 2**). At birth, the calf immune system, although competent, is still naive.[48] The organs of the calf immune system are classified as central (eg, bone marrow and thymus) or peripheral (eg, lymph nodes, spleen, and mucosa-associated lymphoid tissues, including the gut-associated mucosal tissue [GALT]). Within central organs, the immune cells initiate or complete development in gestation, which is in contrast with what occurs in the peripheral organs, where exposure to antigens is required for complete development and activation of immune cells and occurs after the calf is born.[49]

The GALT comprises physical barriers (eg, mucus, epithelium), chemical barriers (eg, antimicrobial peptides [AMPs], secretory IgA), and immunologic barriers (eg, intraepithelial lymphocytes, macrophages, dendritic cells, T and B cells, and natural killer cells) that, together, recognize and act against pathogens[50] (**Fig. 3**). Impairment of these mechanisms of defense could result in hindered protection and facilitation of pathogen overgrowth.[51,52]

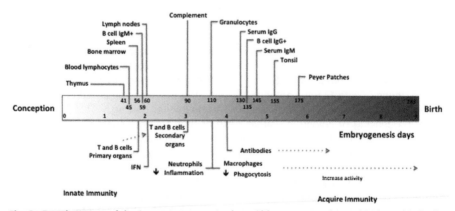

Fig. 2. Development of the immune system in the calf from conception to birth. At birth, the calf immune system, although competent, is still naive. (*Adapted from* Gerald N. Callahan, and Robin M. Yates. Fetal and neonatal immunity. Basic Veterinary Immunology. Boulder, Colorado: University Press of Colorado; 2014.)

Intestinal innate immunity

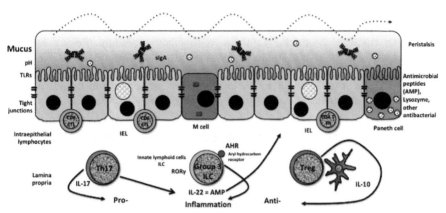

Fig. 3. Microbiota and the intestinal barrier. The gut mucosal immune system involves physical barriers (eg, mucosa, epithelium), chemical barriers (AMP, secretory IgA), and immunologic barriers (intraepithelial lymphocytes, macrophages, dendritic cells, T and B cells, and natural killer cells) that, together, recognize and act against pathogens. The mucosal immune system is best described as a system of cells and cytokines within the mucosa and mesenteric ganglia that are ultimately regulated by the commensal bacteria. IEL, intraepithelial lincogytes; ROR gamma, RAR-related orphan nuclear receptor gamma; Th17, T-helper 17; TLR, Toll-like receptor.

How Does the Microbiota Influence the Development of Tight Junctions in the Gut?

In the gastrointestinal mucosa, a single layer of epithelial cells adhere to one another, through an intercellular junctional complex known as TJs. The structure of the TJ is composed of proteins, including occludin, claudins, zonula occludens, and junctional adhesion molecules. The TJ proteins function in a gate-and-fence manner, which selectively facilitates paracellular transport of nutrients, ions, and water, but prevents diffusion of microorganisms and microbial-derived peptides.[53,54] During the first hours after birth, the calf gut intercellular permeability is high, as shown by its pronounced ability to absorb nutrients, proteins (eg, immunoglobulins), and leukocytes.[55,56] This permeability reduces substantially during the first 24 to 36 hours and continues decreasing over the first month of life.[57,58] Studies investigating the mechanisms of development of the mucosal barrier in calves are limited, but investigations of the whole transcriptome and microRNAome of the small intestine of calves showed that the expression of genes encoding TJ proteins was upregulated during the first week of life.[59] The mechanisms for the increased expression of TJ proteins are not completely understood; however, it has been established that interaction between the mucosal surface and mucosal bacteria (eg, *Lactobacillus* spp and *Bifidobacterium* spp) or bacterial metabolites promotes intestinal barrier integrity via upregulation of TJ proteins.[8,60,61] This could lead to the conclusion that, given the dominance of both *Lactobacillus* spp and *Bifidobacterium* spp in the calf gut during the first days of life, the interactions between these bacteria and the epithelium stimulate and promote the development of TJs.

The TJs are also regulated by dietary components. In human celiac disease, gliadin, a glycoprotein present in wheat, compromises the TJ structure, leading to increased intercellular permeability and subsequent gastrointestinal disease.[62] Similarly, in preweaned calves, abrupt introduction of solid food to the diet increases permeability of the mucosal barrier of the gut associated with downregulated expression of claudin and occludin in the small intestine.[63] This increase in epithelial permeability has been associated with a proinflammatory response, likely related to the interaction between bacteria or bacterial products, pathogen recognition receptors (PRRs), and the release of cytokines with inflammatory effects (ie, tumor necrosis factor [TNF]) by immune cells.[64] These findings suggest that acute dietary changes could influence calf gut homeostasis, predisposing to an inflammatory response that could result in gastrointestinal diseases.

HOW DOES THE MICROBIOTA AFFECT THE SECRETORY COMPONENTS OF THE GUT MUCOSAL IMMUNE SYSTEM IN CALVES?

Mucus is a physical barrier that contributes to the maintenance of gut integrity,[65,66] the abnormal production of which has been associated with gastrointestinal disease.[66,67] The production of mucus in the gut seems to be stimulated by the presence of commensal bacteria. Comparisons between germ-free and conventional-microbiota mice showed that a lack of gut bacteria results in decreased production of mucus.[9,68] Exposure of the epithelium of germ-free animals to lipopolysaccharide and peptidoglycans resulted in normal mucus secretion,[68,69] suggesting that bacteria or bacterial products promote mucus production in the gut.

Intestinal epithelial cell turnover and mucosal metabolic activity are also stimulated by the presence of commensal bacteria on the mucosal surface. Lower rates of epithelial cell turnover and reduction in mucosal metabolic activity were described in germ-free piglets.[70] Similarly, germ-free mice showed abnormalities in the development of mesenteric lymph nodes and had lower antibody production compared with control animals.[71,72] These observations indicate that the structure and functional potential of the early colonizing bacteria affect both the physical and functional development of the gut.

Paneth cells and enterocytes produce and release broad-spectrum AMPs such as defensins, cathelicidins, S100 proteins, and peptidoglycan recognition protein 1.[73,74] These peptides are active against gram-positive and gram-negative bacteria, virus, fungi, and protozoa.[73,74] The production and secretion of AMPs is associated with the presence of both commensal and pathogenic bacteria and seem to play important role in the innate immune response.[10,12,75] However, studies in germ-free animals showed that expression of some AMPs, including α-defensins, seems to be constitutive and does not require bacteria stimulus.[76] Therefore, production and secretion of AMPs occur as a result of diverse mechanisms, acting simultaneously, to avoid bacterial expansion and inflammation.

Dimeric secreted IgA (sIgA), produced by plasma cells, acts by regulating commensal and pathogenic bacteria by promoting symbiotic interactions.[77] The sIgA is the main immunoglobulin produced in calves, with large amounts secreted across the epithelium of the gut.[78] In humans, approximately 50% to 70% of commensal bacteria recovered from feces are coated with sIgA[79] and similar results were reported for calves and pigs.[80] When sIgA reaches the intestinal lumen, it binds to the bacteria, inducing a direct effect of neutralization.[79,80] Then, the sIgA-pathogen complex moves through the gut via peristaltic action, ultimately being eliminated in the feces.[79,80] M cells also capture the sIgA-pathogen complex for presentation to the APCs in Peyer patches.[78] In both cattle and humans, the ratio of sIgA-coated bacteria to total bacteria differs by gut region.[80] These differences can be explained, at least in part, by the bacteria present in the different regions of the gut because some genera are highly coated (eg, Enterobacteriaceae family) and others seem resistant (eg, *Lactobacillus* spp and *Bacteroides* spp).[80,81]

Absence of IgA allows bacterial expansion, with associated local and systemic inflammatory responses.[82] However, resumption of IgA production results in the recovery of normal bacterial composition and eliminates both local and systemic inflammation.[83] This finding is of interest clinically because the proliferation of the Enterobacteriaceae family has been associated with diarrhea in calves.[26,28] However, currently, the role of IgA secretion in the pathogenesis of calf diarrhea and its association with the expansion of this family is unknown and warrants investigation.

How Does the Gut Microbiota Affect the Expression of Toll-Like Receptors in Calves?

Enterocytes and APCs recognize antigens through genetically encoded PRRs.[84] The PRRs, including the Toll-like receptors (TLRs), are capable of recognizing highly conserved pathogen-associated molecular patterns (PAMPs) present in several microorganisms and triggering either proinflammatory or antiinflammatory pathways.[85] Expression of TLRs in the colon of germ-free animals seems to be lower than in normal, healthy individuals,[11] suggesting that interaction between bacteria and TLRs plays some role in maintenance of gut homeostasis and the innate immune response.[86]

Expression of TLRs in the gut of calves is influenced by diet, age, and gut region.[13,59,63] TLRs (measured at the messenger RNA level) were expressed at high levels in the small intestine compared with other regions of the gut during the first weeks of life. For instance, the expression of TLR2 and TLR6 was downregulated with increasing age (ie, 3 weeks vs 6 months).[13] This downregulation was associated with an increase in the abundance of digesta and tissue-associated total bacteria and lactic acid bacteria,[13] suggesting that colonization and establishment of gut commensal bacteria modulates immune response in early life. Introduction of solid food to dairy calves also increases the expression of TLR2 and TLR6, indicating that diet can alter the permeability of the calf gut, allowing contact of bacteria and bacterial products with the mucosal barrier and leading to an enhanced expression of PRRs.[63]

Activation of a proinflammatory cytokine response against intestinal pathogens aids the host in preventing microbial invasion, but an exacerbated inflammatory process can impair the metabolic and hemodynamic homeostasis of the host.[87] Consequently, the immune system has several antiinflammatory mechanisms to counteract the production of proinflammatory cytokines and limit tissue damage. During the first week of the calf's life, expression of both proinflammatory and antiinflammatory cytokines, such as interleukin (IL)-8 and IL-10, respectively, is upregulated in the small intestine.[59] IL-8 activates and recruits neutrophils from the intravascular bed into the interstitial space,[88] whereas IL-10 inhibits the synthesis of proinflammatory molecules (eg, INF-γ, TNFα, IL-6) and suppresses the antigen-presentation ability of APCs.[89] Colonization of the gut of neonates by *Lactobacillus* spp and *Bifidobacterium* spp stimulates the expression of IL-10 by immature dendritic cells, likely to mitigate the proinflammatory response against commensal bacteria.[90] This finding is of clinical interest because *Bifidobacterium* spp are a dominant group of the calf gut during the first weeks of life and increase rapidly throughout the first 8 weeks of life.[26,37,38,91] Therefore, it is possible that the colonization of the calf gut by *Lactobacillus* spp and *Bifidobacterium* spp promotes a regulatory immune response, perhaps to avoid exacerbated inflammatory response.

The upregulation of IL-10 is consistent with the suppression of the proinflammatory response of the host and the induction of immune regulation observed during early bacterial colonization of the calf's gut.[92] For instance, TLR6 expression was increased in the small intestine of calves in the first week of life, which positively correlated with the tissue-associated bacteria content.[13] In calves, stimulation of TLR6 in immature dendritic cells leads to Treg development. Similarly, an increase in expression in both the jejunum and ileum of genes related to Tregs (eg, FOXP3) from day 0 to day 7 has been identified.[53] This upregulation of Tregs in the small intestine during the neonatal period indicates a possible microbiota-dependent adaptive immune response.

Based on the current knowledge regarding the development of the calf microbiota and the gut immune system, it is clear that the gut bacteria play a fundamental role in immune regulation of calves during early life. However, more studies investigating how changes in the normal microbiota composition can affect later-in-life immune responses and disease resistance are necessary.

UTERINE MICROBIOTA AND THE IMMUNE SYSTEM

The transition to lactation is a challenging period for high-producing dairy cows. This period is characterized by a marked decrease in immune function.[93] Simultaneously, physical barriers (ie, the cervix) are breached at parturition, which allows rapid colonization of the uterus by bacteria.[94] In addition to ascending colonization, recent evidence points to hematogenous transfer of pathogens from the gut as an alternative route of uterine colonization and infection.[95] Prevention of diseases is therefore highly dependent on recognition and elimination of pathogenic bacteria by the immune system. However, with the decrease in immune function and the large bacterial challenge, the immune system is overwhelmed and uterine diseases such as metritis, clinical endometritis, and subclinical endometritis occur.[96,97] The causes of uterine disease are multifactorial and depend on elements related to the host, the pathogen, and the environment.[94] This article presents information regarding the local and systemic immunologic alteration and the uterine microbial changes that predispose cows to develop uterine disease in the postpartum period.

How Do Abnormal Uterine Immune Responses Predispose to the Development of Uterine Disease in Postpartum Cattle?

Innate immunity is the most important defense system of the bovine uterus, with neutrophils being the main phagocytic cells.[98] Resident tissue macrophages and dendritic cells control neutrophil recruitment.[99,100] Resident macrophages and endometrial cells are also involved in the initial recognition of invading pathogens and the initiation of the immune response.[99,100] These cells produce and release proinflammatory cytokines and chemokines, including TNFα, IL-1, IL-6, and IL-8, leading to a massive influx of leukocytes into the uterine tissue and lumen, which are responsible for most of the bacterial clearance after uterine infection.[98,101–103] However, during the transition into lactation, dairy cows experience a reduction in leukocyte function, including a reduction in neutrophil phagocytosis and killing capacity, and a reduction in cytokine production and proliferation by mononuclear cells.[93,104,105] This reduction is particularly evident in cows that develop metritis and endometritis.[104–106] This immunosuppression is associated with downregulation of proinflammatory cytokines by macrophages and endometrial cells[100,101] and a decreased production of TNFα by E coli–stimulated monocytes.[100] Chemotaxis of neutrophils to the sites of placental attachment, IL-8 production,[107] and the influx of neutrophils into the uterine lumen are similarly reduced.[103]

Several factors might account for the reduction in the immune function of postpartum cows, including depletion of energy storages and calcium concentrations and an increase in nonesterified fatty acid (NEFA) and beta-hydroxyl butyrate acid concentrations.[108,109] Glucose[110–112] and calcium[113–115] are essential for chemotaxis, phagocytosis, and microbial killing,[110–112,116] and NEFAs affect proliferation of mononuclear cells and oxidative bursts of neutrophils in cell culture, which negatively influences the killing of bacteria.[117–120] The NEFAs have both immunostimulatory and immunosuppressive effects on the immune function, depending on the degree of saturation.[109] Primarily, saturated fatty acids have a stimulatory effect on the immune system, whereas unsaturated fatty acids have an inhibitory effect.[109] In early lactation, there is an increase in the circulating concentration of unsaturated fatty acids, which may contribute to the immunosuppression observed in this period. By-products of bacterial metabolism, such as proteins, short-chain fatty acids, and as-yet uncharacterized metabolites, also have cytotoxic effects on leukocytes by suppressing leukocyte phagocytosis and killing ability.[121–123] Nonetheless, the individual effect of these metabolites and minerals can be shown, but the complex interaction between the whole host and bacterial metabolome and innate immune function has not been evaluated.

In cows, vascular degeneration occurs shortly after calving, allowing blood to leak into the uterine lumen, facilitating exchange of metabolites between blood and uterus.[106,124] Current knowledge of the association between the peripheral blood leukocyte and tissue leukocyte function and the uterine bacteria is limited. Therefore, investigating the metabolome of blood and uterus from calving through establishment of metritis would allow the identification of metabolites that affect leukocyte function and expansion of the uterine bacteria leading to disease. A recent study evaluated the serum metabolome of healthy and metritic cows and identified several metabolites that accurately discriminated cows from each group.[125] The metabolites that differed between cows were products of protein metabolism, such as the amino acids valine, leucine, ornithine, serine, and glutamic acid. In addition, none of the carbohydrate metabolism products, such as butyrate, acetate, and propionate, were associated with the development of metritis. These findings are of interest because they may show that bacteria and their products and the host metabolome play a role in development of uterine disease in cattle. In addition, they highlight the need for more metagenomic studies to expand the understanding of the development of uterine disease in cattle.

How Do Changes in Uterine Microbiota Predispose to the Development of Uterine Disease in Postpartum Cattle?

The uterus of the dairy cow is unique in that virtually all cows are infected with bacteria postpartum, and failure to control pathogenic bacterial growth leads to the establishment of disease.[94,126] Traditionally, bacterial culture has been used to characterize the uterine bacteria of postpartum cows with uterine disease, particularly cows with endometritis.[127,128] E coli, T pyogenes, Fusobacterium necrophorum, and Prevotella melaninogenica are the most common bacteria isolated from cows with endometritis, whereas Streptococcus spp, Staphylococcus spp, and Bacillus spp, are commonly isolated from healthy cows.[103,129–131] Studies targeting specific bacteria using polymerase chain reaction assays showed an involvement of E coli, especially strains possessing specific virulence factors (fimH, hlyA, cdt, kpsMII, ibeA, and astA), in the pathogenesis of metritis.[132,133] Of interest, colonization of the uterus by

E coli possessing fimH is a risk factor for the expansion of *F necrophorum*.[133] This interaction between uterine bacteria during the pathogenesis of the disease is synergistic because *E coli* seems to facilitate the uterine colonization by *Bacteroides* spp, *Porphyromonas* spp, and *Fusobacterium* spp.[103,132,133]

Recent work using NGS to study uterine diseases in cattle showed that the uterine microbiota establishes within 20 minutes of calving, with 28 phyla and 824 genera of bacteria having been identified.[95,126] The uterine microbiota changes dramatically from calving until the diagnosis of metritis, with a reduction in the relative abundance Proteobacteria (mainly *Coxiella*) and an increase in the relative abundance of Bacteroidetes (mainly *Bacteroides* and *Porphyromonas*) and Fusobacteria (mainly *Fusobacterium*) in cows that developed metritis (**Fig. 4**). During the first 2 days postpartum (DPP) the uterine bacteria are identical between healthy cows and cows that later develop metritis. However, after 2 DPP the uterine bacteria changes in metritic cows and these changes are characterized by expansion of *Bacteroides* spp, *Porphyromonas* spp, and *Fusobacterium* spp.[126,134–138] (see **Fig. 4**). Then, these bacterial groups seem to act synergistically among themselves and with other bacteria to facilitate the development of metritis in dairy cows.[95,126,138] These findings indicate that uterine dysbiosis occurs from calving to 2 DPP in cattle and seems to play an important role in the development of metritis.[126] They also further support that the uterine environment or the host defense mechanisms, or both, change in the first 2 DPP and becomes more conducive to the proliferation of pathogenic bacteria in cows that later develop metritis (see **Fig. 4**).

Future studies involving the analysis of the bacteria, the host and bacterial metabolome, and the host immune function are required to better understand the complex

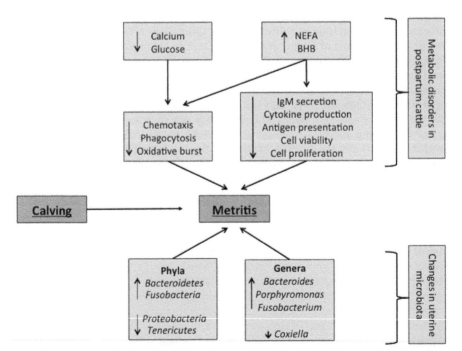

Fig. 4. Metabolic disorders, immune system alterations, and uterine microbiota changes predisposing cattle to the development of metritis in the early postpartum period. BHB, beta-hydroxybutyrate.

interactions that lead to immunosuppression, microbial dysbiosis, and disease establishment in postpartum dairy cattle.[139–141] This approach is being used in human medicine with the Integrative Human Microbiome Project, and a similar approach in animals is needed in order to advance the understanding of factors that influence animal health and disease.

MICROBIOTA AND IMMUNE SYSTEM OF THE MAMMARY GLAND

Several body sites previously thought to be free of bacteria, such as the uterus and mammary glands, are now suggested to have a normal resident microbiota because of the advance of NGS technology. However, some of this remains controversial. There is strong evidence regarding the important role that bacteria from different body sites play in the local and systemic immune system; however, the existence of resident mammary gland bacteria remains a topic of discussion. The current knowledge regarding whether there are resident bacteria of the mammary gland of cattle, how this microbiota may influence udder health, and how it can affect the health of the calves is discussed here.

Paradigm: Is There a Resident Microbiota Inhabiting the Bovine Mammary Gland?

Whether or not the bovine mammary gland is colonized by a core microbiota is the focus of discussion following several studies using NGS, which found bacterial DNA present in milk samples aseptically collected.[142–145] Some researchers claim that the immune system of the udder is not compatible with an inherent resident bacteria, mainly based on the argument that the mammary gland epithelium is very different from the intestinal mucosa, which have a mucus layer with high concentrations of sIgA and AMPs and the presence of organized lymphoid formations.[146] As such, this approach considers all bacteria living in the mammary gland as pathogens. This view is in contrast with the fact that the bovine mammary gland is constantly exposed to bacterial agents living on the teat skin and in the milk canal[147] that are regularly successful in reaching the cisterna, as shown by the innate immune response found in milking cows represented by the presence of somatic cells.

Bacterial DNA reported in studies investigating bacterial communities of low-biomass environments, such as the udder, could be a matter of contamination during the sampling procedure, a known limitation inherent to NGS methods.[148] However, the differences in microbial composition reported between breeds,[149] geographic location,[42] and seasons of the year[144] suggest that there are bacteria (resident or not) and that the relationship between those organisms and the udder immune system deserves close attention.

Another inherent limitation of the NGS technologies relates to the ability to detect DNA but not to address bacterial viability. Nevertheless, it is possible that only the simple presence of antigens (from dead bacteria) could be a factor capable of triggering a local immune response, because infusion of PAMPs was associated with strong inflammatory response in the mammary gland.[150] Therefore, the question that remains to be answered is whether there is protective microbiota that is harmless to the udder that stimulates a protective immune response while concurrently competing with pathogenic organisms.

How Does Microbiota Affect the Mammary Gland Health?

The bacteria and the immune system are constantly interacting in a way such that one modulates the other. In general, greater intestinal richness and diversity are associated with health.[151,152] Likewise, the mammary glands of healthy cattle have a greater richness compared with samples from cows with subclinical or clinical mastitis.[142–144] Much attention is given to understand the impact of the gut bacteria on the immune system.[151] However, the ideal bacterial composition and how changes in management, environment, and genetic selection can affect the local immune response and, thus, susceptibility to mastitis has yet to be determined in the bovine species. Milk antibodies have an immune modulatory effect on gut microbiota,[153] so it is reasonable to assume that different concentrations of immune elements would also affect the bacterial composition in the mammary gland. Therefore, the changes during the lactation cycle (ie, dry period, colostrum with high IgG level, transition milk, and regular milk with more IgA) are likely to select for different organisms that can thrive in that particular environment.[154] Recent evidence suggests that intestinal bacteria can colonize the mammary gland via hematogenous spread by macrophages.[155] Additional support for this route of spread has been shown in laboratory animals[156] as well as cattle.[157] However, it is unlikely that these pioneer bacteria play a role in the development of the mammary gland epithelium, as they do in the intestinal mucosa, but they may be important for regulation of local immunity.

More detailed investigations designed to address overall changes, and the influence of local immune system components on the milk microbiota, are necessary. Efforts should also be focused on the impact of different bacteria on the mammary immune response. This focus might allow the development of new probiotic products to improve immune response, resistance to udder infection, and therefore animal performance.[145,158]

Does the Mammary Gland Microbiota Affect the Gut Health of Preweaned Calves?

It is also important to mention that the interaction between the mammary gland microbiota and immune system goes beyond mastitis predisposition and milk quality, because it can affect gut health in calves, and it might have serious lifelong implications on gut health of neonates. For example, mice exposed to breast milk–derived secretory IgA had different bacterial patterns during adulthood and different expression of intestinal genes related to inflammation regulation compared with those that did not receive IgA.[153] As such, the stimulation of the appropriate immune components in the milk could increase protection against enteropathogens in calves, which would have a significant impact on animal performance.

In addition, in other species the mammary gland microbiota seems to be important in facilitating milk digestion and regulation of the intestinal immune system in neonates.[159] In calves, the colonization with these bacteria is probably less expressive in the development of the gut immune system compared with bacteria acquired from the birth canal and the environment.

SUMMARY

The interaction of the microbiota and the host mucosal immune system plays an important role in the maintenance of host homeostasis and prevention against pathogenic microorganisms. In cattle, several studies have investigated the direct interaction between bacteria from the gut, uterus, and mammary gland with the local immune system. At the mucosal surface, these interactions are essential to generating an appropriate tolerance to commensal bacteria, avoiding pathogen colonization, and stimulating local innate immunity. Multidisciplinary research investigating factors that can affect the development of the mucosal immune system is required to broaden the current knowledge base regarding how microorganisms and bovines coevolved resulting from, or leading to, reciprocally beneficial interactions. In the near future, microbiota manipulation is likely to be used to achieve a balanced immune reaction to increase resistance to diseases and enhance animal performance.

REFERENCES

1. Willing BP. The role of the immune system in regulating the microbiota. Gut Microbes 2010;1(4):213–23.
2. Hooper LV, Littman DR, Macpherson AJ. Interaction between the microbiota and the immune system. Science 2012;336(6086):1268–73.
3. Gensollen T, Iyer SS, Kasper DL, et al. How colonization by microbiota in early life shapes the immune system. Science 2016;352(6285):539–44.
4. Mack DR, Michail S, Wei S, et al. Probiotics inhibit enteropathogenic E. coli adherence in vitro by inducing intestinal mucin gene expression. Am J Physiol 1999;276(4):941–50.
5. Riedel CU, Foata F, Philippe D, et al. Anti-inflammatory effects of bifidobacteria by inhibition of LPS-induced NF-kappaB activation. World J Gastroenterol 2006; 12(23):3729–35.
6. Audy J, Mathieu O, Belvis J, et al. Transcriptomic response of immune signalling pathways in intestinal epithelial cells exposed to lipopolysaccharides, Gram-negative bacteria or potentially probiotic microbes. Benef Microbes 2012;3(4): 273–86.
7. Anderson RC, Cookson AL, McNabb WC, et al. Lactobacillus plantarum DSM 2648 is a potential probiotic that enhances intestinal barrier function. FEMS Microbiol Lett 2010;309(2):184–92.
8. Ewaschuk JB, Diaz H, Meddings L, et al. Secreted bioactive factors from Bifidobacterium infantis enhance epithelial cell barrier function. Am J Physiol Gastrointest Liver Physiol 2008;295(5):1025–34.
9. Szentkuti L, Riedesel H, Enss ML, et al. Pre-epithelial mucus layer in the colon of conventional and germ-free rats. Histochem J 1990;22(9):491–7.
10. Kato LM, Kawamoto S, Maruya M, et al. The role of the adaptive immune system in regulation of gut microbiota. Immunol Rev 2014;260(1):67–75.
11. Huhta H, Helminen O, Kauppila JH, et al. The expression of toll-like receptors in normal human and murine gastrointestinal organs and the effect of microbiome and cancer. J Histochem Cytochem 2016;64(8):470–82.
12. Turner JR. Intestinal mucosal barrier function in health and disease. Nat Rev Immunol 2009;9(11):799–809.
13. Malmuthuge N, Fries P, Griebel PJ, et al. Regional and age dependent changes in gene expression of toll-like receptors and key antimicrobial defence molecules throughout the gastrointestinal tract of dairy calves. Vet Immunol Immunopathol 2012;146(1):18–26.
14. Mackie RI, Sghir A, Gaskins HR. Developmental microbial ecology of the neonatal gastrointestinal tract. Am J Clin Nutr 1999;69(5):1035S–45S.
15. Malmuthuge N, Griebel PJ, Guan L, et al. Taxonomic identification of commensal bacteria associated with the mucosa and digesta throughout the gastrointestinal tracts of preweaned calves. Appl Environ Microbiol 2014;80(6):2021–8.
16. Collado MC, Sanz Y. Quantification of mucosa-adhered microbiota of lambs and calves by the use of culture methods and fluorescent in situ hybridization coupled with flow cytometry techniques. Vet Microbiol 2007;121(3–4):299–306.
17. Uyeno Y, Shigemori S, Shimosato T. Effect of probiotics/prebiotics on cattle health and productivity. Microbes Environ 2015;30(2):126–32.

18. Zambrano-Nava S, Boscón-Ocando J, Nava J. Normal bacterial flora from vaginas of Criollo Limonero cows. Trop Anim Health Prod 2011;43(2):291–4.

19. Laguardia-Nascimento M, Branco KM, Gasparini MR, et al. Vaginal microbiome characterization of nellore cattle using metagenomic analysis. PLoS One 2015; 10(11):e0143294.

20. Bicalho MLS, Santin T, Rodrigues M, et al. Dynamics of the microbiota found in the vaginas of dairy cows during the transition period: Associations with uterine diseases and reproductive outcome. J Dairy Sci 2017;100(4):3043–58.

21. Ellinger DK, Muller LD, Glantz PJ. Influence of feeding fermented colostrum and Lactobacillus acidophilus on fecal flora of dairy calves. J Dairy Sci 1980;63(3): 478–82.

22. Malmuthuge N, Chen Y, Liang LA, et al. Heat-treated colostrum feeding promotes beneficial bacteria colonization in the small intestine of neonatal calves. J Dairy Sci 2015;98:8044–53.

23. Fischer AJ, Song Y, He Z, et al. Effect of delaying colostrum feeding on passive transfer and intestinal bacterial colonization in neonatal male Holstein calves. J Dairy Sci 2018;101(4):3099–109.

24. Grønvold AM, Mao Y, L'Abée-Lund TM, et al. Fecal microbiota of calves in the clinical setting: effect of penicillin treatment. Vet Microbiol 2011;153(3–4): 354–60.

25. Oultram J, Phipps E, Teixeira AG, et al. Effects of antibiotics (oxytetracycline, florfenicol or tulathromycin) on neonatal calves' faecal microbial diversity. Vet Rec 2015;177(23):598.

26. Gomez DE, Arroyo LG, Poljak Z, et al. Implementation of an algorithm for selection of antimicrobial therapy for diarrhoeic calves: Impact on antimicrobial treatment rates, health and faecal microbiota. Vet J 2017;226:15–25.

27. Weese JS, Jelinski M. Assessment of the fecal microbiota in beef calves. J Vet Intern Med 2017;31(1):176–85.

28. Gomez DE, Arroyo LG, Costa MC, et al. Characterization of the fecal bacterial microbiota of healthy and diarrheic dairy calves. J Vet Intern Med 2017;31(3): 928–39.

29. Petersen C, Round JL. Defining dysbiosis and its influence on host immunity and disease. Cell Microbiol 2014;16(7):1024–33.

30. Doré E, Paré J, Cuté G, et al. Risk factors associated with transmission of Mycobacterium avium subsp. paratuberculosis to calves within dairy herd: a systematic review. J Vet Intern Med 2012;26(1):32–45.

31. Mayer M, Abenthum A, Matthes JM, et al. Development and genetic influence of the rectal bacterial flora of newborn calves. Vet Microbiol 2012;161(1–2): 179–85.

32. Fecteau G, Baillargeon P, Higgins R, et al. Bacterial contamination of colostrum fed to newborn calves in Québec dairy herds. Can Vet J 2002;43(7):523–7.

33. Mylrea PJ. The bacterial content of the small intestine of young calves. Res Vet Sci 1969;10(4):394–5.

34. Karney TL, Johnson MC, Ray B. Changes in the lactobacilli and coliforms populations in the intestinal tract of calves from birth to weanling. J Anim Sci 1986; 63:446–7.

35. Vlkova E, Trojanova I, Rada V. Distribution of bifidobacteria in the gastrointestinal tract of calves. Folia Microbiol (Praha) 2006;51(4):325–8.

36. Vlkova E, Rada V, Trojanova, et al. Occurrence of bifidobacteria in faeces of calves fed milk or a combined diet. Arch Anim Nutr 2008;62(5):359–65.

37. Smith HW. The development of the flora of the alimentary tract in young animals. J Pathol Bacteriol 1965;90(2):495–513.

38. Song Y, Malmuthuge N, Steele MA, et al. Shift of hindgut microbiota and microbial short chain fatty acids profiles in dairy calves from birth to pre-weaning. FEMS Microbiol Ecol 2018;94(3):1–15.

39. Fischer AJ, Malmuthuge N, Guan LL, et al. The effect of heat treatment of bovine colostrum on the concentration of oligosaccharides in colostrum and in the intestine of neonatal male Holstein calves'. J Dairy Sci 2018;101(1):401–7.

40. Lukas F, Koppova I, Kudrna V, et al. Postnatal development of bacterial population in the gastrointestinal tract of calves. Folia Microbiol (Praha) 2007;52(1): 99–104.

41. Klein-Jöbstl D, Schornsteiner E, Mann E, et al. Pyrosequencing reveals diverse fecal microbiota in Simmental calves during early development. Front Microbiol 2014;5:622.

42. Oikonomou G, Bicalho ML, Meira E, et al. Microbiota of cow's milk; distinguishing healthy, sub-clinically and clinically diseased quarters. PLoS One 2014;9(1): e85904.

43. Alipour MJ, Jalanka J, Pessa-Morikawa T, et al. The composition of the perinatal intestinal microbiota in cattle. Sci Rep 2018;8(1):10437.

44. Dias J, Marcondes MI, Motta de Souza S, et al. Bacterial community dynamics across the gastrointestinal tracts of dairy calves during preweaning development. Appl Environ Microbiol 2018;84(9) [pii:e02675-17].

45. Jost T, Lacroix C, Braegger CP, et al. New insights in gut microbiota establishment in healthy breast fed neonates. PLoS One 2012;7(8):e44595.

46. Costa MC, Stampfli HR, Allen-Vercoe E, et al. Development of the faecal microbiota in foals. Equine Vet J 2016;48(6):681–8.

47. Edrington TS, Dowd SE, Farrow RF, et al. Development of colonic microflora as assessed by pyrosequencing in dairy calves fed waste milk. J Dairy Sci 2012; 95(8):4519–25.

48. Barrington GM, Parish SM. Bovine neonatal immunology. Vet Clin North Am Food Anim Pract 2001;17(3):463–76.

49. Felippe MJ. The immune system. In: Felippe MJ, editor. Equine clinical immunology. Ames (IA): Wiley Blackwell; 2015. p. 1–10.

50. Sansonetti PJ. War and peace at mucosal surfaces. Nat Rev Immunol 2004; 4(12):953–64.

51. Arrieta MC, Bistritz L, Meddings JB. Alterations in intestinal permeability. Gut 2006;55(10):1512–20.

52. Groschwitz KR, Hogan SP. Intestinal barrier function: molecular regulation and disease pathogenesis. J Allergy Clin Immunol 2009;124(1):3–20.

53. Rajasekaran SA, Beyenbach KW, Rajasekaran AK. Interactions of tight junctions with membrane channels and transporters. Biochim Biophys Acta 2008;1778(3): 757–69.

54. Sawada N, Murata M, Kikuchi K, et al. Tight junctions and human diseases. Med Electron Microsc 2003;36(3):147–56.

55. Bush LJ, Staley TE. Absorption of colostral immunoglobulins in newborn calves. J Dairy Sci 1980;63(4):672–80.

56. Besser TE, Gay CC. The importance of colostrum to the health of the neonatal calf. Vet Clin North Am Food Anim Pract 1994;10(1):107–17.

57. Araujo G, Yunta C, Terré M, et al. Intestinal permeability and incidence of diarrhea in newborn calves. J Dairy Sci 2015;98(10):7309–17.

58. Castro J. Calf intestinal health: assessment and dietary interventions for its improvement [PhD thesis]. Champaign (IL): University of Illinois at Urbana-Champaign; 2014.

59. Liang G, Malmuthuge N, Bao H, et al. Transcriptome analysis reveals regional and temporal differences in mucosal immune system development in the small intestine of neonatal calves. BMC Genomics 2016;17(1):602.

60. Miyauchi E, O'Callaghan J, Buttó LF, et al. Mechanism of protection of transepithelial barrier function by Lactobacillus salivarius: strain dependence and attenuation by bacteriocin production. Am J Physiol Gastrointest Liver Physiol 2012; 303(9):1029–41.

61. Sultana R, McBain AJ, O'Neill CA. Strain-dependent augmentation of tight-junction barrier function in human primary epidermal keratinocytes by Lactobacillus and Bifidobacterium lysates. Appl Environ Microbiol 2013;79(16):4887–94.

62. Schuppan D. Current concepts of celiac disease pathogenesis. Gastroenterology 2000;119(1):234–42.

63. Malmuthuge N, Li M, Goonewardene LA, et al. Effect of calf starter feeding on gut microbial diversity and expression of genes involved in host immune responses and tight junctions in dairy calves during weaning transition. J Dairy Sci 2013;96(5):3189–200.

64. Marchiando AM, Graham WV, Turner JR. Epithelial barriers in homeostasis and disease. Annu Rev Pathol 2010;5:119–44.

65. Okumura R, Takeda K. Maintenance of intestinal homeostasis by mucosal barriers. Inflamm Regen 2018;2(38):5.

66. Bergstrom KS, Kissoon-Singh V, Gibson DL, et al. Muc2 protects against lethal infectious colitis by disassociating pathogenic and commensal bacteria from the colonic mucosa. PLoS Pathog 2010;6(5):e1000902.

67. Zarepour M, Bhullar K, Montero M, et al. The mucin Muc2 limits pathogen burdens and epithelial barrier dysfunction during Salmonella enterica serovar Typhimurium colitis. Infect Immun 2013;81(10):3672–83.

68. Enss ML, Grosse-Siestrup H, Schmidt-Wittig U, et al. Changes in colonic mucins of germfree rats in response to the introduction of a "normal" rat microbial flora. Rat colonic mucin. J Exp Anim Sci 1992;35(3):110–9.

69. Enss ML, Schmidt-Wittig U, Müller H, et al. Response of germfree rat colonic mucous cells to peroral endotoxin application. Eur J Cell Biol 1996;71(1): 99–104.

70. Willing BP, Van Kessel AG. Enterocyte proliferation and apoptosis in the caudal small intestine is influenced by the composition of colonizing commensal bacteria in the neonatal gnotobiotic pig. J Anim Sci 2007;85(12):3256–66.

71. Bauer H, Horowitz RE, Levenson SM, et al. The response of the lymphatic tissue to the microbial flora. Studies on germfree mice. Am J Pathol 1963;42:471–83.

72. Macpherson AJ, Gatto D, Sainsbury E, et al. A primitive T cell-independent mechanism of intestinal mucosal IgA responses to commensal bacteria. Science 2000;288(5474):2222–6.

73. Sperandio B, Fischer N, Sansonetti PJ. Mucosal physical and chemical innate barriers: Lessons from microbial evasion strategies. Semin Immunol 2015; 27(2):111–8.

74. Zasloff M. Antimicrobial peptides in health and disease. N Engl J Med 2002; 347(15):1199–200.

75. Rescigno M, Iliev ID. Interleukin-23: linking mesenteric lymph node dendritic cells with Th1 immunity in Crohn's disease. Gastroenterology 2009;137(5): 1566–70.

76. Putsep K, Axelsson LG, Boman A, et al. Germ-free and colonized mice generate the same products from enteric prodefensins. J Biol Chem 2000;275(51):40478–82.

77. Nakajima A, Vogelzang A, Maruya M, et al. IgA regulates the composition and metabolic function of gut microbiota by promoting symbiosis between bacteria. J Exp Med 2018;215(8):2019–34.

78. Macpherson AJ, Hunziker L, McCoy K, et al. IgA responses in the intestinal mucosa against pathogenic and non-pathogenic microorganisms. Microbes Infect 2001;3(12):1021–35.

79. van der Waaij LA, Limburg PC, Mesander G, et al. In vivo IgA coating of anaerobic bacteria in human faeces. Gut 1996;38(3):348–54.

80. Tsuruta T, Inoue R, Tsukahara T, et al. Commensal bacteria coated by secretory immunoglobulin A and immunoglobulin G in the gastrointestinal tract of pigs and calves. Anim Sci J 2012;83(12):799–804.

81. Tsuruta T, Inoue R, Iwanaga T, et al. Development of a method for the identification of S-IgA-coated bacterial composition in mouse and human feces. Biosci Biotechnol Biochem 2010;74(5):968–73.

82. Cunningham-Rundles C. Physiology of IgA and IgA deficiency. J Clin Immunol 2001;21(5):303–9.

83. Shroff KE, Meslin K, Cebra JJ. Commensal enteric bacteria engender a self-limiting humoral mucosal immune response while permanently colonizing the gut. Infect Immun 1995;63(10):3904–13.

84. Gaudino SJ, Kumar P. Cross-talk between antigen presenting cells and t cells impacts intestinal homeostasis, bacterial infections, and tumorigenesis. Front Immunol 2019;6(10):360.

85. Belkaid Y. Regulatory T cells and infection: a dangerous necessity. Nat Rev Immunol 2007;7(11):875–88.

86. Rakoff-Nahoum S, Paglino J, Eslami-Varzaneh F, et al. Recognition of commensal microflora by toll-like receptors is required for intestinal homeostasis. Cell 2004;118(2):229–41.

87. Chen L, Deng H, Cui H, et al. Inflammatory responses and inflammation-associated diseases in organs. Oncotarget 2017;9(6):7204–18.

88. Stillie R, Farooq SM, Gordon JR, et al. The functional significance behind expressing two IL-8 receptor types on PMN. J Leukoc Biol 2009;86:529–43.

89. Iyer SS, Cheng G. Role of interleukin 10 transcriptional regulation in inflammation and autoimmune disease. Crit Rev Immunol 2012;32(1):23–63.

90. Smits HH, Engering A, van der Kleij D, et al. Selective probiotic bacteria induce IL-10-producing regulatory T cells in vitro by modulating dendritic cell function through dendritic cell-specific intercellular adhesion molecule 3-grabbing non-integrin. J Allergy Clin Immunol 2005;115(6):1260–7.

91. Malmuthuge N, Griebel PJ, Guan LL. The gut microbiome and its potential role in the development and function of newborn calf gastrointestinal tract. Front Vet Sci 2015;2:36.

92. Weng M, Walker WA. The role of gut microbiota in programming the immune phenotype. J Dev Orig Health Dis 2013;4(3):203–14.

93. Kehrli ME Jr, Goff JP. Periparturient hypocalcemia in cows: effects on peripheral blood neutrophil and lymphocyte function. J Dairy Sci 1989;72:1188–96.

94. Sheldon IM, Dobson H. Postpartum uterine health in cattle. Anim Reprod Sci 2004;82(83):295–306.

95. Jeon SJ, Cunha F, Vieira-Neto A, et al. Blood as a route of transmission of uterine pathogens from the gut to the uterus in cows. Microbiome 2017;5(1):109.

96. LeBlanc SJ. Postpartum uterine disease and dairy herd reproductive performance: A review. Vet J 2008;176:102–14.

97. Galvão KN. Postpartum uterine diseases in dairy cows. Anim Reprod 2012;9: 290–6.

98. Hussain AM. Bovine uterine defense mechanisms: a review. Zentralbl Veterinarmed B 1989;36:641–51.

99. Paape MJ, Bannerman DD, Zhao X, et al. The bovine neutrophil: Structure and function in blood and milk. Vet Res 2003;34:597–627.

100. Galvão KN, Felippe MJ, Brittin SB, et al. Evaluation of cytokine expression by blood monocytes of lactating Holstein cows with or without postpartum uterine disease. Theriogenology 2012;77(2):356–72.

101. Galvão KN, Santos NR, Galvão JS, et al. Association between endometritis and endometrial cytokine expression in postpartum Holstein cows. Theriogenology 2011;76(2):290–9.

102. Tzianabos AO. Polysaccharide immunomodulators as therapeutic agents: structural aspects and biologic function. Cli Microbiol Rev 2000;13:523–33.

103. Gilbert RO, Santos NR. Dynamics of postpartum endometrial cytology and bacteriology and their relationship to fertility in dairy cows. Theriogenology 2016;85(8):1367–74.

104. Hammon DS, Evjen IM, Dhiman TR, et al. Neutrophil function and energy status in Holstein cows with uterine health disorders. Vet Immunol Immunopathol 2006; 113(1–2):21–9.

105. Galvão KN, Santos JE. Recent advances in the immunology and uterine microbiology of healthy cows and cows that develop uterine disease. Turk J Vet Anim Sci 2014;38:577–88.

106. Jeon SJ, Cunha F, Ma X, et al. Uterine microbiota and immune parameters associated with fever in dairy cows with metritis. PLoS One 2016;11:e0165740.

107. Kimura KJ, Goff P, Kehrli ME Jr, et al. Decreased neutrophil function as a cause of retained placenta in dairy cattle. J Dairy Sci 2002;85(3):544–50.

108. Goff JP, Horst RL. Physiological changes at parturition and their relationship to metabolic disorders. J Dairy Sci 1997;80(7):1260–8.

109. Ingvartsen KL, Moyes K. Nutrition, immune function and health of dairy cattle. Animal 2013;7(Suppl 1):112–22.

110. Kuehl FA Jr, Egan RW. Prostaglandins, arachidonic acid, and inflammation. Science 1980;210:978–84.

111. Weisdorf DJ, Craddock PR, Jacob HS. Glycogenolysis versus glucose transport in human granulocytes: Differential activation in phagocytosis and chemotaxis. Blood 1982;60(4):888–93.

112. Weisdorf DJ, Craddock PR, Jacob HS. Granulocytes utilize different energy sources for movement and phagocytosis. Inflammation 1982;6(3):245–56.

113. Grinstein S, Klip A. Calcium homeostasis and the activation of calcium channels in cells of the immune system. Bull N Y Acad Med 1989;65(1):69–79.

114. Vig M, Kinet JP. Calcium signaling in immune cells. Nat Immunol 2009; 10(1):21–7.

115. Nunes P, Demaurex N. The role of calcium signaling in phagocytosis. J Leukoc Biol 2010;88(1):57–68.

116. Galvão KN, Flaminio MJ, Brittin SB, et al. Association between uterine disease and indicators of neutrophil and systemic energy status in lactating Holstein cows. J Dairy Sci 2010;93(7):2926–37.

117. Hoeben D, Heyneman R, Burvenich C. Elevated levels of beta-hydroxybutyric acid in periparturient cows and in vitro effect on respiratory burst activity of bovine neutrophils. Vet Immunol Immunopathol 1997;58(2):165–70.
118. Scalia D, Lacetera N, Bernabucci U, et al. In vitro effects of nonesterified fatty acids on bovine neutrophils oxidative burst and viability. J Dairy Sci 2006; 89(1):147–54.
119. Grinberg N, Elazar S, Rosenshine I, et al. Beta-hydroxybutyrate abrogates formation of bovine neutrophil extracellular traps and bactericidal activity against mammary pathogenic Escherichia coli. Infect Immun 2008;76(6):2802–7.
120. Ster C, Loiselle MC, Lacasse P. Effect of postcalving serum nonesterified fatty acids concentration on the functionality of bovine immune cells. J Dairy Sci 2012;95(2):708–17.
121. Ingham HR, Sisson PR, Tharagonnet D, et al. Inhibition of phagocytosis in vitro by obligate anaerobes. Lancet 1977;2(8051):1252–4.
122. Ruder CA, Sasser RG, Williams RJ, et al. Uterine infections in the postpartum cow. II. Possible synergistic effect of Fusobacterium necrophorum and Corynebacterium pyogenes. Theriogenology 1981;15(6):573–80.
123. Tan ZL, Nagaraja TG, Chengappa MM. Fusobacterium necrophorum infections: virulence factors, pathogenic mechanism and control measures. Vet Res Commun 1996;20(2):113–40.
124. Archbald LF, Schultz RH, Fahning M, et al. A sequential histological study of the post-partum bovine uterus. J Reprod Fertil 1972;29(21):133–6.
125. Hailemariam D, Mandal R, Saleem F, et al. Identification of predictive biomarkers of disease state in transition dairy cows. J Dairy Sci 2014;97(5):2680–93.
126. Jeon SJ, Vieira-Neto A, Gobikrushanth M, et al. Uterine microbiota progression from calving until establishment of metritis in dairy cows. Appl Environ Microbiol 2015;81(18):6324–32.
127. Sheldon IM, Noakes DE, Rycroft AN, et al. Influence of uterine bacterial contamination after parturition on ovarian dominant follicle selection and follicle growth and function in cattle. Reproduction 2002;123(6):837–45.
128. Williams EJ, Fischer DP, Pfeiffer DU, et al. Clinical evaluation of postpartum vaginal mucus reflects uterine bacterial infection and the immune response in cattle. Theriogenology 2005;63(1):102–17.
129. Bonnett BN, Martin SW, Gannon VP, et al. Endometrial biopsy in Holstein-Friesian dairy cows. III. Bacteriological analysis and correlations with histological findings. Can J Vet Res 1991;55(2):168–73.
130. Bondurant RH. Inflammation in the bovine female reproductive tract. J Anim Sci 1999;77(Suppl 2):101–10.
131. Huszenicza G, Fodor M, Gacs M, et al. Uterine bacteriology, resumption of ovarian activity and fertility in postpartum cows kept in large-scale dairy herds. Reprod Domest Anim 1999;34(3–4):237–45.
132. Bicalho RC, Machado VS, Bicalho ML, et al. Molecular and epidemiological characterization of bovine intrauterine Escherichia coli. J Dairy Sci 2010; 93(12):5818–30.
133. Bicalho ML, Machado VS, Oikonomou G, et al. Association between virulence factors of Escherichia coli, Fusobacterium necrophorum, and Arcanobacterium pyogenes and uterine diseases of dairy cows. Vet Microbiol 2012;157(1–2): 125–31.
134. Knudsen LR, Karstrup CC, Pedersen HG, et al. An investigation of the microbiota in uterine flush samples and endometrial biopsies from dairy cows during the first 7 weeks postpartum. Theriogenology 2016;86(2):642–50.

135. Bicalho ML, Machado VS, Higgins CH, et al. Genetic and functional analysis of the bovine uterine microbiota. Part I: Metritis versus healthy cows. J Dairy Sci 2017;100(5):3850–62.

136. Cunha F, Jeon SJ, Daetz R, et al. Quantifying known and emerging uterine pathogens, and evaluating their association with metritis and fever in dairy cows. Theriogenology 2018;114:25–33.

137. Sicsic R, Goshen T, Dutta R, et al. Microbial communities and inflammatory response in the endometrium differ between normal and metritic dairy cows at 5-10 days post-partum. Vet Res 2018;49(1):77.

138. Galvão KN, Higgins CH, Zinicola M, et al. Effect of pegbovigrastim administration on the microbiome found in the vagina of cows postpartum. J Dairy Sci 2019;102(4):3439–51.

139. Segata N, Boernigen D, Tickle TL, et al. Computational metaomics for microbial community studies. Mol Syst Biol 2013;9:666–80.

140. Franzosa EA, Hsu T, Sirota-Madi A, et al. Sequencing and beyond: integrating molecular 'omics' for microbial community profiling. Nat Rev Microbiol 2015; 13(6):360–72.

141. Aguiar-Pulido V, Huang W, Suarez-Ulloa V, et al. Metagenomics, metatranscriptomics, and metabolomics approaches for microbiome analysis. Evol Bioinform Online 2016;12(Suppl 1):5–16.

142. Oikonomou G, Machado VS, Santisteban C, et al. Microbial diversity of bovine mastitic milk as described by pyrosequencing of metagenomic 16s rDNA. PLoS One 2012;7:e47671.

143. Kuehn JS, Gorden PJ, Munro D, et al. Bacterial community profiling of milk samples as a means to understand culture-negative bovine clinical mastitis. PLoS One 2013;8(4):e61959.

144. Metzger SA, Hernandez LL, Skarlupka JH, et al. A cohort study of the milk microbiota of healthy and inflamed bovine mammary glands from dryoff through 150 days in milk. Front Vet Sci 2018;5:247.

145. Derakhshani H, Fehr KB, Sepehri S, et al. Invited review: Microbiota of the bovine udder: Contributing factors and potential implications for udder health and mastitis susceptibility. J Dairy Sci 2018;101(12):10605–25.

146. Rainard P. Mammary microbiota of dairy ruminants: fact or fiction? Vet Res 2017; 48(1):25.

147. Braem G, De Vliegher S, Verbist B, et al. Culture-independent exploration of the teat apex microbiota of dairy cows reveals a wide bacterial species diversity. Vet Microbiol 2012;157(3–4):383–90.

148. Kim D, Hofstaedter CE, Zhao C, et al. Optimizing methods and dodging pitfalls in microbiome research. Microbiome 2017;5(1):52.

149. Cremonesi P, Ceccarani C, Curone G, et al. Milk microbiome diversity and bacterial group prevalence in a comparison between healthy Holstein Friesian and Rendena cows. PLoS One 2018;13(10):e0205054.

150. Bougarn S, Cunha P, Harmache A, et al. Muramyl dipeptide synergizes with Staphylococcus aureus lipoteichoic acid to recruit neutrophils in the mammary gland and to stimulate mammary epithelial cells. Clin Vaccine Immunol 2010; 17(11):1797–809.

151. Qian LJ, Kang SM, Xie JL, et al. Early-life gut microbial colonization shapes Th1/Th2 balance in asthma model in BALB/c mice. BMC Microbiol 2017;17(1):135.

152. Clemente JC, Pehrsson EC, Blaser MJ, et al. The microbiome of uncontacted Amerindians. Sci Adv 2015;1(3) [pii:e1500183].

153. Rogier EW, Frantz AL, Bruno ME, et al. Secretory antibodies in breast milk promote long-term intestinal homeostasis by regulating the gut microbiota and host gene expression. Proc Natl Acad Sci U S A 2014;111(8):3074–9.
154. Derakhshani H, Plaizier JC, De Buck J, et al. Association of bovine major histocompatibility complex (BoLA) gene polymorphism with colostrum and milk microbiota of dairy cows during the first week of lactation. Microbiome 2018; 6(1):203.
155. Perez PF, Doré J, Leclerc M, et al. Bacterial imprinting of the neonatal immune system: lessons from maternal cells? Pediatrics 2007;119:e724–32.
156. Fernández L, Langa S, Martín V, et al. The human milk microbiota: origin and potential roles in health and disease. Pharmacol Res 2013;69(1):1–10.
157. Young W, Hine BC, Wallace OA, et al. Transfer of intestinal bacterial components to mammary secretions in the cow. PeerJ 2015;3:e888.
158. Arroyo R, Martín V, Maldonado A, et al. Treatment of infectious mastitis during lactation: antibiotics versus oral administration of Lactobacilli isolated from breast milk. Clin Infect Dis 2010;50(12):1551–8.
159. Martín R, Langa S, Reviriego C, et al. The commensal microflora of human milk: new perspectives for food bacteriotherapy and probiotics. Trends Food Sci Technol 2004;15(3–4):121–7.

Nutraceuticals
An Alternative Strategy for the Use of Antimicrobials

Michael A. Ballou, PhD*, Emily M. Davis, MS,
Benjamin A. Kasl, DVM

KEYWORDS

- Health • Immune • Nutraceutical • Probiotic • Prebiotic • Phytonutrient
- Polyunsaturated fatty acid

KEY POINTS

- Nutraceutical is a term derived from nutrition and pharmaceutical. There are many compounds that improve immune responses and reduce the risk of disease through different mechanisms of action.
- Probiotics are the supplementation of viable microorganisms that offer potential health benefits to the animal. Probiotics are predominately supplemented to improve gastrointestinal health, rumen fermentation, or nutrient utilization.
- Prebiotics are a group of indigestible carbohydrates that function to improve the growth of commensal bacteria. Some fractions (eg, β-glucans and mannanoligosaccharides) have direct immunomodulatory, gram-negative pathogen binding, or hydrophobic mycotoxin absorption capacities.
- Phytonutrients are a group of compounds isolated from plants with potential therapeutic applications given their intrinsic antioxidative, anti-inflammatory, and antimicrobial properties.
- Polyunsaturated fatty acids influence the degree of inflammation. Generally, increasing the supplementation of omega-3 fatty acid sources decreases inflammation, whereas supplementation of omega-6 fatty acids increases inflammation. How much inflammation is needed at any specific physiologic stage is less understood in ruminant species.

INTRODUCTION

Public concerns regarding the potential association between zoonotic multidrug-resistant bacterial strains and antibiotic use in food animals has prompted significant regulatory changes to on-farm antimicrobial availability and use.[1] Producers and

Disclosure: M.A. Ballou has equity ownership in MB Nutritional Sciences, LLC. The rest of the authors have nothing to disclose.
Department of Veterinary Sciences, Texas Tech University, Lubbock, TX 79409, USA
* Corresponding author.
E-mail address: michael.ballou@ttu.edu

veterinarians alike face increasingly limited options to therapeutically treat diseased animals. As a result, microbial and plant-based compounds and their derivatives received increased research and commercial attention in the past few decades. Nutraceuticals, as many of them are known, is a hybrid of nutrition and pharmaceuticals. They consist of natural compounds and/or microbes that offer potentially advantageous effects related to ruminant health and productivity, including improved feed efficiency, milk production, and disease resistance through immune modulation or decreased disease pressure.[1–3]

Nutraceuticals are a broad group of compounds that can be classified in several ways. Some of the more common classifications are based on the mechanism of action, chemical nature, or the feed source of the compound. In this review, we discuss the general mechanisms of action of common nutraceutical classes that are currently available to be used in ruminants. We classify and discuss each nutraceutical as either a *probiotic*, *prebiotic*, *phytonutrient* (eg, polyphenol, spices/essential oils), or *polyunsaturated fatty acid*. Finally, nutraceuticals are a rapidly developing field and it is important to note that these compounds lack governmental regulatory oversight by the Food and Drug Administration given their classification as "dietary supplements." Therefore, product label statements regarding composition, dosage, effectiveness, and quality are not necessarily independently validated or standardized.

PROBIOTICS

Probiotics, also known as direct-fed microbials, can improve health in many animal species. Common probiotic microorganisms currently used commercially include *Lactobacillus* sp. and other lactic acid-producing bacteria, *Bifidobacterium* sp., *Bacillus* sp., and *Saccharomyces cerevisiae*. Important considerations when supplementing probiotics include the dose (colony-forming units [CFU]), the duration of supplementation, and the age of the animal. A significant portion of the research on probiotic supplementation in ruminants focused on the health benefits to the gastrointestinal tract (GIT), which makes teleologic sense because these microorganisms may directly influence microbial communities and cellular function within the GIT. Most of the health benefits described in **Table 1** report reduced incidence or duration of scours. Ancillary benefits of probiotics, both direct and indirect, in other organ systems including the respiratory tract, urogenital tract, and mammary gland have also been investigated, but are only briefly discussed in this review.

The dynamics of the GIT vary between individual animals, diets, ages, environment, and management factors. Therefore, there is a significant amount of complexity involved in evaluating and comparing the efficacy of these probiotic strategies on their ability to affect health and performance. Typically, a probiotic must contain live microorganisms (usually bacteria and/or yeast) and produce one or more of the following desirable outcomes[66,67]:

- Regulate GIT microbial communities
- Prevent adherence or colonization of potential pathogens in the GIT
- Produce antimicrobial or bactericidal products against potential pathogens
- Maintain host GIT integrity including improved barrier defenses
- Improve mucosal adaptive immune responses
- Regulate GIT inflammation
- Improve ruminal fermentation and nutrient utilization

The application of probiotics in neonates is more common, which makes sense because the GIT and immune system are both developing rapidly and the risk for

Table 1
Effects of probiotics and prebiotics on the immune function, health, and performance of calves, dairy cows, and feedlot steers

Animal	Strain/Type	Dose	Duration/Frequency	Health/Production Status	Outcome	Reference
Calf	Probiotic	10^9 CFU/d multistrain	8 wk	High risk	Decreased scours and therapy	Timmerman et al,[4] 2005
Calf	Probiotic	10^9 CFU/d LAB 6 strains	8 wk	High risk	Decreased scours and therapy	Timmerman et al,[4] 2005
Calf	Probiotic	10^8 CFU/d LAB, *Enterococcus faecium, B bifidum, S thermophilus*	90 d	Low risk	Decreased scours	Mokhber-Dezfouli et al,[5] 2007
Calf	Probiotic	10^7 CFU/d *Lactobacillus acidophilus* and *L plantarum*	15 wk	Low risk	Increased white blood cell counts, increased IgG concentration	Al-Saiady,[6] 2010
Calf	Probiotic	Meta-analysis on LAB	Range 14–187 d	Low risk	Decreased scours	Signorini et al,[7] 2012
Calf	Probiotic	2.0×10^9 CFU/d *L acidophilus* and *Enterococcus faecium*	21 d	Moderate *Salmonella enteria* challenge	Reduced systemic inflammation, decreased mucosal damage, increased villi height:crypt depth in the duodenum and ileum	Liang et al,[8]
Calf	Probiotic	10^{10} CFU challenge EHEC *E coli* then 10^{10} CFU probiotic *E coli*	35 d	8–10-wk-old calves	Decreased *E. coli* O157:H7 GIT growth and fecal shedding	Tkalcic et al,[9] 2003
Calf	Probiotic + yeast	10^9 CFU/d *L acidophilus, E faecium, Saccharomyces cerevisiae*	56 d	High risk	Decreased neutrophil oxidative burst, increased lymphocyte counts, decreased haptoglobin, decreased scours	Davis,[10] 2018
Calf	Probiotic + yeast	10^8 CFU/d LAB, 10^6 CFU/d *S cerevisiae*, 10^8 CFU/d LAB	24 wk	Low risk	Decreased scours	Agarwal et al,[11] 2002
Calf	Yeast	10^9 CFU/d *S cerevisiae*	2×/d for 84 d	High risk	Decreased scours	Galvao et al,[12] 2005

(continued on next page)

Table 1
(continued)

Animal	Strain/Type	Dose	Duration/Frequency	Health/Production Status	Outcome	Reference
Calf	BG	5 mL/d 50% BG extract	56 d	High risk	Increased neutrophil counts, decreased neutrophil functionality, decreased haptoglobin	Davis,[10] 2018
Calf	BG	113 g/d of a 1.8% BG + vitamin C	28 d	Transport stress	Increased neutrophil counts at d 28	Eicher et al,[13] 2010
Calf	BG	150 g/d of a 70% BG + vitamin C	28 d	Transport stress	Decreased white blood cells and neutrophil phagocytosis	Eicher et al,[13] 2010
Calf	MOS + Bs	3 g/hd/d MOS + 10^9 CFU *Bacillus subtilis*	56 d	High risk	Decreased lymphocyte counts and haptoglobin	Davis,[10] 2018
Calf	MOS	7 g/hd/d MOS	From 5 to 56 d	Low risk	Reduced antibiotic treatments and cost of scours	Kara et al,[14] 2015
Calf	MOS	4 g/hd/d MOS	30 d	Low risk	Decreased fecal scores and fecal coliform counts	Ghosh & Mehla,[15] 2012
Calf	MOS	4 g/hd/d MOS	5 wk	Low risk	Decreased probability of scours	Heinrichs et al,[16] 2003
Calf	MOS	4 or 6 g/hd/d MOS	56 d	Low risk	No changes	Hill et al,[17] 2008
Calf	FOS	4 or 8 g/hd/d FOS	56 d	Low risk	No changes	Hill et al,[17] 2008
Calf	FOS	3 or 6 g/hd/d FOS	168 d	Low risk	Increased carcass weight	Grand et al,[18] 2013
Calf	GOS	3.4% GOS DM in milk replacer	84 d	Low risk	Increased days with high fecal scores, increased epithelium growth in the SI, increased LAB and *Bifidobacterium* abundance in the SI	Castro et al,[19] 2016

Animal	Type	Dosage	Duration	Stage	Effects	Reference
Dairy cow	Probiotic	50 g/d Lactobacillus casei and L plantarum of 1.3 × 10^9 CFU/g	30 d	Lactating	Decreased SCC, no change in milk components but increased overall milk production at 15 and 30 d of the study (75 and 90 DIM)	Xu et al,[20] 2017
Dairy cow	Probiotic	10, 15, or 20 g/d Saccharomyces cerevisiae and LAB, no CFU listed	60 d	Early to mid lactation	Increased milk yield, FCM, solids, and profit	Shreedhar et al,[21] 2016
Dairy cow	Probiotic	10 g/hd/d probiotics, no CFU listed	21 d	Early lactation	Increased total milk yield and fat	Musa et al,[22] 2017
Dairy cow	Probiotic + yeast	10, 15, or 20 g/hd/d Lactobacillus, S cerevisiae, Propionibacterium, no CFU listed	6 wk	Lactating	Increased milk production with 20 g/d (most cost-effective), tendency to increase milk fat and protein	Vibhute et al,[23] 2011
Dairy cow	Yeast	9 mL/hd/d commercial yeast product in the water, no CFU listed	10 wk	30 DIM	Increased rumen pH, decreased BHBA, increased milk production, decreased milk protein yield	Rossow et al,[24] 2014
Dairy cow	Yeast	3 g/hd/d of 6.0 × 10^9 CFU live yeast	5 periods of 45 d	Lactating	Increased nutrient utilization in the rumen, increased milk yield, protein, and fat	Rossow et al,[25] 2018
Dairy cow	Yeast	2.5 g/d of 2.5 × 10^{10} CFU S cerevisiae	105 d	Lactating	Increased milk production	Maamouri et al,[26] 2014
Dairy cow	Yeast	40 g/d of 5.0 × 10^{11} CFU S cerevisiae	90 d	3rd lactation, early in lactation	Increased milk yield and fat, decreased SCC	Dailidaviciene et al,[27] 2018
Dairy cow	Synbiotic	1.0 × 10^7 CFU/kg diet L casei + 10 g/hd/d Dextran	1 y	Lactating	Decreased SCC, decreased mastitis, decreased adverse impacts of heat stress, increased milk production and components	Yasuda et al,[28] 2007

(continued on next page)

Table 1
(continued)

Animal	Strain/Type	Dose	Duration/Frequency	Health/Production Status	Outcome	Reference
Dairy cow	Synbiotic	10 g/d of 5.0×10^9 CFU/g *Saccharomyces cerevisiae* and a mix of 10^7 CFU *L casei, Streptococcus faecium, L acidophilus.*	75 d	Lactating	Increased milk fat, decreased SCC	Sretenovic et al,[29] 2008
Feedlot steer	Probiotic	10^9 CFU/d LAB	2 y	Feedlot	Decreased fecal shedding of *E coli* O157:H7	Peterson et al,[30] 2007
Feedlot steer	Probiotic	10^8 CFU/d *E coli*	90 d	Feedlot	Decreased fecal shedding of *E coli* O157:H7	Schamberger et al,[31] 2004
Feedlot steer	Probiotic	10^9 LAB+ 10^9 *Propionibacterium freudenreichii*	9 mo	Feedlot	Decreased fecal shedding of *E coli* and *Salmonella*	Tabe et al,[32] 2008
Feedlot steer	Probiotic	10^9 CFU/d LAB	141 d	Feedlot	Decreased fecal shedding of *E coli,* decreased shedding by 80% at slaughter, only 3.4% of hides positive at harvest	Younts-Dahl et al,[33] 2005
Feedlot steer	Probiotic	10^8 CFU/d, 10^7 CFU/d LAB	141 d	Feedlot	Decreased fecal shedding of *E coli*	Younts-Dahl et al,[33] 2005
Feedlot steer	Probiotic	10^9 CFU/d LAB NPC 747	45–108 d	Feedlot	Decreased fecal prevalence of *E coli;* 1.6% prevalence on hides	Brashears et al,[34] 2003
Feedlot steer	Probiotic	10^9 CFU/d LAB NPC 750	45–108 d	Feedlot	Decreased fecal prevalence of *E coli;* 0% prevalence on hides	Brashears et al,[34] 2003
Feedlot steer	MOS	0.2% MOS in diet, DM	24 d	Feedlot	Decreased haptoglobin and endotoxin translocation from the GIT to circulation	Jin et al,[35] 2014

Concentrations of prebiotics are not standardized, so comparisons among studies are not recommended. Some prebiotics included a carrier that may or may not influence the outcome.

Abbreviations: BG, β-glucan; CFU, colony-forming units; EHEC, enterohemorrhagic *E coli*; FCM, fat corrected milk; FOS, fructooligosaccharide; GOS, galactoo-ligosaccharide; LAB, lactic acid-producing bacteria; MOS, mannanoligosaccharide; SI, small intestine

GIT disease is greater in the neonate. There is a shift in the microbial ecology in the GIT in early life. The neonatal GIT is colonized by many facultative anaerobic bacteria that are common in the environment, including a lot of the family of *Enterobacteriaceae* that include many strains of pathogenic *Escherichia coli* and *Salmonella* sp. There is a shift to more strict anaerobic bacteria as the animal ages with reduced abundance of *Enterobacteriaceae*.[68] Many of the probiotic microorganisms supplemented are either strict anaerobes or facultative anaerobes that commonly increase in abundance as an animal increases in age and are more often lactic acid-producing bacteria. Some of the logic is that speeding up this microbial progression will reduce GIT disease, especially by *Enterobacteriaceae*, because the GIT environment is less conducive to their colonization.

Probiotics can help maintain a beneficial host relationship and colonize the lumen and outer epithelium of the lower GIT creating competition for space on the mucosal surface as well as for nutrients on the mucosa that allow for bacterial adherence and growth (**Fig. 1**). The more "beneficial" bacteria present on the mucosa taking up space and nutrients the less that is available for pathogenic bacteria and potentially other enteric disease-causing microorganisms such as rotavirus, coronavirus, *Cryptosporidium*, and *Eimeria*. This mechanism is often referred to as competitive exclusion. Furthermore, increased lactic acid concentrations in the lower GIT reduces lumen pH and may help limit establishment of pathogenic *Enterobacteriaceae*.[69]

Another mechanism of action through which probiotics may influence health and performance of animals is via interaction with the GIT mucosal immune system (see **Fig. 1**). There are specialized cells in the GIT epithelium known as M cells that constantly sample contents from the GIT and deliver antigens to the lymphocyte-rich Peyer's patches. Maintenance of the commensal microbial structure of the GIT

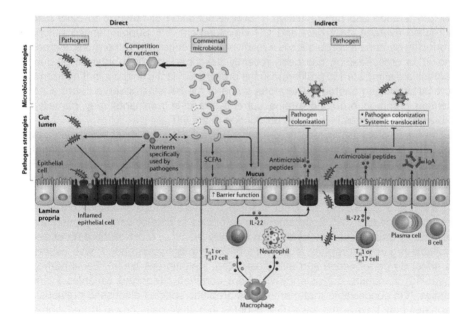

Fig. 1. Mechanisms of action of commensal microbiota and putative probiotics on immune defenses in mucosal tissues. (*From* Kamada et al. Role of the gut microbiota in immunity and inflammatory disease. Nature Reviews Immunology 2013; 13:321-335; with permission.)

helps regulate the inflammatory response in the small intestine to prevent an overreaction to the commensal microbiome and potentially other enteric pathogens.[70] The presence of secretory immunoglobulin A (IgA), antimicrobial peptides, and other regulatory leukocyte responses at the GIT mucosa is an important mechanism that regulates proinflammatory responses, which are essential to maintaining GIT integrity and function. Liang et al. (in press) supplemented Jersey bull calves with 2 strains of lactic acid-producing bacteria and challenged them at 7 days of age with a moderate dose of *Salmonella enterica* serotype Typhimurium. Calves supplemented with probiotic bacteria had reduced systemic inflammation and less mucosal damage as demonstrated by greater villi height:crypt depth in both the duodenum and ileum compared with the unsupplemented, challenged calves.[8] Localized proinflammatory responses are considered beneficial in most tissues; however, in the GIT mucosa, an excessive proinflammatory response may compromise the integrity of the GIT barrier and further exacerbate the pathogenesis of the disease.

Most of the mechanisms of action of probiotics discussed are to decrease the colonization of pathogenic microorganisms or directly improve GIT mucosal immune responses. However, supplementing probiotic species that either produce or stimulate the production of more butyrate have the potential to alter GIT mucosal defenses (see **Fig. 1**). Butyrate is one of the short-chain fatty acids produced by bacteria in the rumen and intestines. Butyrate is a preferred energy source for GIT epithelium that results in the proliferation and differentiation of epithelial cells in the rumen and both the small and large intestines. Butyrate can affect barrier development of the small intestine by increasing tight junction protein expression and exhibiting immunomodulatory effects on enterocytes and mucosal surfaces of the GIT by increasing neutrophil migration.[71,72] Current research suggests that butyrate has anti-inflammatory, antioxidant, and anticancer functions along with promoting epithelial cell proliferation and differentiation.[73] Supplementation of butyrate to dairy heifers increased average daily gain and GIT development.[74,75] Supplementing butyrate-producing bacteria as probiotics is a relatively novel concept. Furthermore, a process known as cross-feeding has been recently described in which butyrate-producing bacteria are stimulated to proliferate in the presence of lactic acid originating from lactic acid-producing bacteria. Therefore, some of the benefits observed from supplementing common probiotic strains currently used in ruminants may partially be explained by changes in butyrate production in the GIT.

The use of probiotics in mature ruminants (eg, feedlot cattle or lactating dairy cows) can affect the rumen and lower GIT. Some probiotic microorganisms bypass the reticuloruminal and abomasal compartments and exert beneficial effects in the lower GIT, likely through similar mechanisms of action as discussed above for preweaned calves. Supplementing feedlot cattle with lactic acid-producing bacteria decreased *E coli* O157:H7 and *Salmonella* sp. fecal shedding, as well as contamination on carcass hides postharvest.[9,30–34] Supplementing probiotics to feedlot cattle as a preharvest food safety strategy is now a common industry practice. Most of the data currently available regarding probiotic supplementation in dairy cow rations have assessed its effect on performance and milk quality (eg, somatic cell count). Fecal pathogen shedding or manure consistency were not commonly reported variables in these studies. It is conceivable that many of the probiotic species discussed previously in neonates may have some lower GIT benefits in mature dairy cows. In fact, some of the performance benefits such as increased milk production may be partially attributable to improvements in GIT health. Furthermore, supplementing probiotics to mature dairy cows seems to have the greatest health and economic benefits during stressful events, most notably the transition period.

The mechanisms of action of orally delivered probiotics on GIT health are more straightforward than how oral probiotics may improve immunity against infections in nonmucosal tissues (eg, mammary gland). The mucosal immune system is a complex network of mucosal surfaces spanning the gastrointestinal, respiratory, and urogenital tracts. Immune responses generated at one mucosal location can transfer to other mucosal surfaces through trafficking and recirculation of effector and memory leukocytes; however, this likely does not include the mammary gland. The paucity of data and the lack of a clear mechanism of action do not support the notion that oral administration of probiotics improves mammary gland health. Rainard and Foucras[76] discussed the potential direct effects of either intramammary infusion or topical application of probiotics, either lactic acid-producing bacteria or *Bacillus* sp., that can inhibit the growth of mastitis causing pathogens in a teat dip as a more promising route of administration to improve mammary gland health. Intramammary infusion of a live lactic acid-producing bacteria culture increased the secretion of proinflammatory cytokines interleukin-8 (IL-8) and IL-1 and attracted neutrophils to the mammary gland.[77] The authors suggested application of this intramammary infusion for the treatment of mastitis because of the production of a broad-spectrum bacteriocin against gram-positive bacteria and a sustained innate immune response.

Finally, a common probiotic application in ruminants is to supplement probiotics, either bacterial or fungal, to improve rumen function and health. The primary mechanisms of action are to stimulate total rumen bacterial population densities, shift or stabilize the balance of rumen bacterial populations, utilize lactic acid, and reduce the risk for ruminal acidosis, and maintain a low oxygen rumen environment.[78–81] Newbold and colleagues[78] designed well-controlled experiments to elucidate the mechanisms by which live yeast supplements may increase rumen bacterial population densities. Oxygen utilization by live yeast supplements seems to be an important mechanism improving the growth of rumen bacteria. Silberberg and colleagues[81] supplemented a live yeast during repeated rumen acidosis challenges and reported improvements in rumen pH, a more stabilized rumen bacteria population, and less systemic inflammation. Another microbial strategy to aid in the prevention of rumen acidosis is a bolus inoculation with lactic acid-utilizing bacteria such as *Megasphaera elsdenii*. Arik and colleagues[82] administered a bolus of lactic acid-utilizing bacteria to the rumen of Holstein heifers with *M elsdenii* for 2 consecutive days during a subacute ruminal acidosis challenge. They observed the *M elsdenii*-treated heifers had a slowed decrease in rumen pH, decreased concentrations of lactic acid-producing bacteria (*Streptococcus bovis*), and increased protozoa counts. These studies support the notion that microbial supplementation strategies can improve rumen function and health.

PREBIOTICS

Prebiotics are indigestible carbohydrates, including many oligosaccharides and fructans, that can improve animal health through a variety of mechanisms. One common mode of action is that they serve as an energy source for commensal or probiotic bacteria in both the rumen and the lower GIT.[83] Synbiotic is the term used when a prebiotic is fed with a probiotic and the effect together is greater than if either is fed alone (see **Fig. 1**). However, the focus of prebiotics in this review is more on their immunomodulatory effects, ability to bind gram-negative bacterial pathogens, and adsorbing certain mycotoxins.

Prebiotics are commonly found in plants, milk, or the cell wall of fungi (yeast and mushrooms). They are found in natural feedstuffs as well as in various extracts. Food sources for galactooligosaccharides include soybeans and milk, whereas fructooligosaccharides are found in vegetables and plants. Prebiotics isolated from yeast cell walls include mannan-oligosaccharides (MOS) and β-glucans (BGs). The composition, availability, and physical chemistry of a prebiotic in a feedstuff or in an extract influences its ability to improve the health of an animal. For example, a prebiotic extract of yeast cell wall may be very different from another extract of yeast cell wall, even if they are extracted from the same strain of yeast.[84] Methods of extraction (eg, enzymatic, solvents, temperature, and time) and additional processing techniques (eg, deproteination) can significantly influence the functional properties of an extract. Making comparisons among various prebiotics are difficult in that many extracts are blended with other ingredients, so 1 g of "extract A" is likely not equivalent to 1 g of "extract B." Therefore, caution should be taken when reviewing the dose of a prebiotic in **Table 1** and when making comparisons among published studies involving different extracts.

The in vitro binding of yeast cell wall extracts with MOS showed that MOS binds to the type 1 fimbriae expressed on many gram-negative bacteria such as pathogenic *Salmonella* sp. and *E coli*.[84] These mannose -specific filaments, or type 1 fimbriae, bind to MOS and prevent pathogenic bacteria from binding to the epithelium and colonizing the GIT. Thus, supplementing yeast cell wall extracts with MOS may be a useful prevention strategy for those animals impacted by greater exposure to gram-negative pathogenic bacteria.[10] Because adhesion of pathogenic bacteria to host mucosal surfaces is generally required for an infection in the GIT, the binding of MOS to these fimbriae decreases potential pathogenic adherence to the host GIT mucosa. The impacts of MOS on specific immune responses are not well characterized. Furthermore, complicating interpretation of data is that MOS extracts are predominately yeast cell wall extracts that also contain various glucan fractions including BGs. Therefore, many of the immunomodulatory effects described in the next paragraph are possible when yeast cell wall extracts are supplemented and likely attributed to the BG fraction of the extract.

β-Glucans are cell wall fractions usually isolated from fungal sources and have potential immunomodulatory effects. The β-1,3-glucans are able to bind to Dectin-1 receptors on monocytes, macrophages, and neutrophils, and, to a lesser extent on dendritic and T-cell surfaces.[85] Ligation of the Dectin-1 receptor when animals are supplemented a fungal extract can cause a slight activation of various leukocyte responses and is currently considered the mechanism of action for a positive immune response. Oral supplementation of BG fractions or yeast cell wall extracts can increase phagocytosis and oxidative burst capacities of immune cells as well as activate an inflammatory response through a nuclear factor κB-mediated pathway. Oral supplementation of BG also affects systemic immune responses in addition to local GIT immune responses. The mechanism of action of BGs is thought to be mediated through specialized M cells that sample intestinal lumen contents. This increased awareness of the immune system allows for mediated inflammation and an enhanced ability of macrophages, neutrophils, and dendritic cells to identify, engulf, and destroy pathogenic bacteria before they have the opportunity to establish an infection in the host.[10,86]

As discussed previously, yeast cell wall extracts contain varying levels of both MOS and BG, and are commonly supplemented to ruminants and other livestock for potential immunomodulatory effects, binding of gram-negative bacteria, or adsorbing hydrophobic mycotoxins. The quantity of MOS and BG that bypasses the rumen is not well understood. However, it does seem that an appreciable, biological amount of MOS and BG does influence lower GIT because supplementing yeast cell wall extracts reduced stress-related disease, improved mammary gland health, and increased milk production.[87,88] Supplementation strategies of yeast cell wall extracts seem to be most effective during periods of stress or increased pathogen exposure. Another application for yeast cell wall extracts is to alleviate some of the negative effects of hydrophobic mycotoxins such as zearalenone. Jouany and colleagues[89] reported that BG interacted with zearalenone, in an "adsorption type" chemical interaction. Both Pereyra and colleagues[90] and Fruhauf and colleagues[91] reported that commercial yeast cell wall extracts with the greatest MOS and BG content adsorbed zearalenone to the greatest extent but were not effective at adsorbing aflatoxin, a hydrophilic mycotoxin. Therefore, a common mycotoxin strategy is to combine a mineral clay and a yeast cell wall extract to gain a more broad-spectrum mycotoxin adsorption capability.

PHYTONUTRIENTS

Phenolic compounds represent a family of phytonutrients with potential therapeutic food animal applications given their intrinsic antioxidative and anti-inflammatory properties (Table 2). In nature, plants synthesize polyphenols as both a defense mechanism against exogenous pathogens and for cellular protection against ultraviolet irradiation. Rich sources of phenolic compounds fed to ruminants include a multitude of industrial fruit and vegetable coproducts, such as citrus, pomegranate, green tea, grape, and green vegetable processing residues. Following consumption, the rumen microbiome can significantly degrade polyphenols and decrease host bioavailability. However, a proportion of dietary polyphenols will bypass ruminal degradation and enter the GIT. Following intestinal absorption, phenolic compounds enter the peripheral circulation where they may exert their bioactive effects on inflammation, oxidative status, and immune function (Fig. 2).[92,93]

Chemically, flavonoids are hydroxylated polyphenolic compounds consisting of a 15-carbon chain bound to an oxygenated heterocyclic ring structure.[92,93] Published studies on the immune effects of feeding flavonoid metabolites specifically to ruminants were limited predominantly to grape, pomegranate, and green tea derivatives.

Byproducts from wine and fruit-juicing industries include pomace, which consists of residual grape pulp, seeds, skin, and stems. Grape pomace contains high concentrations of flavonoid derivatives and tannins, thus acting as a potential reservoir of dietary antioxidant, anti-inflammatory, and antimicrobial phenolic compounds.[45] Supplementing grape seed and pomace extracts can reduce mRNA abundancy of fibroblast growth factor 21 (FGF21), a stress hormone associated with hepatic fatty acid oxidation and ketogenesis, in transition dairy cows.[50] Grape polyphenols lowered leukocyte mRNA expression of superoxide dismutase, an endogenous free radical scavenger, in postpartum dairy cows. This effect suggests the ability of grape polyphenols to decrease superoxide dismutase expression as a consequence of their endogenous antioxidant capacity.[46]

Pomegranate byproducts (eg, seeds, pulp, and peels) contain a potent source of polyphenols, predominantly flavonoids, phenolic acids, and tannins, as well as stereoisomers of vitamin E. Together, these compounds reduce reactive oxygen species and chelate metal ions to induce potentially beneficial immunomodulatory effects in ruminants.[49,94] Dairy calves supplemented with pomegranate extracts had increased in vitro synthesis of the lymphocyte-derived cytokines interferon-γ and IL-4, as well as greater total immunoglobulin G (IgG), in response to ovalbumin vaccination. By improving aspects of both humoral and cell-mediated immunity, calves supplemented with polyphenols may have an improved immune response following vaccination.[42] Hydrolysable tannins may be able to reduce intraluminal oxidation thereby increasing

Table 2
Effects of phytonutrients on the immune function, health, and performance of calves, dairy cows, sheep, and goats

Animal	Strain/Type	Dose	Duration/Frequency	Health/Production Status	Outcome	Reference
Calf	Oregano	1%, 1.5%, or 2% oregano oil in MR	4 d to weaning	Low risk, 4 d of age to 5 mo	Increased IgG concentrations, decreased fecal score, reduced Enterobacteriaceae shedding	Ozkaya[36] 2018
Calf	Oregano	100 ppm/hd/d	120 d	Low risk, 30–150 d of age calves	No reduction in Eimeria oocyst shedding	Grandi et al,[37] 2016
Calf	Oregano	12.5 mg/kg	15 d	Preweaned	Decreased incidence, severity, and duration of scours	Katsoulos et al,[38] 2017
Calf	EO	Multiple doses 0–281 mg/calf/d	24 wk	Low risk	Reduced health scores, scours, and antibiotic treatment	Soltan,[39] 2009, and Oh et al,[40] 2017
Calf	Pomegranate	140 mg polyphenols/g DM; about 5%–20% total DMI	8 wk	Postweaned; apparently healthy; low risk; 11 mo old	Increased DMI, tendency for increased weight gain	Shabtay et al,[41] 2008
Calf	Pomegranate	5 and 10 g/d top-dressed onto starter	70 d	Apparently healthy; low risk; 0–70 d old	Increased peripheral cytokine synthesis (IFN-γ, IL-4), improved IgG response to ovalbumin vax, no effect on fecal scores or rectal temperatures	Oliveira et al,[42] 2010
Dairy cow	EO (garlic, oregano)	3 mL intravaginally, 12 mL intramammary, 25 mL topical teat dip	Once daily for 3 d, 2× daily for 1 d, and 1 application	Mid to late lactation multiparous Holstein cows, Streptococcus uberus mastitis challenge	No cure of mastitis	Mullen et al,[43] 2108

Dairy cow	EO	0, 100, and 200 mg/d	28 d	Lactating	Increase CD4+ T-cell response to vaccine/immune challenge, tendency to increase milk production	Oh et al,[44] 2016
Dairy cow	Grape	4.5 g/hd/d	75 d	Apparently healthy, mid lactation; low risk	No effect on SCC, tendency to increase milk yield	Nielsen & Hansen,[45] 2004
Dairy cow	Grape	10 g/d mixed into pellets	3 wk pre-/postcalving; 44 total day approx.	Apparently healthy; primiparous, 7 mo pregnant	Lowered leukocyte mRNA expression of SOD during initial 3 wk postpartum; no effect on glutathione peroxidase expression	Colitti & Stefanon et al,[46] 2006
Dairy cow	Green tea	100 µg/mL	12 h	In vitro study; mammary epithelial cells isolated from lactating Holstein cows	Greater cell viability, protein, mRNA abundance of NFE2L2; lower intracellular ROS accumulation in response to H_2O_2 challenge	Ma et al,[47] 2018
Transition dairy cow	Mixture	150 g/d prepartum; 170 g/d postpartum	25 d prepartum/26 d postpartum	Apparently healthy; multiparous, primiparous Holstein transition cows	Lower serum NEFA, lower NEFA:insulin postpartum, improved insulin sensitivity pre-/postpartum, higher total antioxidant capacity prepartum; lower malondialdehyde pre-/postpartum	Hashemzadeh-Cigari et al,[48] 2015

(continued on next page)

Table 2
(continued)

Animal	Strain/Type	Dose	Duration/Frequency	Health/Production Status	Outcome	Reference
Transition dairy cow	Pomegranate	350 g DM/d for seeds only; 1350 g DM/d pulp (seeds + peels blend)	25 d pre-/postpartum	Apparently healthy; multiparous, primiparous Holstein transition cows	Higher total plasma antioxidant capacity, lower TAG/FFA/BHBA at both pre-/ postpartum, pulp blend increased SOD, decreased MDA postpartum, higher FCM yield	Safari et al,[49] 2018
Transition dairy cow	Grape	1% of DM	3 wk prepartum until 9 wk postpartum	Multiparous, primiparous Holstein transition cows	Reduced mRNA expression of FGF21 (liver stress hormone) postpartum, no effect on hepatic inflammatory gene expression, increase daily milk yield, increase daily milk protein yield	Gessner et al,[50] 2015
Transition dairy cow	Green tea	0.175 g/kg feed DM	3 wk prepartum until 9 wk postpartum	Primiparous, multiparous Holstein transition cows	Trend for reduced mRNA (haptoglobin), reduced mRNA (FGF21) postpartum; no difference (TNF), (CRP), higher ECM wk 2–9 postpartum; lower hepatic TAG, cholesterol concentrations wk 1 and 3 postpartum	Winkler et al,[51] 2015

Species	Nutraceutical	Dosage	Duration	Animal	Results	Reference
Sheep	Mixture (4 compounds)	Single ruminal infusion; 10% DMI	1 d	Apparently healthy; 18-mo-old, castrated males	Grape-enhanced total plasma antioxidant capacity; reduced plasma susceptibility to liperoxidation	Gladine et al,[52] 2007
Sheep	Green tea	2, 4, or 6 g/kg feed DM	8 wk	Lambs infected with *Haemonchus contortus* GIT parasites	Decreased serum APPs at all dosages (Hpt, LBP, a1AGP), regulate SAA in dose-dependent manner, higher ADG in infected, supplemented lambs vs. infected only lambs; reduced adult worm burden to uninfected levels at 6 g/kg group	Zhong et al,[53] 2014
Goat	Green tea	2, 3, or 4 g TC/kg DM feed	60 d	Low risk	Reduced plasma glutathione most efficaciously at 2 g dosage; over 3 g dosage reduced plasma protein and globulins (bad)	Zhong et al,[54] 2011
Goat	Green tea	2.0% on weight:weight ratio	90 d	Low risk, castrated male goats	Linear increase average weight gain and feed intake, increased splenic cell growth, reduced intramuscular TBARS	Ahmed et al,[55] 2015

Abbreviations: ADG, average daily gain; APP, acute-phase proteins; BHBA, beta-hydroxybutyric acid; DIM, days in milk; DM, dry matter; DMI, dry matter intake; ECM, energy-corrected milk; EO, essential oil; FCM, fat corrected milk; FFA, free fatty acids; MDA, malondialdehyde; MR, milk replacer; NEFA, nonesterified fatty acid; ROS, reactive oxygen species; SAA, serum amyloid A; SCC, somatic cell count; SOD, superoxide dismutase; TAG, triacylglycerol; TBARS, thiobarbituric acid reactive substances.

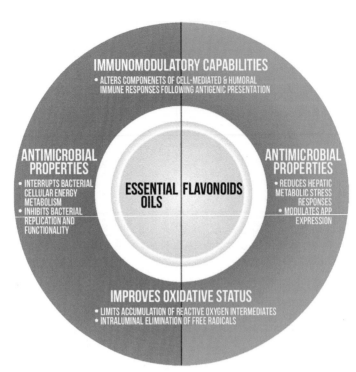

Fig. 2. Mechanisms of action of phytonutrients on immune defenses.

dietary vitamin E bioavailability, suggesting a potential mechanism for antioxidants to improve health.[41]

Green tea leaf extracts, particularly catechins, represent another rich source of phenolic compounds with antioxidant potential. Tea polyphenols reduced accumulations of reactive oxygen intermediates in bovine mammary epithelial cells following a hydrogen peroxide challenge in vivo.[47] Green tea polyphenols also seem to modulate acute-phase protein expression upon parasitic challenge in small ruminant species.[53] Reduced hepatic metabolic stress, coupled with decreased intrahepatic lipid concentrations and acute-phase protein expression, may indicate improved energy status, ultimately leading to improved ruminant health and performance.[51]

Essential oils represent another class of phytonutrients with potential antimicrobial and immunomodulatory capabilities. Essential oils (EOs) provide a plant with its unique color and fragrance. Chemically, EOs are composed of a lipophilic mixture of terpenoids, phenolics, and a variety of low-molecular-weight compounds.[1,95] The antibacterial mode of action of volatile oils is likely multifactorial with hypothesized mechanisms including disruption of biochemical pathways associated with cell membranes and passage of low-molecular-weight EO derivatives across inner plasma membranes of both gram-positive and gram-negative bacteria. By interrupting cellular energy metabolism, EOs can partially inhibit bacterial growth and functionality and have demonstrated microbicidal effects against common food-borne pathogens, rumen bacteria, and gastrointestinal parasites (see **Fig. 2**).[1] Most of the immunologic effects of EOs were investigated in monogastric species. Receptor-mediated responses upon EO supplementation can result in improved mucosal blood flow, altered cytokine and neuropeptide release, and modified immune cell functionality. Volatile oils undergo significant ruminal biodegradation, likely limiting the immunomodulatory and antibacterial effects.[44] Of the published studies of EOs performed specifically on ruminants, oregano, garlic, and *Capsicum oleoresin* oils were shown have potential health and immunomodulatory effects.

Oregano (*Origanum onite* L) oil and its 2 main phenolic derivatives, carvacrol and thymol, offer a potential potent source of antimicrobial and antioxidant capabilities. Oregano oil increased hematologic variables in dairy calves including hemoglobin, packed cell volume, and mean corpuscular volume.[96] Initial experiments have demonstrated potential benefits of using oregano to minimize scours and improve health scores in neonatal ruminants.[38] Dairy calves supplemented with oregano water had increased fecal firmness, reduced *Enterobacteriaceae* shedding, and increased immunoglobulin concentrations.[36] However, adult dairy cattle supplemented with EO products containing either garlic, thyme, or oregano failed to cure experimentally induced *Streptococcus uberis* mastitis following either topical or intramammary administration.[43] Oregano supplementation also failed to reduce *Eimeria* oocyst shedding in dairy heifers.[37]

Garlic (*Allium sativum*) and garlic oils have the capacity to eliminate free radical species and reduce lipid peroxidation in vivo. The effects of garlic oil on immunologic variables in mature ruminants are inconclusive. However, Oh and colleagues[97] recently described the broad immuno-stimulatory effects of garlic oil following intra-abomasal infusion via an increased neutrophil to lymphocyte ratio as well as increased helper (CD4[+]) T-cell proliferation.

Capsaicinoids, bioactive compounds sourced from flowering *Capsicum* plants, demonstrated an ability to modulate the acute-phase response in dairy cows, including in response to an intravenous lipopolysaccharide (LPS) challenge.[3,98] Furthermore, postruminal supplementation of capsaicinoids increased CD4[+] T-cell proliferation.[97] By potentially affecting both the innate and adaptive branches of the immune system, capsaicinoid supplementation may be particularly beneficial during vaccination events.[99] However, more research is needed to validate observations using these EO-based compounds in ruminant species.

POLYUNSATURATED FATTY ACIDS

Dietary fat is more than just calories. The composition of fatty acids in fat sources can influence many cellular functions (**Table 3**). The fatty acid composition of cellular membranes reflects the fatty acid composition of the diet. The physical chemistry of the various fatty acids differs and increasing the incorporation of polyunsaturated fatty acids (PUFAs) can increase the membrane fluidity. Increasing the fluidity of leukocytes can disrupt the organization of cell surface receptors in the plasma membrane, and ultimately alter cellular function.[100–104]

In addition to influencing membrane fluidity, the fatty acid composition of cellular membranes can alter the biosynthesis of various lipid mediators (**Fig. 3**). The eicosanoid family are some of the most well-known bioactive lipid mediators and include prostaglandins, leukotrienes, and thromboxanes. The balance of omega-6 to omega-3 PUFA in cellular membranes influences the quantity and biological potency of the eicosanoids produced. Generally, eicosanoids from omega-3 PUFAs have a reduced affinity for cyclooxygenase enzymes. They also produce many eicosanoids that have a lower biological activity than those produced from omega-6 PUFAs. This led to the concept that omega-3 PUFAs have a greater anti-inflammatory capacity than omega-6 PUFAs.

Preweaned calves fed milk replacer with either 1% or 2% of the total dry matter (DM) replaced as fish oil, which is rich in omega-3 PUFAs, reduced the

Table 3
Effects of polyunsaturated fatty acids on the immune function, health, and performance of calves, dairy cows, and feedlot steers

Animal	Strain/Type	Dose	Duration/Frequency	Health/Production Status	Outcome	Reference
Calf	Fish oil	1% and 2% DM of the milk replacer	42 d	High risk	Reduced inflammatory response to LPS challenge, quadratic effect on secondary antibody response, no effect on fecal scores	Ballou et al,[56] 2008; Ballou & DePeters,[57] 2008
Calf	Fish oil	2% of the DM	14–55 d of life	Low risk	No effect on serum haptoglobin or mitogen-induced IFN-γ secretion, no difference in fecal scores, fish oil decreased starter intake and ADG	McDonnell et al,[58] 2019
Calf	Coconut oil	Replaced 20 or 40% of the lard in milk replacer	56 d	Low risk	Quadratic decrease in fecal scores, no difference in starter intake or ADG	Bowen Yoho et al,[59] 2013
Calf	Linoleic acid	0.48% or 9.0% of the fatty acids in milk replacer as linoleic acid	30 d	Low risk	Caused differential expression of many immune-related hepatic genes	Garcia et al,[60] 2016
Calf	Blend of short- and medium-chain fatty acids and α-linolenic acid	0.46%, 0.51%, 0.19%, and 0.18% of DM as butyric, lauric, myristic, and linolenic acids, respectively, in milk replacer	56 d	Low risk	No difference in fecal score or medication, improved DM digestion and ADG	Hill et al,[61] 2016

Dairy cow	Ca salts of palm oil, safflower oil, or fish oil	n-6 to n-3 ratios of 4, 5, or 6 14 d postpartum to 105 d postpartum	Early lactation	Lower n-6 to n-3 decreased plasma IL-6 and haptoglobin concentrations after a moderate intramammary LPS challenge, no effect on neutrophil phagocytosis or oxidative burst, greater DMI and 3.5% FCM in the n-6 to n-3 ratio of 4	Greco et al,[62] 2015
Dairy cow	Whole flaxseed	10.4% of DM	Calving to 105 DIM	Early lactation	Transient reduction in mitogen proliferation of PBMC, no effect on humoral response, decreased prostaglandin E_2	Lessard et al,[63] 2003
Transition dairy cow	Fish oil	250 g prepartum and 0.92% DM postpartum	3 wk prepartum until 10 d postpartum	Apparently healthy, multiparous Holstein cows	No effect on inflammatory response to a high dose of LPS intramammary, no difference in DMI or milk production	Ballou et al,[64] 2009
Transition dairy cow	Ca salts of palm oil, safflower oil, or fish oil	1.5% of DM	Safflower oil from 30 d prepartum to 35 d postpartum; fish oil 35–160 d postpartum	Apparently healthy, multiparous Holstein cows	Safflower oil increased plasma acute-phase proteins, neutrophil proinflammatory cytokines, neutrophil L-selectin, and neutrophil phagocytic and oxidative burst activities, fish oil decreased neutrophil proinflammatory cytokine	Silvestre et al,[65] 2011

Abbreviations: DIM, days in milk; DM, dry matter; n-3, omega-3 polyunsaturated fatty acids; n-6, omega-6 polyunsaturated fatty acid; PBMC, peripheral blood mononuclear cell.

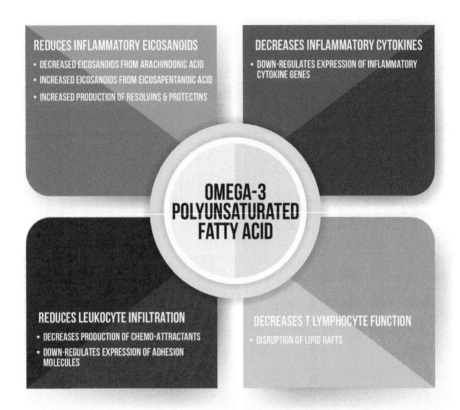

Fig. 3. Mechanisms of action of omega-3 long-chain polyunsaturated fatty acids.

proinflammatory response when challenged with a large dose of LPS to mimic sepsis.[56] In a recent study replacing 2% of the total DM with fish oil fed to preweaned calves did not reduce the serum haptoglobin concentrations or mitogen-induced interferon-γ secretion.[58] In contrast, Garcia and colleagues[60] supplemented preweaned calves with either a low or high omega-6 linoleic acid milk replacer (0.46% or 9.0% of the total fatty acids, respectively) and reported that the high linoleic acid treatment had many differentially expressed genes in the liver that should predict a reduced risk of infection. The linoleic fatty acid compositions used in the study of Garcia and colleagues likely reflect milk diets based on milk fat (low linoleic acid) and those in which the primary fat source is based on lard (high linoleic acid). The exact PUFA composition or balance of omega-6 to omega-3 PUFAs in milk solids that improves immune responses and overall health remains to be determined. Finally, although short-chain fatty acids are not PUFAs it is important to emphasize their importance in GIT development as we discussed previously in the section on probiotics. Supplementing short-chain fatty acids such as butyrate can improve GIT development and calf performance.[61] Furthermore, the effect may be more pronounced in milk replacer diets in which the primary fat source is not milk fat. Milk fat already contains a significant quantity of butyrate; however, the exact concentrations of these short-chain fatty acids to supplement in milk replacer are not known.[59,61]

Supplementing omega-3 PUFAs and altering the omega-6 to omega-3 PUFA ratio to transition and early lactating cows was investigated as a strategy to improve health and production performance. Feeding whole flaxseed as a source of the omega-3 PUFA, specifically α-linolenic acid, from calving until 105 days in milk (DIM) decreased the serum concentrations of the proinflammatory eicosanoid, prostaglandin E_2.[63] Furthermore, decreasing the omega-6 to omega-3 PUFA ratio using calcium salts of fish oil from 14 to 105 DIM decreased the proinflammatory response following a mild intramammary LPS challenge.[62] In contrast, there was no difference in the proinflammatory response in cows when challenged with 10 times the dose of LPS in the mammary gland at 7 DIM whether they were supplemented with fish oil or not.[64] The authors attributed the lack of an effect on the severity of the LPS challenge. Silvestre and colleagues[65] supplemented 1.5% of the total DM as safflower oil as a source of omega-6 PUFA from 30 d prepartum to 35 DIM. Observations included increased plasma acute-phase proteins, neutrophil proinflammatory cytokines, neutrophil L-selectin, and neutrophil phagocytic and oxidative burst capacities during the periparturient period. Furthermore, cows were switched to a breeding diet at 35 DIM that contained 1.5% of the total DM as calcium salts of fish oil and fed through 160 DIM. Supplementing cows with the calcium salts of fish oil decreased neutrophil proinflammatory cytokine secretion. These data further support that the balance of omega-6 to omega-3 PUFAs in the diets of both calves and cows can influence various immune responses. However, it remains to be determined at what age, physiologic stage, and conditions more inflammation is desirable and vice versa when less inflammation is preferred.[105,106]

SUMMARY

Nutraceuticals represent a group of compounds that may help fill that void because they exert some health benefits when supplemented to livestock. There remains significant ambiguity regarding nutraceuticals because this field is evolving at a rapid pace without regulatory oversight. In this review, we broadly classify and discuss nutraceuticals as either probiotics, prebiotics, phytonutrients, or PUFAs. These compounds work through various mechanisms of action including stabilizing commensal microbial communities, improving mucosal immune responses and barrier function, binding or adsorbing potential pathogens or toxins, improving antioxidant capacity, direct antimicrobial activity, and increasing or decreasing systemic immune responses.

REFERENCES

1. Benchaar C, Calsamiglia S, Chaves A, et al. A review of plant-derived essential oils in ruminant nutrition and production. Anim Feed Sci Technol 2008;145(1–4): 209–28.

2. Braun H, Schrapers K, Mahlkow-Nerge K, et al. Dietary supplementation of essential oils in dairy cows: evidence for stimulatory effects on nutrient absorption. Animal 2019;13(3):518–23.

3. Oh J, Wall E, Bravo D, et al. Host-mediated effects of phytonutrients in ruminants: a review. J Dairy Sci 2017;100(7):5974–83.

4. Timmerman HM, Mulder L, Everts H, et al. Health and growth of veal calves fed milk replacers with or without probiotics. J Dairy Sci 2005;88(6):2154–65.

5. Mokhber-Dezfouli MR, Tajik P, Bolourchi M, et al. Effects of probiotics supplementation in daily milk intake of newborn calves on body weight gain, body height, diarrhea occurrence and health condition. Pak J Biol Sci 2007;10(18): 3136–40.

6. Al-Saiady MY. Effect of probiotic bacteria on immunoglobulin G concentration and other blood components of newborn calves. J Anim Vet Adv 2010;9(3): 604–9.

7. Signorini ML, Soto LP, Zbrun, et al. Impact of probiotic administration on the health and fecal microbiota of young calves: a meta-analysis of randomized controlled trials of lactic acid bacteria. Res Vet Sci 2012;93(1):250–8.

8. Liang Y, Hudson RE, Ballou MA. Supplementing neonatal Jersey calves with a blend of probiotic bacteria improves the pathophysiological response to an oral *Salmonella enterica challenge*. Jacobs Journal of Veterinary Science and Research 2019;6(3):050.

9. Tkalcic S, Zhao T, Harmon B, et al. Fecal shedding of enterohemorrhagic *Escherichia coli* in weaned calves following treatment with probiotic *Escherichia coli*. J Food Prot 2003;66(7):1184–9.

10. Davis EM. Impacts of various milk replacer supplements on the health and performance of high-risk dairy calves. Master's thesis. Lubbuck (TX): Texas Tech University; 2018.

11. Agarwal N, Kamra D, Chaudhary L, et al. Microbial status and rumen enzyme profile of crossbred calves fed on different microbial feed additives. Lett Appl Microbiol 2002;34:329–36.

12. Galvao KN, Santos JEP, Coscioni A, et al. Effect of feeding live yeast products to calves with failure of passive transfer on performance and patterns of antibiotic resistance in fecal *Escherichia coli*. Reprod Nutr Dev 2005;44(6):427–40.

13. Eicher SD, Wesley IV, Sharma VK, et al. Yeast cell-wall products containing β-glucan plus ascorbic acid affect neonatal *Bos taurus* calf leukocytes and growth after a transport stressor. J Anim Sci 2010;88(3):1195–203.

14. Kara C, Cihan H, Temizel M, et al. Effect of supplemental mannanoligosaccharides on growth performance, faecal characteristics, and health in dairy calves. Asian-Australas J Anim Sci 2015;28(11):1599–605.

15. Ghosh S, Mehla RK. Influence of dietary supplementation of prebiotics (mannanoligosaccharide) on the performance of crossbred calves. Trop Anim Health Prod 2012;44(3):617–22.

16. Heinrichs AJ, Jones CM, Heinrichs BS. Effects of mannan oligosaccharides or antibiotics in neonatal diets on health and growth of dairy calves. J Dairy Sci 2003;86(12):4064–9.

17. Hill TM, Bateman HG, Aldrich JM, et al. Oligosaccharides for dairy calves. Professional Animal Scientist 2008;24(5):460–4.

18. Grand E, Respondek F, Martineau C, et al. Effects of short-chain fructooligosaccharides on growth and performance of preruminant veal calves. J Dairy Sci 2013;96(2):1094–101.

19. Castro J, Gomez A, White B, et al. Changes in the intestinal bacterial community, short-chain fatty acid profile, and intestinal development of preweaned Holstein calves. 1. Effects of prebiotic supplementation depend on site and age. J Dairy Sci 2016;99(12):9682–702.

20. Xu H, Huang W, Hou Q, et al. The effect of probiotics administration on the milk production, milk components, and fecal bacteria microbiota of dairy cows. Sci Bull (Beijing) 2017;62(11):767–74.

21. Shreedhar JN, Patil M, Kumar P. Effect of probiotics supplementation on milk yield and its composition in lactating Holstein Fresien and Deoni cross bred cows. J Med Bioeng 2016;5(1):19–23.

22. Musa A, Pandey N, Pandy R. Effects of feeding sodium bicarbonate and multi-strain probiotics on milk yield and milk composition of lactating Holstein Frisian crossbred cows. J Pharmacogn Phytochem 2017;6(6):1912–6.

23. Vibhute V, Shelke R, Chavan S, et al. Effect of probiotics supplementation on the performance of lactating crossbred cows. Vet World 2011;4(12):557–61.

24. Rossow H, DeGroff D, Parsons M. Performance of dairy cows administered probiotic in water troughs. Professional Animal Scientist 2014;30(5):527–33.

25. Rossow H, Riordan T, Riordan A. Effects of addition of a live yeast product on dairy cattle performance. J Appl Anim Res 2018;46(1):159–63.

26. Maamouri O, Selmi H, M'hamdi N. Effects of yeast (*Saccharomyces cerevisiae*) feed supplement on milk production and its composition in Tunisian Holstein Fresian cows. Scientia Agriculturae Bohemica 2014;45(3):170–4.

27. Dailidaviciene J, Budreckiene R, Gruzauskas R, et al. The influence of probiotic additives or multienzyme composition on blood biochemical parameters and milk quality of Lithuanian Black-and-White cattle. Arq Bras Med Vet Zootec 2018;70(3):939–45.

28. Yasuda K, Hashikawa S, Sakamoto H, et al. New synbiotic consisting of *Lactobacillus casei* subsp. *casei* and dextran improves milk production in Holstein dairy cows. J Vet Med Sci 2007;69(2):205–8.

29. Sretenovic Lj, Petrovic M, Aleksic S, et al. Influence of yeast, probiotics and enzymes in rations on dairy cow performances during transition. Biotechnology in Animal Husbandry 2008;24(5-6):33–43.

30. Peterson R, Klopfenstein T, Erickson G, et al. Effect of *Lactobacillus acidophilus* strain NP51 on *Escherichia coli* O157:H7 fecal shedding and finishing performance in beef feedlot cattle. Journal of Food Protection 2007;70(2):287–91.

31. Schamberger G, Phillips R, Jacobs J, et al. Reduction of *Escherichia coli* and O157:H7 populations in cattle by addition of Colicin E7-Producing *E. coli* to feed. Appl Environ Microbiol 2004;70(10):6053–60.

32. Tabe E, Oloya J, Doetkott D, et al. Comparative effect of direct-fed microbials on fecal shedding of *Escherichia coli* O157:H7 and *Salmonella* in naturally infected feedlot cattle. J Food Prot 2008;71(3):539–44.

33. Younts-Dahl S, Osborn G, Galyean M, et al. Reduction of *Escherichia coli* O157 in finishing beef cattle by various doses of *Lactobacillus acidophilus* in direct-fed microbials. J Food Prot 2005;68(1):6–10.

34. Brashears M, Galyean M, Loneragan G, et al. Prevalence of *Escherichia coli* O157:H7 and performance by beef feedlot cattle given *Lactobacillus* direct-fed microbials. J Food Prot 2003;66(5):748–54.

35. Jin L, Dong G, Lei G, et al. Effects of dietary supplementation of glutamine and mannan oligosaccharides on plasma endotoxin and acute phase protein concentrations and nutrient digestibility in finishing steers. J Appl Anim Res 2014; 42(2):160–5.

36. Ozkaya S, Erbas S, Ozkan O, et al. Effect of supplementing milk replacer with aromatic oregano (*Oreganum onites* L.) water on performance, immunity and general health profiles of Holstein calves. Anim Prod Sci 2018;58(10):1892–900.

37. Grandi G, Kramer L, Quarantelli A, et al. Influence of oregano essential oil (OEO) on prevalence and oocyst shedding dynamics of naturally acquired *Eimeria* spp. infection in replacement dairy heifers. Ann Anim Sci 2016;16(1):171–9.

38. Katsoulos PD, Karatzia M, Dovas C, et al. Evaluation of the in-field efficacy of oregano essential oil administration on the control of neonatal diarrhea syndrome in calves. Res Vet Sci 2017;115:478–83.

39. Soltan M. Effect of essential oils supplementation on growth performance, nutrient digestibility, health condition of Holstein male calves during pre- and post-weaning periods. Pak J Nutr 2009;8(5):642–52.

40. Oh J, Harper M, Bravo D, et al. Effects of rumen-protected *Capsicum oleoresin* on productivity and responses to a glucose tolerance test in lactating dairy cows. J Dairy Sci 2017;100(3):1888–901.

41. Shabtay A, Eitam H, Tadmor Y, et al. Nutritive and antioxidative potential of fresh and stored pomegranate industrial byproduct as a novel beef cattle feed. J Agric Food Chem 2008;56(21):10063–70.

42. Oliveira R, Narciso C, Bisinotto R, et al. Effects of feeding polyphenols from pomegranate extract on health, growth, nutrient digestion, and immunocompetence of calves. J Dairy Sci 2010;93(9):4280–91.

43. Mullen K, Lyman R, Washburn S, et al. Effect of 3 phytoceutical products on elimination of bacteria in experimentally induced *Streptococcus uberis* clinical mastitis. J Dairy Sci 2018;101(11):10409–13.

44. Oh J, Bravo D, Wall E, et al. Rumen disappearance of capsaicin and dihydro-capsaicin in lactating dairy cows. J Anim Sci 2016;94(5):801.

45. Nielsen B, Hansen H. Effect of grape pomace rich in flavonoids and antioxidants on production parameters in dairy production. J Anim Feed Sci 2004;13(1):535–8.

46. Colitti M, Stefanon B. Effect of natural antioxidants on superoxide dismutase and glutathione peroxidase mRNA expression in leukocytes from periparturient dairy cows. Vet Res Commun 2006;30(1):19–27.

47. Ma Y, Zhao L, Gao M, et al. Tea polyphenols protect bovine mammary epithelial cells from hydrogen peroxide-induced oxidative damage in vitro by activating NFE2L2/HMOX1 pathways. J Dairy Sci 2018;102(2):1658–70.

48. Hashemzadeh-Cigari F, Ghorbani G, Khorvash M, et al. Supplementation of herbal plants differently modulated metabolic profile, insulin sensitivity, and oxidative stress in transition dairy cows fed various extruded oil seeds. Prev Vet Med 2015;118(1):45–55.

49. Safari M, Ghasemi E, Alikhani M, et al. Supplementation effects of pomegranate by-products on oxidative status, metabolic profile, and performance in transition dairy cows. J Dairy Sci 2018;101(12):11297–309.

50. Gessner D, Koch C, Romberg F, et al. The effect of grape seed and grape marc meal extract on milk performance and the expression of genes of endoplasmic reticulum stress and inflammation in the liver of dairy cows in early lactation. J Dairy Sci 2015;98(12):8856–68.

51. Winkler A, Gessner D, Koch C, et al. Effects of a plant product consisting of green tea and curcuma extract on milk production and the expression of hepatic genes involved in endoplasmic stress response and inflammation in dairy cows. Arch Anim Nutr 2015;69(6):425–41.

52. Gladine C, Rock E, Morand C, et al. Bioavailability and antioxidant capacity of plant extracts rich in polyphenols, given as a single acute dose, in sheep made highly susceptible to lipoperoxidation. Br J Nutr 2007;98(4):691–701.

53. Zhong RZ, Li H, Sun H, et al. Effects of supplementation with dietary green tea polyphenols on parasite resistance and acute phase protein response to *Haemonchus contortus* infection in lambs. Vet Parasitol 2014;205(1–2):199–207.

54. Zhong R, Xiao W, Ren G, et al. Dietary tea catechin inclusion changes plasma biochemical parameters, hormone concentrations and glutathione redox status in goats. Asian-Australas J Anim Sci 2011;24(12):1681–9.

55. Ahmed S, Lee J, Mun H, et al. Effects of supplementation with green tea by-products on growth performance, meat quality, blood metabolites and immune cell proliferation in goats. J Anim Physiol Anim Nutr 2015;99(6):1127–37.

56. Ballou M, Cruz G, Pittroff W, et al. Modifying the acute phase response of Jersey calves by supplementing milk replacer with omega-3 fatty acids from fish oil. J Dairy Sci 2008;91(9):3478–87.

57. Ballou MA, DePeters EJ. Supplementing milk replacer with omega-3 fatty acids from fish oil on immunocompetence and health of Jersey calves. J Dairy Sci 2008;91(9):3488–500.

58. McDonnell R, O'Doherty J, Earley B, et al. Effect of supplementation with n-3 polyunsaturated fatty acids and/or β-glucans on performance, feeding behavior and immune status of Holstein Friesian bull calves during the pre- and post-weaning periods. J Anim Sci Biotechnol 2019;10(7):1–17.

59. Bowen Yoho W, Swank V, Eastridge M, et al. Jersey calf performance in response to high-protein, high-fat liquid feeds with varied fatty acid profiles: intake and performance. J Dairy Sci 2013;96(4):2494–506.

60. Garcia M, Greco L, Lock A, et al. Supplementation of essential fatty acids to Holstein calves during late uterine life and first month of life alters hepatic fatty acid profile and gene expression. J Dairy Sci 2016;99(9):7085–101.

61. Hill T, Quigley J, Suarez-Mena F, et al. Effect of milk replacer feeding rate and functional fatty acids on dairy calf performance and digestion of nutrients. J Dairy Sci 2016;99(8):6352–61.

62. Greco L, Neves Neto J, Pedrico, et al. Effects of altering the ratio of dietary n-6 to n-3 fatty acids on performance and inflammatory responses to a lipopolysaccharide challenge in lactating Holstein cows. J Dairy Sci 2015;98(1):602–17.

63. Lessard M, Gagnon N, Petit H. Immune response of postpartum dairy cows fed flaxseed. J Dairy Sci 2003;86(8):2647–57.

64. Ballou MA, Gomes R, Juchem S, et al. Effects of dietary supplemental fish oil during the peripartum period on blood metabolites and hepatic fatty acid compositions and total triacylglycerol concentrations of multiparous Holstein cows. J Dairy Sci 2009;92(2):657–69.

65. Silvestre F, Carvalho T, Francisco N, et al. Effects of differential supplementation of fatty acids during the peripartum and breeding periods of Holstein cows: I. Uterine and metabolic responses, reproduction, and lactation. J Dairy Sci 2011;94(1):189–204.

66. Isolauri E, Sutas Y, Kankaanpaa P, et al. Probiotics: effects on immunity. Am J Clin Nutr 2001;73:444–50.

67. Gaggia F, Mattarelli P, Biavati B. Probiotics and prebiotics in animal feeding for safe food production. Int J Food Microbiol 2010;141:S15–28.

68. Meale SJ, Chaucheyras-Durand F, Berends H, et al. From pre- to postweaning: transformation of the young calf's gastrointestinal tract. J Dairy Sci 2017;100(7):5984–95.

69. Frizzo LS, Soto LP, Zbrun MV, et al. Lactic acid bacteria to improve growth performance in young calves fed milk replacer and spray-dried whey powder. Anim Feed Sci Technol 2010;157(3–4):159–67.

70. Jung C, Hugot J, Barreau F. Peyer's patches: the immune sensors of the intestine. Int J Inflamm 2010;2010:1–12.

71. Bocker U, Nebe T, Herweck F, et al. Butyrate modulates intestinal epithelial cell-mediated neutrophil migration. Clin Exp Immunol 2003;131(53):53–60.

72. Peng L, Li Z, Green R, et al. Butyrate enhances the intestinal barrier by facilitating tight junction assembly via activation of AMP-activated protein kinase in Caco-2 cell monolayers. J Nutr 2009;139:1619–25.

73. Knudsen K, Lerke H, Hedemann, et al. Impact of diet-modulated butyrate production on intestinal barrier function and inflammation. Nutrients 2018;10:1–19.

74. Gorka P, Kowalskim Z, Zabielski R, et al. Invited Review. Use of butyrate to promote gastrointestinal tract development in calves. J Dairy Sci 2018;101(6): 4785–800.

75. Rice E, Aragona K, Moreland S, et al. Supplementation of sodium butyrate to postweaned heifer diets: effects on growth performance, nutrient digestibility, and health. J Dairy Sci 2019;102(4):3121–30.

76. Rainard P, Foucras G. A critical appraisal of probiotics for mastitis control. Front Vet Sci 2018;5:1–13.

77. Beecher C, Daly M, Berry D, et al. Administration of a live culture of *Lactococcus lactis* DPC 3147 into the bovine mammary gland stimulates the local host immune response, particularly IL-1 and IL-8 gene expression. J Dairy Res 2009; 76:340–8.

78. Newbold CJ, Wallace RJ, Chen XB, et al. Different strains of *Saccharomyces cerevisiae* differ in their effects on ruminal bacterial numbers in vitro and in sheep. J Anim Sci 1995;73(6):1811–8.

79. Chaucheyras-Durand F, Fonty G. Establishment of cellulolytic bacteria and development of fermentative activities in the rumen of gnotobiotically reared lambs receiving the microbial additive *Saccharomyces cerevisiae* CNCM I1077. Reprod Nutr Dev 2001;41(1):57–68.

80. Mosoni P, Chaucheyras-Durand F, Bera-Maillet C, et al. Quantification by real-time PCR of cellulolytic bacteria in the rumen of sheep after supplementation of a forage diet with readily fermentable carbohydrates: effect of a yeast additive. J Appl Microbiol 2007;103(6):2676–85.

81. Silberberg M, Chaucheyras-Durand F, Commun L, et al. Repeated acidosis challenges and live yeast supplementation shape rumen microbiota and fermentations and modulate inflammatory status in sheep. Animal 2013;7(12): 1910–20.

82. Arik H, Gulsen N, Hayirli A, et al. Efficacy of *Megasphaera elsdenii* inoculation in subacute ruminal acidosis in cattle. J Anim Physiol Anim Nutr 2018;103(2):416–26.

83. Liu F, Li P, Chen Y, et al. Fructooligosaccharide (FOS) and galactooligosaccharides (GOS) increase *Bifidobacterium* but reduce butyrate producing bacteria with adverse glycemic metabolism in heathy young population. Sci Rep 2017; 11. https://doi.org/10.1038/s41598-017-10722-2.

84. Ganner A, Stoiber C, Uhlik JT, et al. Quantitative evaluation of *E. coli* F4 and *Salmonella typhimurium* binding capacity of yeast derivatives. AMB Express 2013; 3(1):1–12.

85. Taylor PR, Brown GD, Reid DM, et al. The beta-glucan receptor, dectin-1, is predominantly expressed on the surface of cells of the monocyte/macrophage and neutrophil lineages. J Immunol 2002;169(7):3876–82.

86. Gantner BN, Simmons RM, Underhill DM. Dectin-1 mediates macrophage recognition of *Candida albicans* yeast but not filaments. EMBO J 2005;24(6): 1277–86.

87. Nocek J, Holt M, Oppy J. Effects of supplementation with yeast culture and enzymatically hydrolyzed yeast on performance of early lactation dairy cattle. J Dairy Sci 2011;94(8):4046–56.

88. Hall L, Rivera F, Villar F, et al. Evaluation of OmniGen-AF in lactating heat-stressed Holstein cows. 2014. Available at: http://dairy.ifas.ufl.edu/RNS/2014/collier.pdf. Accessed September 12, 2019.

89. Jouany J, Yiannikouris A, Bertin G. The chemical bonds between mycotoxins and cell wall components of *Saccharomyces cerevisiae* have been identified. Archiva Zootechnica 2005;8:26–50.

90. Pereyra C, Cavaglieri L, Chiacchiera S, et al. The corn influence on the adsorption levels of aflatoxin B1 and zearalenone by yeast cell wall. J Appl Microbiol 2013;114(3):655–62.

91. Fruhauf S, Schwartz H, Ottner F, et al. Yeast cell-based feed additives: studies on aflatoxin B1 and zearalenone. Food Addit Contam Part A Chem Anal Control Expo Risk Assess 2012;29(2):217–31.

92. Gessner D, Ringseis R, Eder K. Potential of plant polyphenols to combat oxidative stress and inflammatory processes in farm animals. J Anim Physiol Anim Nutr 2017;101(4):605–28.

93. Kalantar M. The importance of flavonoids in ruminant nutrition. Archives of Animal Husbandry & Dairy Science 2018;1(1). AAHDS.MS.ID.000504.

94. Stover MG, Watson RR. Polyphenols in foods and dietary supplements: role in veterinary medicine and animal health. In: Watson RR, Preedy VR, Zibadi S, editors. Polyphenols in human health and disease. New York: Elsevier; 2014. p. 3–7.

95. Yang W, Benchaar C, Ametaj B, et al. Effects of garlic and juniper berry essential oils on ruminal fermentation and on the site and extent of digestion in lactating cows. J Dairy Sci 2007;90(12):5671–81.

96. Seirafy H, Sobhanirad S. Effects of oregano (*Origanum vulgare*) and thyme (*Thymus vulgaris*) oils on growth performance and blood parameters in Holstein suckling calves. Iran J Appl Anim Sci 2017;7(4):585–93.

97. Oh J, Hristov A, Lee C, et al. Immune and production responses of dairy cows to postruminal supplementation with phytonutrients. J Dairy Sci 2013;96(12):7830–43.

98. Oh J, Giallongo F, Frederick T, et al. Effects of dietary *Capsicum oleoresin* on productivity and immune responses in lactating dairy cows. J Dairy Sci 2015;98(9):6327–39.

99. Lee S, Lillehoj H, Jang S, et al. Effects of dietary supplementation with phytonutrients on vaccine-stimulated immunity against infection with *Eimeria tenella*. Vet Parasitol 2011;181(2):97–105.

100. Leroy J, Sturmey R, Hoeck V, et al. Dietary lipid supplementation on cow reproductive performance and oocyte and embryo viability: a real benefit? Anim Reprod 2013;10(3):258–67.

101. Sun Y, Bu D, Wang J, et al. Supplementing different ratios of short- and medium-chain fatty acids to long-chain fatty acids in dairy cows: changes in milk fat production and milk fatty acids composition. J Dairy Sci 2013;96(4):2366–73.

102. Welter K, Martins C, Vizeu de Palma A, et al. Canola oil in lactating dairy cow diets reduces milk saturated fatty acids and improves its omega-3 and oleic fatty acid content. PLoS One 2016;11(3):1–16.

103. Yang X, Sheng W, Sun G, et al. Effects of fatty acid unsaturation numbers on membrane fluidity and alpha-secretase-dependent amyloid precursor protein processing. Neurochem Int 2010;58(3):321–9.

104. Simons K, Sampaio J. Membrane organization and lipid rafts. Cold Spring Harb Perspect Biol 2011;3(10):1–17.

105. Ballou MA. Growth and Development Symposium: inflammation: role in the etiology and pathophysiology of clinical mastitis in dairy cows. J Anim Sci 2012; 90(5):1466–78.
106. Bradford B, Yuan K, Farney J, et al. Invited Review. Inflammation during the transition to lactation: new adventures with an old flame. J Dairy Sci 2015;98(10): 6631–50.

Colostrum Management for Dairy Calves

Sandra M. Godden, DVM, DVSc[a],*, Jason E. Lombard, DVM, MS[b],
Amelia R. Woolums, DVM, MVSc, PhD[c]

KEYWORDS

- Calf • Colostrum management • Passive immunity • Monitoring

KEY POINTS

- Colostrum management is the single most important management factor in determining calf health and survival.
- Although good progress has been made in the past 20 years, there remains a considerable opportunity for many dairy producers to improve their colostrum management practices, resulting in improved short-term and long-term health and performance of the animals.
- Producers should provide calves with a sufficient volume of clean, high-quality colostrum within the first few hours of life.

INTRODUCTION

The syndesmochorial placenta of the cow separates the maternal and fetal blood supplies, preventing in utero transmission of protective immunoglobulins (Ig) (**Fig. 1**).[1] Consequently, the calf is born agammaglobulinemic and so is almost entirely dependent on the absorption of maternal Ig from colostrum after birth. Achieving early and adequate intake of high-quality colostrum is widely recognized as the single most important management factor in determining the health and survival of neonatal calves.[2–4] The absorption of maternal Ig across the small intestine during the first 24 hours after birth, termed passive transfer, helps to protect the calf against common disease organisms until its own immature immune system becomes functional. In addition to reduced risk for preweaning morbidity and mortality, additional long-term benefits associated with successful passive transfer include reduced mortality in the postweaning period, improved rate of gain, reduced age at first calving,

Disclosures: None.
[a] Department of Veterinary Population Medicine, College of Veterinary Medicine, University of Minnesota, 225 VMC, 1365 Gortner Avenue, St Paul, MN 55108, USA; [b] National Animal Health Monitoring System (NAHMS), USDA:APHIS:VS:CEAH, 2150 Centre Avenue, Building B-2E7, Fort Collins, CO 80526, USA; [c] Department of Pathobiology and Population Medicine, College of Veterinary Medicine, Mississippi State University, Mississippi State, MS 39762, USA
* Corresponding author.
E-mail address: godde002@umn.edu

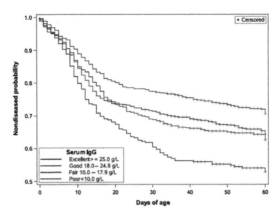

Fig. 1. Nondiseased probability for preweaned heifer calves by days of age and serum IgG concentration categories. Corresponding with serum IgG levels of greater than or equal to 25.0 g/L, 18.0 to 24.9 g/L, 10 to 17.9 g/L, and less than 10.0 g/L were serum total protein categories of greater than or equal to 6.2 g/dL, 5.8 to 6.1 g/dL, 5.1 to 5.7 g/dL, and less than 5.1 g/dL, and Brix score categories of greater than or equal to 9.4%, 8.9% to 9.3%, 8.1% to 8.8%, and less than 8.1%, respectively.[131]

improved first and second lactation milk production, and reduced tendency for culling during the first lactation.[5–8] Benefits from colostrum may be attributed to protective Ig as well as high levels of nutrients and bioactive compounds that stimulate postnatal growth and development.[9]

Calves have historically been defined as having failure of passive transfer (FPT) if the serum IgG concentration is less than 10 g/L when sampled between 24 and 48 hours of age, based on increased mortality risk below this threshold.[10–12] However, this definition of FPT needs to be reevaluated, given that recent studies have described reduced morbidity in calves to be associated with incrementally higher serum IgG levels (**Fig. 1**).[4,12,13] Although the US dairy industry has shown steady improvement in colostrum and calf management over the past few decades, a recent national dairy study reported FPT to affect 15.6% of calves tested,[14] indicating a need for continued efforts to improve colostrum management. This article reviews the process of colostrogenesis and colostrum composition, and discusses the key components of developing a successful colostrum management program. In addition, it discusses methods for monitoring and presents new goals for passive immunity in dairy herds.

COLOSTROGENESIS AND COLOSTRUM COMPOSITION

Bovine colostrum consists of a mixture of lacteal secretions and constituents of blood serum, most notably Ig and other serum proteins, which accumulate in the mammary gland during the prepartum dry period.[15] This process begins several weeks before calving, under the influence of lactogenic hormones including prolactin, and ceases abruptly at parturition. Important constituents of colostrum include Ig, leukocytes, growth factors, hormones, nonspecific antimicrobial factors, and nutrients. Concentrations of many of these components are greatest in the first secretions harvested after calving (first milking colostrum), then decline steadily over the next 6 milkings (transition milk) to reach the lower concentrations routinely measured in saleable whole milk (**Table 1**).[15]

Table 1
Composition of colostrum, transition milk, and whole milk of Holstein cows

Parameter	Colostrum 1	Transition Milk (Milking Postpartum) 2	3	Milk
Specific gravity	1.056	1.040	1.035	1.032
Total solids (%)	23.9	17.9	14.1	12.9
Fat (%)	6.7	5.4	3.9	4.0
Total protein (%)	14.0	8.4	5.1	3.1
Casein (%)	4.8	4.3	3.8	2.5
Albumin (%)	6.0	4.2	2.4	0.5
Immunoglobulins (%)	6.0	4.2	2.4	0.09
IgG (g/100 mL)	3.2	2.5	1.5	0.06
Lactose (%)	2.7	3.9	4.4	5.0
IgGF-I (μg/L)[9]	341	242	144	15
Insulin (μg/L)[9]	65.9	34.8	15.8	1.1
Ash (%)	1.11	0.95	0.87	0.74
Calcium (%)	0.26	0.15	0.15	0.13
Magnesium (%)	0.04	0.01	0.01	0.01
Potassium (%)	0.14	0.13	0.14	0.15
Sodium (%)	0.07	0.05	0.05	0.04
Chloride (%)	0.12	0.1	0.1	0.07
Zinc (mg/100 mL)	1.22	—	0.62	0.3
Manganese (mg/100 mL)	0.02	—	0.01	0.004
Iron (mg/100 g)	0.20	—	—	0.05
Copper (mg/100 g)	0.06	—	—	0.01
Cobalt (μg/100 g)	0.5	—	—	0.10
Vitamin A (μg/100 mL)	295	190	113	34
Vitamin D (IU/g fat)	0.89–1.81	—	—	0.41
Vitamin E (μg/g fat)	84	76	56	15
Thiamine (μg/mL)	0.58	—	0.59	0.38
Riboflavin (μg/mL)	4.83	2.71	1.85	1.47
Biotin (μg/100 mL)	1.0–2.7	—	—	2.0
Vitamin B$_{12}$ (μg/100 mL)	4.9	—	2.5	0.6
Folic acid (μg/100 mL)	0.8	—	0.2	0.2
Choline (mg/mL)	0.7	0.34	0.23	0.13
Ascorbic acid (mg/100 mL)	2.5	—	2.3	2.2

Adapted from Foley, J.A. and D.E. Otterby. Availability, storage, treatment, composition, and feeding value of surplus colostrum: A review. J. Dairy Sci. 1978; 61:1033-1060; with permission and *data from* Hammon, H.M., I.A. Zanker, and J.W. Blum. Delayed colostrum feeding affects IGF-1 and insulin plasma concentrations in neonatal calves. J. Dairy Sci. 2000; 83:85-92.

Immunoglobulins

IgG, IgA, and IgM account for approximately 85% to 90%, 5%, and 7%, respectively, of the total Ig in colostrum, with IgG$_1$ accounting for 80% to 90% of the total IgG.[16]

Although levels are highly variable among cows, one study reported that mean colostral concentrations of IgG, IgA, and IgM were 75 g/L, 4.4 g/L, and 4.9 g/L, respectively.[17] IgG, and IgG$_1$ in particular, is transferred from the blood stream across the mammary barrier into colostrum by a specific transport mechanism; receptors on the mammary alveolar epithelial cells capture IgG$_1$ from the extracellular fluid, and the molecule undergoes endocytosis, transport, and eventually release into the luminal secretions.[16] The alveolar epithelial cells cease expressing this receptor, most likely in response to increasing prolactin concentrations, at the onset of lactation.[18] Smaller amounts of IgA and IgM are largely derived from local synthesis by plasmacytes in the mammary gland.[16] Although not well understood, colostral transfer of IgE also occurs and may be important in providing early protection against intestinal parasites.[19] After absorption into the calf's circulation, the duration of passive immunity from maternal Ig is highly variable and depends to a great extent on the total mass of Ig consumed and absorbed within the first 24 hours of life. The rate of decay of colostral antibodies can be influenced by multiple factors, including active viral infections or vaccination.[20–22]

Maternal Leukocytes

Fresh colostrum contains leukocytes of maternal origin; in cattle, macrophages and lymphocytes (mononuclear cells) make up the largest proportion of maternal colostral leukocytes.[23] Maternal colostral leukocytes enter the tissues of neonates following ingestion or enteral delivery in a variety of species, including rats, sheep, swine, and cattle,[24–26] and feeding colostrum containing maternal leukocytes has been associated with modified neonatal immune responses.[27–31] Blood mononuclear cells from calves fed colostrum containing maternal leukocytes developed the ability to activate cell-mediated immune responses by the time calves were 1 week of age, compared with 3 weeks of age for calves fed leukocyte-free colostrum.[27] Significant differences in percentage and degree of blood mononuclear cell activation were measured in calves receiving colostrum containing maternal leukocytes, compared with calves fed leukocyte-free maternal colostrum or frozen colostrum.[29–31] Both freezing[28] and heat treatment (Godden, unpublished, 2010) of colostrum kill most if not all colostral leukocytes. Blood mononuclear cells from 1-day-old calves fed colostrum containing maternal leukocytes were significantly more responsive to bovine viral diarrhea virus, compared with day-old calves that received frozen colostrum or leukocyte-free colostrum.[28] In contrast, there was no difference between treatment groups in the response to a mycobacterial antigen that the calves' dams had not encountered, suggesting that antigen-specific responses measured in a calf following ingestion of maternal colostral leukocytes are related to specific immune memory in the dam. In support of this, cell-mediated immune responses in piglets that nursed maternal colostrum containing leukocytes were significantly higher if their dams had been vaccinated against the tested antigen than if their dams had not been vaccinated.[32] Although research has not evaluated the degree of difference in responses induced by colostral leukocytes from a calf's own dam versus colostral leukocytes from another cow, cross-fostering experiments in piglets suggest that effects of colostral leukocytes on neonatal cell-mediated immunity are greatest when the colostrum contains leukocytes from the neonate's dam.[33]

Although multiple studies have confirmed that colostral leukocytes modify immune responses in calves in ways that seem relevant to protective immunity, to date research has not clearly shown an unequivocally beneficial effect of colostral leukocytes on practical outcomes such as calf respiratory or enteric morbidity, or induction of specific and measurable protective immunity following vaccination. Colostral leukocytes fed alone are not sufficient to protect calves from fatal disease in the neonatal period,[34] and recent studies comparing proportions of calves affected by naturally occurring diarrhea or respiratory disease after calves consume fresh maternal colostrum containing leukocytes, or frozen colostrum from their own dam[31] or other cows,[35] have shown small or variable differences in disease between the groups. Regarding the effect of colostral leukocytes on vaccine responses, Meganck and colleagues[36] evaluated humoral and cell-mediated responses to tetanus toxoid vaccination at 2, 5, or 10 days of age in calves fed pooled colostral whey with maternal leukocytes added, or calves fed only pooled colostral whey; this work suggested that colostral leukocytes influenced both tetanus toxoid–specific cell-mediated and humoral responses in calves, but the number of calves tested was small, and the effects measured varied substantially for calves vaccinated at 2, 5, or 10 days of age. Langel and colleagues[37] evaluated total (ie, not antigen-specific) monocyte and lymphocyte responses by measuring relative numbers and activation state of calf blood mononuclear cell subsets after routine calfhood vaccination; these investigators found significant differences between groups at certain time points over the months following vaccination. However, the clinical relevance of these differences for immunity against specific pathogens, or resistance to disease, was not defined. In summary, colostral leukocytes modify calf immune responses, and these effects may affect cow health and immunity months or years later. However, to date, effects of colostral leukocytes on practically important health outcomes have not been unequivocally identified, which may in part because it is logistically challenging and expensive to conduct research to measure effects of colostral leukocytes on calf immunity and health, so trials to date may not have included enough calves to provide adequate statistical power to identify small but important health differences.

Nutrients and Nonnutritive Factors

In addition to Ig for passive immunity, colostrum also contains high amounts of nutrients and nonnutritive biologically active factors that stimulate maturation and function of the neonatal gastrointestinal tract (GIT).[9] The total solids content (percentage) in first milking colostrum and whole milk in Holstein cows was reported to average 23.9% and 12.9%, respectively (see **Table 1**). Much of the increase in colostrum solids content is attributed to a more than 4-fold increase in protein content of colostrum versus milk, this being caused by significant increases in both Ig and casein content.[2] The crude fat content of first milking Holstein colostrum (6.7%) is also significantly higher than for milk (3.6%).[15] Energy from fat and lactose in colostrum is critical for thermogenesis and body temperature regulation. Certain vitamins and minerals, including calcium, magnesium, zinc, vitamin A, vitamin E, carotene, riboflavin, vitamin B12, folic acid, choline, and selenium, are also found in increased concentrations in bovine colostrum.[15,38]

Nonnutritive factors found in increased levels in colostrum include, but are not limited to, growth factors, hormones, cytokines, and nonspecific antimicrobial factors. Trypsin inhibitor, a compound found in colostrum in concentrations nearly 100 times greater than in milk, serves to protect Ig and other proteins from proteolytic degradation in the intestine of the neonatal calf. Bioactive components with antimicrobial activity include lactoferrin, lysozyme, and lactoperoxidase.[39–41] Oligosaccharides may provide protection against pathogens by acting as competitive inhibitors for the binding sites on the epithelial surfaces of the intestine.[38] It has also been suggested that certain oligosaccharides in colostrum may contribute to gut microbiome development by serving as a substrate to beneficial microorganisms such as *Bifidobacterium*, although this hypothesis requires further study.[42]

Growth factors in bovine colostrum include transforming growth factor beta-2, growth hormone, and insulin. Colostral insulinlike growth factor I and II may be key to regulating development of the GIT of bovine neonates, including stimulation of mucosal growth, brush-border enzymes, intestinal DNA synthesis, and increased villus size, resulting in enhanced absorptive capacity and glucose uptake.[9,43]

Another intriguing and potentially beneficial factor found in high levels in colostrum may be microRNAs (miRNAs). MiRNAs are short, noncoding RNA molecules that can regulate gene expression at the posttranscriptional level, and could represent one possible method of postnatal signaling from the mother to the neonate. Although studies are needed to describe their functional significance in calves, early research in other species suggests that, once absorbed by the neonate, MiRNAs from colostrum may be important in the differentiation and functional development of the intestinal epithelium,[44] and could also play an important role in the maturation of the neonate's immune system.[45]

These nutrients and nonnutritive factors, combined with benefits of disease protection from Ig, may contribute to the short-term and long-term benefits from improved colostrum intake, including improved rate of gain, reduced age at first calving, improved first and second lactation milk production, and reduced tendency for culling during the first lactation.[5–8] Further research is needed to investigate the concept of epigenetic programming or imprinting effects of colostrum on both short-term and long-term health and performance.[9]

COMPONENTS OF A SUCCESSFUL COLOSTRUM MANAGEMENT PROGRAM

To achieve successful passive transfer, calves must consume a sufficient mass of IgG in colostrum, and then successfully absorb a sufficient portion of IgG into their circulation. In order to achieve acceptable passive transfer (APT) in greater than or equal to 90% of calves fed, using the traditional definition of APT (serum IgG >10 g/L), it has been estimated that a minimum of 150 to 200 g of IgG needs to be delivered to the calf shortly after birth. In order to achieve the more ambitious goals for excellent passive transfer, presented later in this article, the authors estimate that producers need to deliver greater than or equal to 300 g of IgG shortly after birth. The 2 major factors affecting the mass of Ig consumed are the quality and volume of colostrum fed. Factors affecting the absorption of Ig molecules into circulation include the quickness with which the first colostrum feeding is provided after birth, bacterial contamination of colostrum, and metabolic status of the calf. This article next discusses these key factors, strategies for minimizing bacterial contamination of colostrum, the use of colostrum supplements (CSs) and replacers, benefits of multiple feedings, and benefits of extended colostrum or transition milk feeding after intestinal closure.

FACTORS ASSOCIATED WITH COLOSTRUM QUALITY AND YIELD

Although it is recognized that colostrum contains a wide spectrum of important immune and nutritional components, the concentration of IgG in colostrum has traditionally been considered the hallmark for evaluating colostrum quality, with high quality defined as IgG levels greater than 50 g/L. Colostrum IgG levels can vary dramatically among cows; in an observational study that tested 2253 colostrum samples from 104 farms in 13 states, mean colostral IgG level was 74.2 g/L, with the 5th and 95th percentiles ranging from 24.9 to 130.2 g/L. A total of 77.4% of samples had colostrum IgG level greater than 50 g/L.[46] Factors affecting colostrum quality and yield are reviewed next and methods for testing colostrum quality are discussed.

Breed

Comparative studies have reported that there can be a breed effect on colostrum quality.[47,48] In one study, Holstein cows produced colostrum with total Ig content (5.6%) that was lower than for Guernsey (6.3%), Brown Swiss (6.6%), Ayrshire (8.1%), or Jersey (9.0%) breed cows.[48] Breed differences could be caused by genetics and/or dilutional effects.

Age of Dam

Most, but not all, studies report a tendency for older cows to produce higher-quality colostrum, presumably /because of older animals having had a longer period of exposure to farm-specific pathogens.[46,49,50] In a study by Shivley and colleagues,[46] colostrum from first and second lactation cows had similar colostrum quality (73.2 and 71.7 g/L of IgG), whereas colostrum from third lactation and older cows was of higher quality (83.3 g/L IgG). Producers should test and record the quality of all colostrum fed. Producers should not automatically discard colostrum from first calf heifers without first testing, because it may be of very good quality.

Nutrition in the Preparturient Period

Studies have generally reported that Ig content of colostrum is not greatly affected by restricting prepartum maternal nutrition.[51–53] Mann and colleagues[54] reported that feeding a controlled energy diet that met, but did not exceed, energy requirements during the dry period increased colostral IgG but did not affect colostrum yield, compared with diets that offered increased energy. Lacetera and colleagues[55] reported that cows supplemented with injections of selenium and vitamin E in late pregnancy produced a greater volume of colostrum than unsupplemented cows, when all cows were fed a prepartum diet that was deficient in vitamin E and selenium. Aragona and colleagues[56] reported that supplementation with nicotinic acid for 4 weeks prepartum increased IgG concentration in colostrum from 73.8 to 86.8 g/L. More research is needed to investigate whether and how nutrition of the dam during the preparturient period may affect colostrum yield and quality. Producers should feed rations balanced according to National Research Council 2001 guidelines.[57]

Season of Calving

The relationship between season and colostrum quality or volume remains unclear. Although some studies have reported that exposure to high ambient temperatures during late pregnancy is associated with poorer colostrum composition, including lower mean concentrations of colostral IgG and IgA,[49,58] others have reported the opposite.[46] It has been suggested that any negative effects of heat stress on colostrum quality might be associated with reduced dry matter intake or reduced mammary blood flow resulting in impaired transfer of IgG and nutrients to the udder.[58] Season may also have an impact on colostrum yield, although this is less well described. In a year-long study of a 2500-cow Jersey dairy in Texas, colostrum yield was highest in June but declined during the fall and winter months.[59] A low-temperature humidity index and a shortened photoperiod 1 month before and at calving were both highly correlated with reduced colostrum yield. The investigators hypothesized that shortened photoperiod may reduce colostrum production because of its impact on melatonin and prolactin, hormones known to be involved with colostrogenesis. However, a study that experimentally manipulated photoperiod reported no effect of photoperiod during the dry period on colostrum quality or yield.[60] Producers should adopt heat-abatement strategies for prepartum cows and heifers and are advised to bank frozen colostrum to meet needs during low colostrum production months.[59]

Preparturient Vaccination of the Dam

Although vaccination is not likely to increase total IgG in colostrum, a large body of research has established that vaccinating pregnant cows and heifers during the final 3 to 6 weeks preceding calving results in increased concentrations of antigen-specific protective colostral antibodies, and increased passive antibody titers in calves of vaccinated dams, specific for some common pathogens including *Pasteurella haemolytica*, *Salmonella typhimurium*, *Escherichia coli*, rotavirus, and coronavirus.[61–64]

Dry Period Length

Cows with excessively short dry periods (<21 days) produce colostrum with lower IgG concentration.[65] Furthermore, cows with shorter dry periods produce lower yields of colostrum.[59,66] One controlled field study reported cows with a short (40-day) dry period produced 2.2 kg less colostrum than did cows with a conventional (60-day) dry period.[67]

Volume of Colostrum Produced at First Milking

Pritchett and colleagues[68] observed that cows producing less than 8.5 kg of colostrum at first milking were more likely to produce high-quality (>50 g/L) colostrum than higher-producing cows, presumably because of dilutional effects. However, more recent studies report that there is no strong predictable relationship between colostrum IgG concentration and weight of colostrum produced at first milking.[67,69,70]

Delayed Colostrum Collection

Most studies report that the concentration of Ig in colostrum is highest immediately after calving but begins to gradually decrease over time if harvest is delayed.[60,71] In an experimental study, Morin and colleagues[60] reported that colostral IgG concentration decreased by 3.7% during each subsequent hour that milking was delayed after calving, because of postparturient secretion (dilution) by the mammary glands. In another study, delaying harvest of colostrum for 6, 10, or 14 hours after calving resulted in a 17%, 27%, and 33% decrease in colostral IgG concentration, respectively.[72]

Cow-Side Testing of Colostrum Quality

It is difficult to predict, based on such factors such as visual consistency, which colostrum collected will be of high (>50 g/L IgG) versus low quality.[69] The colostrometer, a hydrometer instrument that estimates IgG concentration by measuring specific gravity, can be useful to differentiate high-quality from low-quality colostrum (specific gravity >1.050 approximates IgG >50 g/L). However, factors such as content of fat and colostrum temperature affect the hydrometer reading.[73] More recently, several studies have validated use of the Brix refractometer, an instrument that measures percentage solids in a solution, to indirectly estimate IgG level in colostrum. The Brix refractometer is less affected by temperature and more durable than the glass colostrometer. Studies have reported that a value between 18% and 23% Brix is an appropriate cut point for determining good-quality colostrum (IgG >50 g/L).[74–77] An achievable herd-level goal is to harvest high-quality colostrum (IgG ≥50 g/L or Brix ≥22%) in greater than or equal to 90% of samples tested.

VOLUME OF COLOSTRUM CONSUMED AT FIRST FEEDING

It is recommended that calves be fed 10% to 12% of their body weight (BW) of colostrum at first feeding (3–4 L for a Holstein calf). In one study, mean serum IgG level at 24 hours was significantly higher for calves fed 4 L of colostrum at 0 hours and a further 2 L at 12 hours (serum IgG = 31.1 g/L) compared with calves fed only 2 L of high-quality colostrum at 0 hours and a further 2 L at 12 hours (serum IgG = 23.5 g/L).[78] Another study reported that Brown Swiss calves fed 3.8 L (vs 1.9 L) of colostrum at first feeding experienced significantly higher rates of average daily gain and greater levels of milk production in both the first and second lactations.[8] The method of delivering colostrum deserves consideration. Suckling the dam is the least preferred approach, because delays in suckling and failure to control quality and volume ingested can result in higher rates of FPT.[79] When colostrum is delivered with an esophageal tube feeder, the esophageal groove reflex is not triggered, resulting in fluid being deposited into the forestomachs. However, this is not a significant limitation because outflow of colostrum from the forestomachs to the abomasum and small intestine occurs for the most part within 3 hours.[80] As such, equal and acceptable levels of passive transfer are achieved when colostrum is delivered by nipple bottle or esophageal tube feeder, provided that a sufficient volume of colostrum is delivered.[81,82] One study reported that calves drinking from a nipple bottle consumed an average of only 2.2 L (range, 1–4 L).[83] As such, producers feeding colostrum by nipple bottle should be prepared to deliver any remaining colostrum using a tube feeder, or provide a second bottle feeding within 6 hours, for those calves that do not voluntarily consume their whole allotment. Veterinarians should train staff on how to safely administer colostrum using tube feeders. Equipment sanitation and maintenance are important for both bottles and tube feeders.

EFFICIENCY OF ABSORPTION OF IMMUNOGLOBULINS

The term open gut refers to the unique ability of the neonatal enterocyte to nonselectively absorb intact large molecules, such as Ig, by pinocytosis.[84] From there, Ig molecules are transported across the cell and released into the lymphatics by exocytosis, after which they enter the circulatory system through the thoracic duct.[85] In a process referred to as closure, the absorption of Ig across the intestinal epithelium decreases linearly with time from birth to completely close at approximately 24 hours.[11] Factors affecting the apparent efficiency of absorption (AEA) of Ig for the first colostrum feeding are discussed here, as well as the value of extended colostrum feeding and feeding colostrum or transition milk after gut closure.

Time to First Colostrum Feeding

The efficiency of Ig transfer across the gut epithelium is optimal soon after birth, with a progressive decline in Ig absorption over time until gut closure.[86,87] Delaying the first colostrum feeding can only slightly postpone gut closure (36 hours).[88] In a study that randomized newborn calves to provide the first feeding of colostrum (7.5% BW; approximately 200 g of IgG) at different times, higher efficiency of absorption and maximum serum IgG levels were achieved for calves fed at 45 minutes of age (AEA = 51.8%; IgG = 25.5 g/L), compared with calves fed at 6 hours (AEA = 35.6%; IgG = 18.2 g/L) or 12 hours (AEA = 35.1%; IgG = 18.5 g/L).[87] Earlier feeding also resulted in more rapid bacterial colonization of the intestine with organisms such as *Bifidobacterium* spp. Producers should aim to feed all calves within 1 to 2 hours after birth.

Bacterial Contamination of Colostrum

High levels of bacteria in colostrum, and particularly coliform bacteria, may bind free Ig in the gut lumen and/or directly block uptake and transport of Ig molecules across intestinal epithelial cells, thus interfering with passive transfer.[89] Strategies to minimize bacterial contamination of colostrum are discussed next.

Metabolic Disturbances

Decreased colostral Ig absorption in the first 12 hours has been reported in calves with postnatal respiratory acidosis, associated with prolonged parturition.[90,91] Hypothermia may also be responsible for a delay in Ig absorption.[92] Although hypoxic calves may have delayed IgG absorption initially, studies have reported that there is no difference in overall absorptive capacity between hypoxic and normoxic calves, and that there is no difference in serum IgG concentrations by the time of gut closure.[93,94] Producers should provide adequate supportive care to newborns, including warming and drying calves born during cold weather, and providing supplemental heat, blankets, and deep straw bedding. Pain management, through the provision of a nonsteroidal antiinflammatory, has been shown to improve calf vigor and enhance IgG absorption for low-vigor calves following difficult calvings.[95–97]

Presence of the Dam

Ig absorption was improved when calves were housed with the dam.[98] However, considering that acceptable levels of serum IgG can be achieved without housing the calf with the dam, and given that the latter practice may increase the calf's risk of exposure to pathogens in the dam's environment, it is currently recommended that the calf be removed from the dam within 1 to 2 hours of birth and hand-fed colostrum.[3]

Value of Extended Colostrum Feeding

Although it is well recognized that maximal efficiency of absorption of IgG is achieved when the first colostrum feeding is provided within 2 hours after birth, the neonatal intestine is still permeable to IgG past 12 hours. Providing a second feeding sometime after the first postnatal meal can further increase passive transfer of IgG. In a recent study in which calves were randomly assigned to be fed a second feeding (5% BW) of either colostrum, a 1:1 colostrum/milk mixture, or milk at 12 hours of age, calves achieved a higher maximum serum IgG concentration if they were fed either colostrum (30 g/L) or mixture (25.0 g/L) at the second feeding, compared with milk (22.4 g/L).[99]

Value of Feeding Colostrum or Transition Milk After Gut Closure

Feeding colostrum after the gut has closed still offers benefits, even though Ig absorption no longer occurs. One benefit may be that bioactive compounds, such as hormones or oligosaccharides, may stimulate development of the GIT.[42,100] In one recent study, calves that were transitioned directly onto milk after the first colostrum meal had less overall gastrointestinal mass and less development of villi in the small intestine compared with calves fed either colostrum or transition milk for the first 3 days of life.[100] This improved GIT development could be beneficial for nutrient absorption and gut health. Another benefit may be local protection of the GIT by colostral antibodies. Challenge studies and field trials have reported health and growth benefits from supplementing the milk diet with colostrum for the first 14 days of life. One controlled field trial that added 70 g of colostrum powder containing 10 g of IgG into milk replacer twice daily for 14 days reported improved growth, reduced diarrhea days, and reduced antimicrobial use in treated calves.[101] In another field trial, supplementation of milk replacer with 150 g of bovine colostrum powder containing 32 g of IgG, for the first 14 days, resulted in reductions in diarrhea, respiratory disease, umbilical enlargement, and antibiotic therapy in treated dairy calves.[102] Producers feeding pasteurized whole milk are encouraged to include transition milk in the pool.

STRATEGIES FOR REDUCING BACTERIAL CONTAMINATION OF COLOSTRUM

Although it is an important source of nutrients and immune factors, colostrum can also represent one of the earliest potential exposures of dairy calves to infectious agents, including *Mycoplasma* spp, *Mycobacterium avium* subsp *paratuberculosis*, and *Salmonella* spp.[103,104] Furthermore, high levels of bacteria in colostrum may interfere with Ig absorption.[89] A negative association between colostrum bacteria levels and Ig absorption has been described in several studies.[105–107] Fresh/raw colostrum fed to calves should contain less than,100,000 colony-forming units (cfu)/mL total plate count (TPC) and less than 10,000 cfu/mL total coliform count.[3] However, bacteria levels in colostrum frequently exceed these goals in dairies. In an observational study that tested 827 colostrum samples from 67 farms in 12 states, almost 43% of samples had TPC greater than 100,000 cfu/mL and 17% of samples had greater than 1 million cfu/mL.[104] Strategies for minimizing bacterial contamination of colostrum are discussed next.

Preventing Contamination During Colostrum Harvest, Storage, and Feeding

Producers should avoid feeding colostrum from known infected cows (eg, Johne disease) and should avoid pooling raw colostrum. Contamination during colostrum harvest, storage, or feeding processes can be reduced by properly cleaning and sanitizing udders before harvesting colostrum; milking into a clean, sanitized bucket; and transferring colostrum into clean, sanitized storage or feeding equipment.

Minimizing Bacterial Growth in Stored Colostrum

Bacteria can multiply rapidly if colostrum or milk is stored at warm ambient temperatures. Unless colostrum is to be fed right away, it should be frozen or refrigerated within 1 hour after collection. Colostrum may be frozen for up to 1 year, provided repeated multiple freeze-thaw cycles do not occur. When thawing frozen colostrum, producers should avoid overheating colostrum (avoid temperatures >60°C) or some denaturation of Ig can occur.[108] Options for storing fresh colostrum include refrigeration with or without the use of US Food and Drug Administration–approved preservatives such as potassium sorbate (0.5% final solution in colostrum). In one study, average bacterial counts in raw refrigerated colostrum reached unacceptably high levels (TPC >100,000 cfu/mL) after 2 days of refrigeration. By comparison, average colostrum TPC remained less than,100,000 cfu/mL for 6 days of refrigeration when colostrum was preserved with potassium sorbate.[109]

Heat-Treated Colostrum

Although pasteurization at higher temperatures can damage Ig, colostrum may be safely heat treated (HT) using a lower-temperature, longer-time approach (60°C [140 F] for 60 minutes), maintaining IgG levels and fluid characteristics while eliminating important pathogens, including *E coli*, *Salmonella enteritidis*, and *Mycoplasma bovis*, and significantly reducing risk of exposure to *M avium* subsp. *paratuberculosis*.[108,110,111] Calves fed HT colostrum have improved efficiency of IgG absorption, presumably caused by reduced bacterial interference with IgG absorption.[105,112] In a field study of 1071 newborn calves in 6 Midwest dairy herds, calves fed HT colostrum had higher serum IgG level (18.0 g/L) and reduced risk for diarrhea (30.9%) compared with calves fed fresh colostrum (15.4 g/L; 36.5%).[106] Possibly contributing to these health benefits, Malmuthuge and colleagues[113] reported that feeding HT colostrum enhanced GIT colonization with *Bifidobacterium* but reduced colonization with *E coli* within the first 12 hours. If refrigerated in a clean covered container, the shelf life of HT colostrum is at least 8 days.[114] Goals for bacteria levels in HT colostrum are TPC less than 20,000 cfu/mL and coliform count less than 100 cfu/mL, respectively.

USE OF COLOSTRUM SUPPLEMENTS OR REPLACEMENT PRODUCTS

Although feeding high-quality, clean maternal colostrum is considered the gold standard, the use of high-quality CSs or colostrum replacements (CRs) may be attractive to producers for a variety of reasons, including availability, consistency, convenience, and as a means of breaking the transmission cycle of pathogens such as *M avium* ssp. *paratuberculosis*.[115] Supplements typically contain less than or equal to 60 g of IgG per dose and are intended to supplement (not replace) existing colostrum. There is no added benefit of feeding CS if already feeding 3 to 4 L of high-quality maternal colostrum.[116] By comparison, CR products are designed to completely replace maternal colostrum. They should provide a minimum of 100 g of IgG per pack and should also provide sufficient levels of nutrients to the calf to support metabolic needs in the first day of life. In Canada and the United States, CS and CR products may be licensed through the Canadian Food Inspection Agency, Canadian Center for Veterinary Biologics (Ottawa, ON), or through the US Department of Agriculture (USDA) Center for Veterinary Biologics (CVB; Ames, IA), respectively. In addition to other requirements, licensed products must originate from bovine colostrum; must be processed using accepted protocols to guarantee efficacy, safety, purity, and potency (minimum IgG content); and every serial made for sale and distribution must be tested for purity and potency.[117,118] Many products that are not CVB-licensed are produced in the United States, using a variety of manufacturing techniques, and with Ig sources including spray-dried bovine colostrum, milk, whey, bovine serum, or plasma. Nonlicensed products are not legally able to claim to supply IgG or to purport to be used for the prevention of FPT, although their use for this purpose is widespread in the United States.

A major consideration when feeding CR products is delivering an adequate dose of IgG to the calf. Many products provide only 100 to 150 g of IgG per pack, although some products provide label directions that suggest feeding increased masses of IgG, at the discretion of the producer. Although not true of all products, studies have shown that several commercially available CR products, when administered at a high enough IgG mass (150–200 g of IgG) within a few hours after birth, can provide acceptable serum IgG concentrations when using a conventional goal for APT (eg, $\geq$90% of calves with serum IgG $\geq$10 g/L).[119–122] However, if producers hope to achieve the more ambitious goals for passive transfer that are proposed in relation to monitoring, the authors suggest that they may need to deliver at least 300 g of IgG in a CR product. Research is required to investigate this hypothesis. Apart from dose, there can also be differences among CR products in Ig absorption, with studies generally reporting greater AEA percentage for lacteal-derived CR compared with serum-derived or plasma-derived CR.[123,124] Because of variable performance among products, veterinarians should review results of peer-reviewed controlled trials when recommending CR products to producers.

ON-FARM MONITORING AND GOALS FOR PASSIVE TRANSFER

A dairy's colostrum management program is one of very few processes in the animal health world that can be easily evaluated and should be routinely reviewed by veterinarians. Although serum IgG measured via radial immunodiffusion (RID) assay is considered the gold standard for evaluating passive transfer in calves,[11] it is expensive and generally requires that samples be tested at a laboratory. Other analytes, such as serum total protein (STP), have been extensively validated, are easily measured at the farm level, and are more economical than measuring IgG directly.[125,126] STP levels in healthy calves should be evaluated from blood samples collected from 24 hours after the first colostrum feeding to 10 days of age.[127] The earlier in this sampling window that samples are collected, the more accurately the results reflect true IgG absorption and the less likely it is for results to be influenced by IgG distribution/decay or dehydration. The use of a standard optical refractometer to measure STP or an optical or digital Brix refractometer, both of which are field friendly, is becoming more common. Optical refractometer values of 5.0 to 5.5 g/dL and Brix readings of 8.1% to 8.5% have been used as the cutoff for FPT.[3,128–131]

The individual calf standard for FPT (serum IgG <10 g/L) has been used for more than 35 years and is mainly based on a decreased risk of mortality when values are greater than or equal to 10 g/L.[7,10,12] Although strategies to evaluate colostrum management programs have traditionally been based on the individual calf standard, McGuirk and Collins[3] proposed sampling a minimum of 12 healthy calves and defined a successful program as one in which 80% of calves had an STP value of 5.5 g/dL or higher. From a study by Calloway and colleagues,[128] Tyler proposed (Personal Communication, 2002) that a successful passive transfer program was one in which 90% of sampled calves test 5.0 to 5.2 g/dL or higher.[132] However, one concern with this approach to setting goals includes the notion that "failure" should be used to describe calves with no measurable IgG, whereas "adequate" does not convey whether an optimal amount of IgG has been absorbed by the calf. In addition, a single cutoff that expresses failure versus adequate passive transfer is too simplistic, because it fails to recognize that increasing concentrations of IgG or STP are associated with reducing morbidity risk and improved calf performance. Studies by Furman-Fratczak and colleagues[13] and Windeyer and colleagues[12] showed that dairy calves with serum IgG levels greater than or equal to 15 g/L and STP greater than or equal to 5.7 g/dL, respectively, experienced lower rates of respiratory disease. In beef calves, Dewell and colleagues[133] reported lower morbidity rates when serum IgG level was greater than or equal to 24 g/L. Based on these and other studies, including the USDA National Animal Health Monitoring System's Dairy 2014 study,[4,46] a reevaluation of the FPT individual and herd-based cut points was conducted. A group of calf experts from the United States and Canada convened in 2018 to review and propose revised individual and herd-based evaluation standards. The proposed consensus standard is based on the association of lower morbidity and higher values of serum IgG, because mortality risk is associated with serum IgG values less than 10 g/L. The proposed standard includes 4 categories: excellent, good, fair, and poor. These categories can be applied to individual calves and to the operation for herd-based evaluation based on the percentage of calves that should be represented in each category (**Table 2**). Because serum IgG level is not commonly measured, equivalent STP and Brix levels are provided for the 4 categories. The proposed consensus standard is meant to set higher goals for calf health in the US dairy industry.

Producers feeding CR products should be aware that the relationship between STP and serum IgG can vary dramatically for calves fed different CR products, depending

Table 2
Proposed categories for immunoglobulin G levels and equivalent total protein and Brix measurements, and percentage of calves recommended in each category

Proposed Categories	Proposed IgG Levels (g/L)	Equivalent STP Levels (g/dL)	Equivalent Serum Brix Levels (%)	Proposed Calves in Each Category (%)
Excellent	≥25.0	≥6.2	≥9.4	>40
Good	18.0–24.9	5.8–6.1	8.9–9.3	~30
Fair	10.0–17.9	5.1–5.7	8.1–8.8	~20
Poor	<10.0	<5.1	<8.1	<10

on manufacturing techniques, the Ig source, level of inclusion, and level of absorption of Ig and non-Ig proteins. As such, the STP and Brix cut points suggested for monitoring passive transfer in calves fed maternal colostrum are frequently inaccurate for calves fed CR. Veterinarians are encouraged to use STP or serum Brix measures to monitor the effectiveness of a CR feeding program only if independently conducted studies are available describing the relationship between STP or serum Brix measures and serum IgG for the specific commercial CR product in use on the farm. If this information is not available for specific CR products, veterinarians are advised to periodically submit frozen serum samples for laboratory analysis of IgG using direct methods such as RID.

SUMMARY

Colostrum management is the single most important management factor in determining calf health and survival. Although good progress has been made in the past 20 years, there remains a considerable opportunity for many dairy producers to improve their colostrum management practices, resulting in improved short-term and long-term health and performance of the animals. Producers should provide calves with a sufficient volume of clean, high-quality colostrum within the first few hours of life. Additional benefits may be captured by providing multiple feedings and by extended feeding of colostrum or transition milk after gut closure. Colostrum replacers are useful tools if clean, high-quality maternal colostrum is not available. Ongoing monitoring helps producers to more quickly identify and correct problems within the colostrum management program.

REFERENCES

1. Arthur GH. The development of the conceptus. In: Arthur GH, Nokes DE, Pearson H, et al, editors. Pregnancy and parturition in veterinary reproduction and obstetrics. 7th edition. Philadelphia: W.B. Saunders; 1996. p. 51–109.

2. Davis CL, Drackley JK. The development, nutrition, and management of the young calf. 1st edition. Ames (IA): Iowa State University Press; 1998. p. 179–206.

3. McGuirk SM, Collins M. Managing the production, storage and delivery of colostrum. Vet Clin North Am Food Anim Pract 2004;20:593–603.

4. Urie NJ, Lombard JE, Shivley CB, et al. Preweaned heifer management on US dairy operations: Part V. Factors associated with morbidity and mortality in preweaned dairy heifer calves. J Dairy Sci 2018;101:9229–44.

5. Robison JD, Stott GH, DeNise SK. Effects of passive immunity on growth and survival in the dairy heifer. J Dairy Sci 1988;71:1283–7.

6. DeNise SK, Robison JD, Stott GH, et al. Effects of passive immunity on subsequent production in dairy heifers. J Dairy Sci 1989;72:552–4.
7. Wells SJ, Dargatz DA, Ott SL. Factors associated with mortality to 21 days of life in dairy heifers in the United States. Prev Vet Med 1996;29:9–19.
8. Faber SN, Faber NE, McCauley TC, et al. Case study: Effects of colostrum ingestion on lactational performance. Applied Animal Scientist 2005;21:420–5.
9. Hammon HM, Steinhoff-Wagner J, Flor J, et al. Lactation Biology Symposium: Role of colostrum and colostrum components on glucose metabolism in neonatal calves. J Anim Sci 2013;91:685–95.
10. Gay CC. Failure of passive transfer of colostral immunoglobulins and neonatal disease in calves: a review. In Proc. 4th Int. Symp. Neonatal Dis. Veterinary Infectious Disease Organization, Saskatoon, SK, Canada. October 3–5, 1983. p. 346–62.
11. Weaver DM, Tyler JW, VanMetre DC, et al. Passive transfer of colostral immunoglobulins in calves. J Vet Intern Med 2000;14:569–77.
12. Windeyer MC, Leslie KE, Godden SM, et al. Factors associated with morbidity, mortality, and growth of dairy heifer calves up to 3 months of age. Prev Vet Med 2014;113:231–40.
13. Furman-Fratczak K, Rzasa A, Stefaniak T. The influence of colostral immunoglobulin concentration in heifer calves' serum on their health and growth. J Dairy Sci 2011;94:5536–43.
14. Urie NJ, Lombard JE, Shivley CB, et al. Preweaned heifer management on US dairy operations: Part I. Descriptive characteristics of preweaned heifer raising practices. J Dairy Sci 2018;101:9168–84.
15. Foley JA, Otterby DE. Availability, storage, treatment, composition, and feeding value of surplus colostrum: A review. J Dairy Sci 1978;61:1033–60.
16. Larson BL, Heary HL Jr, Devery JE. Immunoglobulin production and transport by the mammary gland. J Dairy Sci 1980;63:665–71.
17. Newby TJ, Stokes CR, Bourne FJ. Immunological activities of milk. Vet Immunol Immunopathol 1982;3:67–94.
18. Barrington GM, Besser TE, Gay CC, et al. Effect of prolactin on in vitro expression of the bovine mammary immunoglobulin G_1 receptor. J Dairy Sci 1997;80: 94–100.
19. Thatcher EF, Gershwin LJ. Colostral transfer of bovine immunoglobulin E and dynamics of serum IgE in calves. Vet Immunol Immunopathol 1989;20:325–34.
20. Kirkpatrick J, Fulton RW, Burge LJ, et al. Passively transferred immunity in newborn calves, rate of antibody decay, and effect on subsequent vaccination with modified live virus vaccine. Bov Pract (Stillwater) 2001;35:47–54.
21. Kirkpatrick JG, Step DL, Payton ME, et al. Effect of age at the time of vaccination on antibody titers and feedlot performance in beef calves. J Am Vet Med Assoc 2008;233:136–42.
22. Chamorro MF, Walz PH, Haines DM, et al. Comparison of levels and duration of detection of antibodies to bovine viral diarrhea virus 1, bovine viral diarrhea virus 2, bovine respiratory syncytial virus, bovine herpesvirus 1, and bovine parainfluenza virus 3 in calves fed maternal colostrum or a colostrum-replacement product. Can J Vet Res 2014;78:81–8.
23. Duhamel GE, Bernoco D, Davis WC, et al. Distribution of T and B lymphocytes in mammary dry secretions, colostrum and blood of adult dairy cattle. Vet Immunol Immunopathol 1987;14:101–22.
24. Sheldrake RF, Husband AJ. Intestinal uptake of intact maternal lymphocytes by neonatal rats and lambs. Res Vet Sci 1985;39-10:15.

25. Tuboly S, Bernáth S, Glávits R, et al. Intestinal absorption of colostral lymphoid cells in newborn piglets. Vet Immunol Immunopathol 1988;20:75–85.

26. Liebler-Tenorio EM, Riedel-Caspari G, Pohlenz JF. Update of colostral leukocytes in the intestinal tract of newborn calves. Vet Immunol Immunopathol 2002;85:33–40.

27. Reber AJ, Hippen AR, Hurley DJ. Effects of the ingestion of whole colostrum or cell-free colostrum on the capacity of leukocytes in newborn calves to stimulate or respond in one-way mixed leukocyte cultures. Am J Vet Res 2005;66: 1854–60.

28. Donovan D, Reber A, Gabbard J, et al. Effect of maternal cells transferred with colostrum on cellular response to pathogen antigens in neonatal calves. Am J Vet Res 2007;68:778–82.

29. Reber AJ, Donovan DC, Gabbard J, et al. Transfer of maternal colostral leukocytes promotes development of the neonatal immune system I. Effects on monocyte lineage cells. Vet Immunol Immunopathol 2008a;123:186–96.

30. Reber AJ, Donovan DC, Gabbard J, et al. Transfer of maternal colostral leukocytes promotes development of the neonatal immune system Part II. Effects on neonatal lymphocytes. Vet Immunol Immunopathol 2008b;123:305–13.

31. Langel SN, Wark WA, Garst SN, et al. Effect of feeding whole compared with cell-free colostrum on calf immune status: The neonatal period. J Dairy Sci 2015;98:3729–40.

32. Bandrick M, Ariza-Nieto C, Baidoo SK, et al. Colostral antibody-mediated and cell-mediated immunity contributes to innate and antigen-specific immunity in piglets. Dev Comp Immunol 2014;43:114–20.

33. Bandrick M, Pieters M, Pijoan C, et al. Effect of cross-fostering on transfer of maternal immunity to Mycoplasma hyopneumoniae to piglets. Vet Rec 2011; 168:100.

34. Riedel-Caspari G, Schmidt FW, Marquardt J. The influence of colostral leukocytes on the immune system of the neonatal calf. IV. Effects on bactericidity, complement and interferon; synopsis. Dtsch Tierarztl Wochenschr 1991;98: 395–8.

35. Novo SMF, dos Reis Costa JF, Baccili CC, et al. Effect of maternal cells transferred with colostrum on the health of neonate calves. Res Vet Sci 2017;112: 97–104.

36. Meganck V, Opsomer G, Piepers S, et al. Maternal colostral leukocytes appear to enhance cell-mediated recall response, but inhibit humoral recall response in prime-boost vaccinated calves. J Reprod Immunol 2016;113:68–75.

37. Langel SN, Wark WA, Garst SN, et al. Effect of feeding whole compared with cell-free colostrum on calf immune status: Vaccination response. J Dairy Sci 2016;99:3979–94.

38. Przybylska J, Albera E, Kankofer M. Antioxidants in bovine colostrum. Reprod Domest Anim 2007;42:402–9.

39. Pakkanen R, Aalto J. Growth factors and antimicrobial factors of bovine colostrum. Int Dairy J 1997;7:285–97.

40. Shah NP. Effects of milk-derived bioactives: an overview. Br J Nutr 2000; 84(Suppl. 1):S3–10.

41. Elfstrand L, Lindmark-Månsson H, Paulsson M, et al. Immunoglobulins, growth factors and growth hormone in bovine colostrum and the effects of processing. Int Dairy J 2002;12:879–87.

42. Fischer AJ, Malmuthuge N, Guan LL, et al. Short communication: The effect of heat treatment of bovine colostrum on the concentration of oligosaccharides in

colostrum and in the intestine of neonatal male Holstein calves. J Dairy Sci 2018; 101:401–7.

43. Blum JW, Baumrucker CR. Insulin-like growth factors (IGFs), IGF binding proteins, and other endocrine factors in milk: Role in the newborn. In: Bösze Z, editor. Bioactive components of milk. New York: Springer; 2008. p. 397–422.

44. Chen T, Xie MY, Sun JJ, et al. Porcine milk-derived exosomes promote proliferation of intestinal epithelial cells. Sci Rep 2016;6:33862.

45. Izumi H, Kosaka N, Shimizu T, et al. Time-dependent expression profiles of microRNAs and mRNAs in rat milk whey. PLoS One 2014;9(2):e88843.

46. Shivley CB, Lombard JE, Urie NJ, et al. Preweaned heifer management on US dairy operations: Part II. Factors associated with colostrum quality and passive transfer status of dairy heifer calves. J Dairy Sci 2018;101:9168–84.

47. Guy MA, McFadden TB, Cockrell DC, et al. Regulation of colostrum formation in beef and dairy cows. J Dairy Sci 1994;77:3002–7.

48. Muller LD, Ellinger DK. Colostral immunoglobulin concentrations among breeds of dairy cattle. J Dairy Sci 1981;64:1727–30.

49. Morin DE, Constable PD, Maunsell FP, et al. Factors associated with colostral specific gravity in dairy cows. J Dairy Sci 2001;84:937–43.

50. Tyler JW, Steevens BJ, Hostetler DE, et al. Colostrum immunoglobulin concentrations in Holstein and Guernsey cows. Am J Vet Res 1999;60:1136–9.

51. Blecha GK, Bulls RC, Olson DP, et al. Effects of prepartum protein restriction in the beef cow on immunoglobulin content in blood and colostral whey and subsequent immunoglobulin absorption by the neonatal calf. J Anim Sci 1981;53: 1174–80.

52. Hough RL, McCarthy FD, Kent HD, et al. Influence of nutritional restriction during late gestation on production measures and passive immunity in beef cattle. J Anim Sci 1990;68:2622–7.

53. Nowak W, Mikuła R, Zachwieja A, et al. The impact of cow nutrition in the dry period on colostrum quality and immune status of calves. Pol J Vet Sci 2012; 15:77–82.

54. Mann S, Leal Yepes FA, Overton TR, et al. Effect of dry period dietary energy level in dairy cattle on volume, concentration of immunoglobulin G, insulin, and fatty acid composition of colostrum. J Dairy Sci 2016;99:1515–26.

55. Lacetera N, Bernabucci U, Ronchi B, et al. Effects of selenium and vitamin E administration during a late stage of pregnancy on colostrum and milk production in dairy cows, and on passive immunity and growth of their offspring. Am J Vet Res 1996;57:1776–80.

56. Aragona KM, Chapman CE, Pereira ABD, et al. Prepartum supplementation of nicotinic acid: Effects on health of the dam, colostrum quality, and acquisition of immunity in the calf. J Dairy Sci 2016;99:3529–38.

57. NRC. Nutrient requirements of dairy cattle. 7th edition. Washington, DC: National Academy Press; 2001.

58. Nardone A, Lacetera N, Bernabucci U, et al. Composition of colostrum from dairy heifers exposed to high air temperatures during late pregnancy and the early postpartum period. J Dairy Sci 1997;80:838–44.

59. Gavin K, Neibergs H, Hoffman A, et al. Low colostrum yield in Jersey cattle and potential risk factors. J Dairy Sci 2018;101:6388–98.

60. Morin DE, Nelson SV, Reid ED, et al. Effect of colostral volume, interval between calving and first milking, and photoperiod on colostral IgG concentrations in dairy cows. J Am Vet Med Assoc 2010;237:420–8.

61. Jones PW, Collins P, Aitkin MM. Passive protection of calves against experimental infection with *Salmonella typhimurium*. Vet Rec 1988;123:536–41.

62. Waltner-Toews D, Martin SW, Meek AH, et al. A field trial to evaluate the efficacy of a combined rotavirus-coronavirus *Escherichia coli* vaccine in dairy cattle. Can J Comp Med 1985;49:1–9.

63. Hodgins DC, Shewen PE. Preparturient vaccination to enhance passive immunity to the capsular polysaccharide of *Pasteurella haemolytica* A1. Vet Immunol Immunopathol 1996;50:67–77.

64. McNulty MS, Logan EF. Effect of vaccination of the dam on rotavirus infection in young calves. Vet Rec 1987;120:250–2.

65. Dixon FJ, Weigle WO, Vazquez JJ. Metabolism and mammary secretion of proteins in the cow. Lab Invest 1961;10:216–37.

66. Rastani RR, Grummer RR, Bertics SJ, et al. Reducing dry period length to simplify feeding transition cows: Milk production, energy balance and metabolic profiles. J Dairy Sci 2005;88:1004–14.

67. Grusenmeyer DJ, Ryan CM, Galton DM, et al. Shortening the dry period from 60 to 40 days does not affect colostrum quality but decreases colostrum yield by Holstein cows. J Dairy Sci 2006;89(Suppl. 1):336.

68. Pritchett LC, Gay CC, Besser TE, et al. Management and production factors influencing Immunoglobulin G_1 concentration in colostrum from Holstein cows. J Dairy Sci 1991;74:2336–41.

69. Maunsell FP, Morin DE, Constable PD, et al. Use of mammary gland and colostral characteristics for prediction of colostral IgG_1 concentration and intramammary infection in Holstein cows. J Am Vet Med Assoc 1999;214:1817–23.

70. Baumrucker CR, Burkett AM, Magliaro-Macrina AL, et al. Colostrogenesis: Mass transfer of immunoglobulin G1 into colostrum. J Dairy Sci 2010;93:3031–8.

71. Conneely M, Berry DP, Sayers R, et al. Factors associated with the concentration of immunoglobulin G in the colostrum of dairy cows. Animal 2013;7:1824–32.

72. Moore M, Tyler JW, Chigerwe M, et al. Effect of delayed colostrum collection on colostral IgG concentration in dairy cows. J Am Vet Med Assoc 2005;226:1375–7.

73. Pritchett LC, Gay CC, Hancock DD, et al. Evaluation of the hydrometer for testing immunoglobulin G_1 concentrations in Holstein colostrum. J Dairy Sci 1994;77:1761–7.

74. Chigerwe M, Hagey JV. Refractometer assessment of colostral and serum IgG and milk total solids concentrations in dairy cattle. BMC Vet Res 2014;10:178.

75. Bielmann V, Gillan J, Perkins NR, et al. An evaluation of Brix refractometry instruments for measurement of colostrum quality in dairy cattle. J Dairy Sci 2010;93:3713–21.

76. Quigley JD, Lago A, Chapman C, et al. Evaluation of the Brix refractometer to estimate immunoglobulin G concentration in bovine colostrum. J Dairy Sci 2013;96:1148–55.

77. Bartier AL, Windeyer MC, Doepel L. Evaluation of on-farm tools for colostrum quality measurement. J Dairy Sci 2015;98:1878–84.

78. Morin DE, McCoy GC, Hurley WL. Effects of quality, quantity, and timing of colostrum feeding and addition of a dried colostrum supplement on immunoglobulin G_1 absorption in Holstein bull calves. J Dairy Sci 1997;80:747–53.

79. Edwards SA, Broom DM. The period between birth and first suckling in dairy calves. Res Vet Sci 1979;26:255–6.

80. Lateur-Rowet HJM, Breukink HJ. The failure of the oesophageal groove reflex, when fluids are given with an oesophageal feeder to newborn and young calves. Vet Q 1983;5:68–74.

81. Godden SM, Haines DM, Konkol K, et al. Improving passive transfer of immuno-globulins in calves II: Interaction between feeding method and volume of colostrum fed. J Dairy Sci 2009;92:1758–64.

82. Desjardins-Morrissette M, van Niekerk JK, Haines D, et al. The effect of tube versus bottle feeding colostrum on immunoglobulin G absorption, abomasal emptying, and plasma hormone concentrations in newborn calves. J Dairy Sci 2018;101:4168–79.

83. Chigerwe M, Coons DM, Hagey JV. Comparison of colostrum feeding by nipple bottle versus oroesophageal tubing in Holstein dairy bull calves. J Am Vet Med Assoc 2012;241:104–9.

84. Broughton CW, Lecce JG. Electron microscopic studies of the jejunal epithelium from neonatal pigs fed different diets. J Nutr 1970;100:445–9.

85. Staley TE, Corles CD, Bush LJ, et al. The ultrastructure of neonatal calf intestine and absorption of heterologous proteins. Anat Rec 1972;172:559–79.

86. Besser TE, Garmedia AE, McGuire TC, et al. Effect of colostral immunoglobulin G1 and immunoglobulin M concentrations on immunoglobulin absorption in calves. J Dairy Sci 1985;68:2033–7.

87. Fisher AJ, Song Y, He Z, et al. Effect of delaying colostrum feeding on passive transfer and intestinal bacterial colonization in neonatal male Holstein calves. J Dairy Sci 2018;101:3099–109.

88. Stott GH, Marx DB, Menefee BE, et al. Colostral immunoglobulin transfer in calves I. Period of absorption. J Dairy Sci 1979;62:1632–8.

89. James RE, Polan CE, Cummins KA. Influence of administered indigenous micro-organisms on uptake of [iodine-125] gamma-globulin in vivo by intestinal segments of neonatal calves. J Dairy Sci 1981;64:52–61.

90. Besser TE, Szenci O, Gay CC. Decreased colostral immunoglobulin absorption in calves with postnatal respiratory acidosis. J Am Vet Med Assoc 1990;196:1239–443.

91. Vermorel M, Vernet J, Dardillat C, et al. Energy metabolism and thermoregulation in the newborn calf; Effect of calving conditions. Can J Anim Sci 1989;69:113–22.

92. Olson DP, Papasian CJ, Ritter RC. The effects of cold stress on neonatal calves II. Absorption of colostral immunoglobulins. Can J Comp Med 1980;44:19–23.

93. Tyler H, Ramsey H. Hypoxia in neonatal calves: Effect on intestinal transport of immunoglobulins. J Dairy Sci 1991;74:1953–6.

94. Drewry JJ, Quigley JD, Geiser DR, et al. Effect of high arterial carbon dioxide tension on efficiency of immunoglobulin G absorption in calves. Am J Vet Res 1999;60:609–14.

95. Murray CF, Haley DB, Duffield TF, et al. A field study to evaluate the effects of meloxicam NSAID therapy and calving assistance on newborn calf vigor, improvement of health and growth in pre-weaned Holstein calves. Bov Pract 2015a;49:1–12.

96. Murray CF, Duffield TF, Haley DB, et al. The effect of Meloxicam NSAID therapy on the change in vigor, suckling reflex, blood gas measures, milk intake and other variables in newborn dairy calves. J Vet Sci Anim Husbandry 2016;3:1–14.

97. Godden S, Knauer W, Gapinski C, et al. Effect of implementing a novel calf vitality scoring system and early intervention program on pain management in

newborn calves. ADSA Discover Conference: Effects of Stress on Health and Production of Dairy Cows. Chicago, IL, October 30–November 1, 2018.

98. Selman IE, McEwan AD, Fisher EW. Studies on dairy calves allowed to suckle their dams at fixed times post-partum. Res Vet Sci 1971;12:1–6.

99. Pletts S, Pyo J, He S, et al. Effect of extended colostrum feeding on serum IgG in newborn calves. J Anim Sci 2018;96(Suppl. S3):182.

100. Pyo J, Pletts S, Romao J, et al. The effects of extended colostrum feeding on gastrointestinal tract growth of the neonatal dairy calf. J Anim Sci 2018; 96(Suppl. 3):170–1.

101. Berge ACB, Besser TE, Moore DA, et al. Evaluation of the effects of oral colostrum supplementation during the first fourteen days on the health and performance of preweaned calves. J Dairy Sci 2009;92:286–95.

102. Chamorro MF, Cernicchiaro N, Haines DM. Evaluation of the effects of colostrum replacer supplementation of the milk replacer ration on the occurrence of disease, antibiotic therapy, and performance of pre-weaned dairy calves. J Dairy Sci 2017;100:1378–87.

103. Streeter RN, Hoffsis GF, Bech-Nielsen S, et al. Isolation of *Mycobacterium paratuberculosis* from colostrum and milk of subclinically infected cows. Am J Vet Res 1995;56:1322–4.

104. Walz PH, Mullaney TP, Render JA, et al. Otitis media in preweaned Holstein dairy calves in Michigan due to *Mycoplasma bovis*. J Vet Diagn Invest 1997; 9:250–4.

105. Johnson J, Godden S, Molitor T, et al. The effect of feeding heat treated colostrum on passive transfer of immune and nutritional parameters in dairy calves. J Dairy Sci 2007;90:5189–98.

106. Godden SM, Smolenski DJ, Donahue M, et al. Heat-treated colostrum and reduced morbidity in preweaned dairy calves: Results of a randomized trial and examination of mechanisms of effectiveness. J Dairy Sci 2012;95:4029–40.

107. Morrill KM, Conrad E, Lago A, et al. Nationwide evaluation of quality and composition of colostrum on dairy farms in the United States. J Dairy Sci 2012;95: 3997–4005.

108. McMartin S, Godden S, Metzger L, et al. Heat-treatment of bovine colostrum I: Effects of temperature on viscosity and immunoglobulin G. J Dairy Sci 2006;89: 2110–8.

109. Stewart S, Godden S, Bey R, et al. Preventing bacterial contamination and proliferation during the harvest, storage and feeding of fresh bovine colostrum. J Dairy Sci 2005;88:2571–8.

110. Godden S, McMartin S, Feirtag J, et al. Heat-treatment of bovine colostrum II: Effects of heating duration on pathogen viability and immunoglobulin G. J Dairy Sci 2006;89:3476–83.

111. Donahue M, Godden SM, Bey R, et al. Heat treatment of colostrum on commercial dairy farms decreases colostrum microbial counts while maintaining colostrum immunoglobulin G concentrations. J Dairy Sci 2012;95:2697–702.

112. Kryzer AA, Godden SM, Schell R. Heat-treated (in single aliquot or batch) colostrum outperforms non-heat-treated colostrum in terms of quality and transfer of immunoglobulin G in neonatal Jersey calves. J Dairy Sci 2015;98:1870–7.

113. Malmuthuge N, Chen Y, Liang G, et al. Heat-treated colostrum feeding promotes beneficial bacteria colonization in the small intestine of neonatal calves. J Dairy Sci 2015;98:8044–53.

114. Bey R, Godden S, Lillegaard H, et al. Improving cleanliness and shelf-life of refrigerated colostrum using heat-treatment and chemical preservatives. Proc.

Annu. Meet. Minnesota Dairy Health Management Conference. St. Paul, MN, May 15–17, 2007.

115. Pithua P, Godden SM, Wells SJ, et al. Efficacy of feeding a plasma-derived commercial colostrum replacer for the prevention of transmission of *Mycobacterium avium* subsp. *paratuberculosis* in Holstein calves. J Am Vet Med Assoc 2009; 234:1167–76.

116. Francisco SFA, Quigley JD. Serum immunoglobulin concentrations after feeding maternal colostrum or maternal colostrum plus colostral supplement to dairy calves. Am J Vet Res 1993;54:1051–4.

117. USDA. United States Department of Agriculture. Center for Veterinary Biologics Policy, Evaluation, and Licensing - Reviewer's Manual. 2018. Available at: https://www.aphis.usda.gov/aphis/ourfocus/animalhealth/sa_vet_biologics/sa_biologics_regulations/ct_vb_pelmanual_toc. Accessed December 6, 2018.

118. USDA. United States Department of Agriculture. Ames (IA): Center for Veterinary Biological Products; 2018. Veterinary Biologics. Available at: https://www.aphis.usda.gov/aphis/ourfocus/animalhealth/veterinary-biologics. Accessed December 6, 2018.

119. Godden SM, Haines DM, Hagman D. Improving passive transfer of immunoglobulins in calves. I: Dose effect of feeding a commercial colostrum replacer. J Dairy Sci 2009;92:1750–7.

120. Morrill KM, Marston SP, Whitehouse NL, et al. Anionic salts in the prepartum diet and addition of sodium bicarbonate to colostrum replacer, and their effects on immunoglobulin G absorption in the neonate. J Dairy Sci 2010;93:2067–75.

121. Foster DM, Smith GW, Sanner TR, et al. Serum IgG and total protein concentrations in dairy calves fed two colostrum replacement products. J Am Vet Med Assoc 2006;229:1282–5.

122. Lago AI, Socha M, Geiger A, et al. Efficacy of colostrum replacer versus maternal colostrum on immunological status, health and growth of preweaned dairy calves. J Dairy Sci 2018;101:1344–54.

123. Place N, Bents A, Leslie K, et al. Relationship between serum total protein and serum IgG in Holstein calves fed either a plasma- or lacteal-derived colostrum replacer. In Proceedings of the 43rd Annu Conf of the AABP. Albuquerque, NM, August 19–21, 2010. p. 193.

124. Priestley D, Bittar JH, Ibarbia L, et al. Effect of feeding maternal colostrum, a plasma-derived, or a colostrum-derived colostrum replacer on passive transfer of immunity, health, and performance of preweaning heifer calves. J Dairy Sci 2013;96:3247–56.

125. Buczinski S, Gicquel E, Fecteau G, et al. Systematic review and meta-analysis of diagnostic accuracy of serum refractometry and Brix refractometry for the diagnosis of inadequate transfer of passive immunity in calves. J Vet Intern Med 2018;32:474–83.

126. Elsohaby I, McClure JT, Waite LA, et al. Using serum and plasma samples to assess failure of transfer of passive immunity in dairy calves. J Dairy Sci 2019;102:567–77.

127. Wilm J, Costa JHC, Neave HW, et al. Technical note: Serum total protein and immunoglobulin G concentrations in neonatal dairy calves over the first 10 days of age. J Dairy Sci 2018;101:6430–6.

128. Calloway CD, Tyler JW, Tessman RK, et al. Comparison of refractometers and test endpoints in the measurement of serum protein concentration to assess passive transfer status in calves. J Am Vet Med Assoc 2002;221:1605–8.

129. Elsohaby I, McClure JT, Keefe GP. Evaluation of digital and optical refractometers for assessing failure of transfer of passive immunity in dairy calves. J Vet Intern Med 2015;29:721–6.

130. Deelen SM, Ollivett TL, Haines DM, et al. Evaluation of a Brix refractometer to estimate serum immunoglobulin G concentration in neonatal dairy calves. J Dairy Sci 2014;97:3838–44.

131. Hernandez D, Nydam DV, Godden SM, et al. Brix refractometry in serum as a measure of failure of passive transfer compared to measured immunoglobulin G and total protein by refractometry in serum from dairy calves. Vet J 2016; 211:82–7.

132. Godden S. Colostrum management for dairy calves. Vet Clin North Am Food Anim Pract 2008;24:19–39.

133. Dewell RD, Hungerford LL, Keen JE, et al. Association of neonatal serum immunoglobulin G1 concentration with health and performance in beef calves. J Am Vet Med Assoc 2006;228:914–21.

Vaccinating Calves in the Face of Maternal Antibodies
Challenges and Opportunities

M. Claire Windeyer, BSc, DVM, DVSc*, Lisa Gamsjäger, Mag.med.vet

KEYWORDS

- Vaccination • Passive immunity • Maternal antibodies • Neonatal calf
- Disease prevention

KEY POINTS

- Research investigating vaccination in the face of maternal antibodies (IFOMA) is highly variable, the results often differing. To better inform evidence-based vaccination recommendations, additional studies are needed, particularly those that examine clinically relevant outcomes in representative populations of calves.
- Parenteral vaccination IFOMA is unlikely to result in seroconversion, and other immune responses are inconsistent. However, the presence of antibodies may be prolonged, immunologic memory may be induced, and a reduction in clinical signs has been observed in some challenge studies.
- Intranasal vaccination IFOMA is able to circumvent interference by maternal antibodies in certain circumstances and may provide some short-term disease-sparing effects. Anamnestic responses may be generated upon later antigen exposure.
- The optimal vaccination strategy for preweaned calves will depend on herd-level factors, such as maternal vaccination, colostrum management, and disease challenge. Herds with poor transfer of passive immunity may particularly benefit from early calfhood vaccination.

OUTLINING THE CHALLENGE

Animals possess most components of a mature immune system at birth; however, soluble portions exist in lesser concentrations than are necessary for an optimal immune response, and cellular portions are generally naive and may be in a quiescent state.[1–3] Furthermore, the syndesmochorial placentation of the bovine means calves are typically born agammaglobulinemic.[2,4] Because of the protective environment of the

Disclosure Statement: Dr M.C. Windeyer and coworkers were recipients of the Zoetis Investment in Innovation Fund in 2018. Drs M.C. Windeyer and L. Gamsjäger collaborate with the Saskatoon Colostrum Company Ltd.
Department of Production Animal Health, University of Calgary Faculty of Veterinary Medicine, 11877 85th Street NW, Calgary, Alberta T3R 1J3, Canada
* Corresponding author.
E-mail address: c.windeyer@ucalgary.ca

uterus, calves have little chance to develop an adaptive immune response before birth. They are born immunologically naive, and therefore, depend on innate and passive immunity to protect them from infectious diseases during the early stages of life[1,2,5] (**Fig. 1**A).

Transfer of passive immunity (TPI) via timely ingestion of sufficient volumes of good-quality colostrum is a crucial component of neonatal calf health and survival and is covered in detail elsewhere in this issue. Neonatal TPI is assessed by measuring serum immunoglobulin G (IgG) concentrations or other surrogate parameters (eg, serum total protein) in calves between 1 and 7 days of age.[5,6] The optimal cut point to define failed TPI is still being debated,[7–9] but it is generally accepted that calves with failed TPI are at increased risk of morbidity and mortality, have reduced growth, and are a costly issue for both the beef and the dairy industries.[10]

Total serum IgG has historically been the major focus of the conversation about TPI in neonatal calves, so little is known about specific antibody titers, their proportions in the makeup of total IgG, and their individual impacts on calf health and growth. Only a few studies have reported initial specific maternal antibody titers against important respiratory and gastrointestinal pathogens in neonatal calves.[11–16] It is challenging to draw any broad conclusions from these studies except that the initial specific maternal antibody titers vary greatly, depending on a variety of factors, including farm-level practices, such as dam vaccination and colostrum management, individual calf-level factors, such as dystocia and vigor, and study-level factors, such as geography, inclusion criteria, and study design. Clinically, this means research reported in the literature is unlikely to be externally valid, and each calf is likely to begin life with a different maternal antibody profile in their systemic circulation.

To further complicate the matter, maternal antibodies may be present in the calf's circulation for varying periods of time, depending on the specific pathogen, initial dose of antibodies ingested and absorbed by the calf (see **Fig. 1**A, B), and degree to which disease challenge accelerates catabolism of antibodies.[4,17,18] The half-lives of specific maternal antibodies against common viral pathogens range between 13 and 36 days.[13,19–23] Various studies have attempted to investigate the age by which maternal antibodies become undetectable in calves. Average ages range from 5 to 6.5 months for bovine respiratory syncytial virus (BRSV)[14,21]; 2 to 10 months for bovine herpesvirus type 1 (BHV1)[14,20,21,23]; 5 to 6 months for parainfluenza virus type 3 (PIV3)[14,21]; and 3 to 7.5 months for bovine viral diarrhea virus (BVDV).[14,19,21–23] Because specific maternal antibody titers are rarely measured outside of research and can be highly variable between and within herds,[14] the actual duration of protective passive immunity against a specific pathogen cannot be feasibly known in the field.[4] Furthermore, the exact antibody titer that would be protective against a particular disease depends on the pathogen involved, the degree of challenge, and other host, pathogen, and environmental factors that influence the epidemiologic triad (**Fig. 1**).

Ideally, calves would be vaccinated before the point when maternal antibodies have decayed past protective levels and would mount an effective immune response in time to provide continual protection against disease challenge, eliminating any window of susceptibility[1,24] (see **Fig. 1**A). In western Canada, 96% of cow-calf producers recently reported vaccinating beef calves at least once before weaning, mostly before or at the time of turnout to summer pasture,[25] when most calves would be about 1 to 3 months of age. This number is an increase from previous studies in the same region,[26,27] although the more recent study surveyed beef producers that were recruited through their relationship with a veterinary practice, so it may overestimate the proportion of producers using calfhood vaccination practices nationally. Interestingly, 13% of those producers reported vaccinating calves at birth, mostly with intranasal (IN) vaccines against either

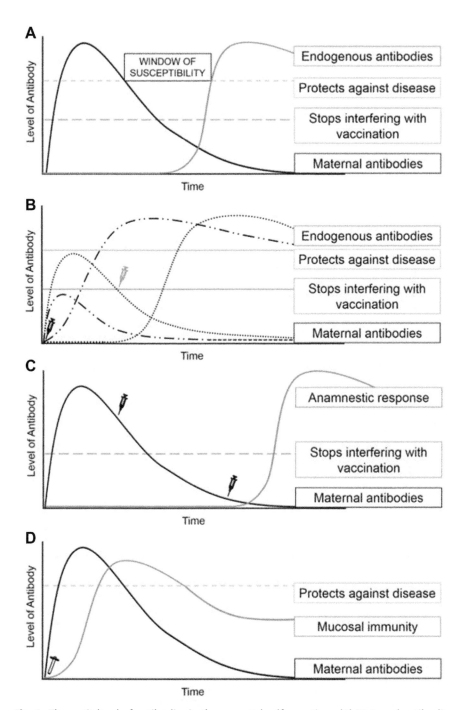

Fig. 1. Theoretic level of antibodies in the neonatal calf over time. (*A*) Maternal antibodies (*solid black line*) acquired via TPI decrease over time. Ideally, adequate TPI protects against disease (*short dashed light gray line*); however, interference with humoral responses (*solid gray line*) to parenteral vaccination is likely until the level of maternal antibodies drops

viral or bacterial respiratory pathogens (9%) but also with oral vaccines against diarrhea pathogens (3%) and parenteral vaccines against clostridial pathogens (3%).[25] In 2007 in the United States, less than 12% of beef producers vaccinated calves before 21 days of age, whereas 62% vaccinated calves between 21 days and weaning.[28] More recent numbers are not yet available, but between 1992 and 2007, the frequency of vaccination seemed to be increasing for respiratory pathogens (ie, BRSV, BHV1, PIV3, BVDV, *Histophilus somni*, and *Pasteurella multocida* [PM]), whereas it was decreasing (ie, brucellosis, clostridial diseases, digestive pathogens) or staying approximately the same (ie, leptospirosis, infectious bovine keratoconjunctivitis) for other pathogens.[25,29] The proportion of dairy herds reporting preweaning vaccination of calves has been increasing in recent years from fewer than 35% of operations vaccinating calves before weaning in 1991 to almost 50% in 2013.[30,31] It is important to note that dairy calves are typically weaned much earlier than beef calves, so maternal antibody titers would be expected to be higher during the preweaning period of dairy calves compared with the latter part of the preweaning period of beef calves.

To summarize, calves are born immunologically naive and depend on TPI in the form of colostral IgG for protection against infectious agents during early life. The amount of specific maternal antibodies that calves receive is highly variable, and the duration of protection is difficult to predict accurately in the field. Growing numbers of cattle producers are implementing preweaning vaccination programs with a goal of providing continuity of immunity. As outlined in the following sections, studies on vaccinating calves in the face of maternal antibodies (IFOMA) can be conflicting and difficult to summarize. Nonetheless, they do provide some guidance for the development of evidence-based strategies to vaccinate calves IFOMA with the intent to improve calf health and survival.

EFFECTS OF MATERNAL ANTIBODIES ON IMMUNE RESPONSES

For many years, the prevailing theory was that vaccinating calves IFOMA was ineffective because maternal antibodies blocked the calves' immune response to injectable vaccines[24] (see **Fig. 1**A). For this reason, TPI was considered a "double-edge sword": it was accepted that TPI was essential for calf health and survival but also that it impeded the ability of parenteral vaccines to consistently and effectively immunize young calves. The exact mechanism by which maternal antibodies interfere with vaccination is still not clearly understood; however, multiple proposed theories have been reviewed in depth elsewhere.[24]

Lack of Seroconversion Following Parenteral Vaccination in the Face of Maternal Antibodies

Numerous studies have demonstrated that calves vaccinated parenterally IFOMA are unlikely to exhibit seroconversion, which is defined as a 4-fold increase in antibody titer and has traditionally been used as the major criterion for successful vaccination.

(*long dashed gray line*), leaving calves vulnerable to disease (window of susceptibility). (*B*) Calves with inadequate (*dotted black line*) or failed (*long dash and dotted black line*) TPI are susceptible to disease (*solid light gray line*) but may produce endogenous antibodies in response to vaccination (*solid gray line*) early in life. (*C*) Parenteral vaccination IFOMA (*solid black line*) may not induce an initial humoral response (*dashed gray line*), but an anamnestic response (*solid gray line*) may occur upon administration of a booster vaccine. (*D*) IN vaccination IFOMA (*solid black line*) can induce a mucosal immune response (*solid gray line*) that provides some short-term disease-sparing effects (*dashed gray line*).

When 8 commercial parenteral multivalent viral vaccines were compared, 6-month-old beef calves that were seropositive at vaccination had lower seroconversion rates to the respective viruses compared with seronegative calves.[32] At this age, it would be expected that the levels of maternal antibody would be insufficient to interfere with vaccination, but 42% to 89% of calves were seropositive, and this impacted seroconversion. Dairy calves between the ages of 50 and 183 days of age that were vaccinated with a parenteral multivalent modified live viral (MLV) vaccine had a significantly lower probability of seroconverting when seropositive at vaccination compared with calves that were seronegative for BVDV1 and BRSV, but there was no difference in seroconversion risk for BVDV2.[21] A complete lack of seroconversion in neonatal, BRSV-seropositive calves that were vaccinated subcutaneously (SC) at 3 to 9 days of age with an MLV vaccine that included BRSV was reported.[12] Similarly, a lack of antibody response after parenteral administration of an inactivated BRSV, PIV3, and mannheimia haemolytica (MH) vaccine to seropositive beef calves at 14 and 42 days of age was also recently described.[16]

These examples are just some of the many examples of research that show parenteral vaccination IFOMA is unlikely to be deemed efficacious if seroconversion is used as the primary outcome measure.[17,33]

Effects of Vaccination in the Face of Maternal Antibodies on Rate of Antibody Decay

Although it has often been demonstrated that high levels of maternal antibodies may interfere with a calf's humoral response to vaccination, other reports suggest that perhaps the use of seroconversion as the measurement of vaccine response for young calves should be reevaluated.

Fulton and colleagues[23] found that parenteral vaccination IFOMA rarely resulted in seroconversion; however, the mean apparent half-lives of BHV1-, PIV3-, and BVDV-specific antibodies were significantly greater in vaccinated calves compared with nonvaccinates. Furthermore, parenteral vaccination against BVDV before 45 days of age delayed the age at which antibodies were undetectable, but this was dependent on the prevaccination titer of maternal antibodies.[22] In that study, calves categorized as having an intermediate level of maternal antibodies against BVDV1 or a low level against BVDV2 took longer to become seronegative if they were vaccinated, but vaccinating calves with high levels of maternal antibodies did not prolong the presence of BVDV antibodies. Calves vaccinated with a parenteral multivalent MLV vaccine at 4 to 5 weeks of age showed increased BVDV1 antibody titers at 9 and 12 weeks postvaccination that were significantly different than age-matched unvaccinated controls, and calves similarly vaccinated at 7 to 8 weeks of age had slower decay of antibodies against BVDV2 compared with age-matched controls 6 to 12 weeks after vaccination.[34] In that study, calves vaccinated at 1 to 2 weeks were not different from their age-matched controls nor were there any differences between vaccination groups for the other pathogens (BRSV, BHV1, and PIV3) regardless of age at vaccination. Vaccination with a parenteral multivalent MLV vaccine at 2 weeks, 5 weeks, or both was not significantly associated with the rate of antibody decline for BRSV, BHV1, PIV3, BVDV1, or BVDV2 in dairy calves from birth to 3 months of age.[13] Interestingly, in that study, being treated for respiratory disease was associated with a reduced decay of BRSV-specific antibodies only for calves in the bottom 10th percentile of initial BRSV antibody titers, which suggests that calves with low initial antibody titers did produce endogenous antibodies as a result of natural exposure to BRSV but not from vaccination.

Together, these studies imply that although vaccination IFOMA does not consistently result in seroconversion, calves may produce endogenous specific antibodies in response to antigen exposure. However, detection of these antibodies may be challenging and inconsistent and is likely influenced by the initial levels of maternal antibodies and age at vaccination. A calf that possesses high levels of maternal antibodies would need to generate substantial amounts of endogenous antibodies to result in a 4-fold or even detectable increase in antibody titer. Therefore, humoral responses by the calf may be difficult to detect even if they do occur. Perhaps seroconversion should be redefined in neonates to account for a prolonged antibody decline as opposed to simply a 4-fold increase in titer, but what exactly would constitute an appropriate measure of humoral response to vaccination IFOMA remains undefined.

Cell-Mediated Immune Responses in Young Calves

Quantifying antibody titers before and after vaccination provides only a limited view of specific humoral immunity and ignores the potentially diverse kinds of immune responses that can be generated by vaccination IFOMA. There is variable evidence that cell-mediated immune responses (CMI) may be generated in young calves even if there is no evidence of a humoral response.

Calves with maternal antibodies against BHV1 were described as lacking antibody responses to IN inoculation with BHV1 but developed CMI as detected with a BHV1-specific interferon-gamma (IFN-γ) assay.[20] Despite the presence of passively acquired BVDV antibodies, inoculation with BVDV2 or vaccination with an MLV vaccine against BVDV1 and BVDV2 at 2 to 5 weeks of age both resulted in T-cell responses without any evidence of a humoral response.[35] In that study, calves vaccinated with a killed BVDV vaccine showed neither response. In contrast, calves vaccinated parenterally with a 10-way killed vaccine containing BHV1, BVDV1, and BVDV2 at 5 months of age had a mean BHV1- and BVDV-specific in vitro IFN-γ concentration that was significantly greater than unvaccinated calves at 7 days after challenge, and a significant disease-sparing effect was reported.[36] However, the calves in the latter study were seronegative at vaccination. Seropositive calves vaccinated IFOMA with a parenteral multivalent MLV vaccine at 1 to 2 weeks, 4 to 5 weeks, or 7 to 8 weeks of age and challenged 12 weeks later with BVDV2 showed variable but extensive evidence of activation (CD25 expression, IFN-γ, and interleukin-4 production) of CD4$^+$, CD8$^+$, and $\gamma\delta$ T cells.[34] Activation markers were often higher among vaccinated calves compared with their age-matched unvaccinated controls when peripheral blood mononuclear cells were stimulated with BVDV1 or BVDV2, both prechallenge and postchallenge, but similar evidence of CMI was seldom observed for BRSV, BHV1, or PIV3. In another study, when passively immune calves were vaccinated with an MLV vaccine containing BHV1, BRSV, PIV3, BVDV1, and BVDV2 at 2 or 70 days of age via either IN or SC administration, no effects on CMI were identified.[37]

Based on these studies and others, it seems calves may be capable of generating a CMI when immunized IFOMA, but that it depends on calf age, level of maternal antibodies, and type of antigenic challenge. Although CMI is the principle immune response desired for protection against viral diseases, few studies report the impacts of vaccination IFOMA on CMI. Additional studies investigating the impacts of vaccination IFOMA on CMI are required.

Anamnestic Responses from Priming in the Face of Maternal Antibodies

Immunologic memory that results in an anamnestic immune response is a key component of disease protection and the fundamental purpose of vaccination. There is evidence that calves vaccinated IFOMA may be primed to have an anamnestic response to later vaccination or disease exposure, even if they have no demonstrable primary response[19,35,38] (see **Fig. 1**C); however, this anamnestic response depends on a variety of factors and does not consistently occur.[39,40]

Calves vaccinated IFOMA at 7 weeks of age with parenteral MLV or killed BVDV1 and BVDV2 vaccines showed no detectable increases in antibody titers initially but had an anamnestic response upon revaccination 14 weeks later with an MLV vaccine against BVDV2.[35] These findings are consistent with some studies[19,38] but conflict with others.[12,37] Humoral and CMI responses to booster vaccination against BHV1, BRSV, PIV3, BVDV1, and BVDV2 at weaning were not different between calves that had or had not been vaccinated IFOMA.[37] Similarly, BRSV-seropositive calves vaccinated at the age of 3 to 9 days with an MLV vaccine containing BRSV did not seroconvert nor was there any evidence of an anamnestic humoral or CMI response following challenge at 11 weeks of age.[12] On the other hand, calves vaccinated with a parenteral multivalent MLV vaccine showed an anamnestic response to BVDV challenge 12 weeks after vaccination when they were initially vaccinated at 4 to 5 or 7 to 8 weeks of age but not at 1 to 2 weeks of age.[34]

These studies demonstrate that although primary responses may not be observed when vaccinating calves IFOMA, in some situations immunologic memory can be generated, depending on the specific pathogen and vaccine being used (see **Fig. 1**C). Differences among studies, including how the memory responses are assessed (eg, humoral immunity vs CMI), study design (eg, age of the calves, time between vaccination, adjuvant), and confounding variables (eg, breed, nutrition, exposure to wild-type pathogens) likely play an important role in the variability in study outcomes. In general, it appears calves vaccinated IFOMA can sometimes be primed for an anamnestic immune response upon reexposure to the antigen, although the underlying immune mechanisms and factors that influence them remain largely unknown.

Immune Responses to Disease Challenge

Although various assays for humoral and CMI responses do provide useful information about the impact of vaccination IFOMA, protection against disease is the most relevant outcome that can be measured.

Calves inoculated with BVDV2 that mounted CMI but not humoral responses were protected against developing clinical signs of acute BVD upon a second challenge with BVDV2.[35] Calves vaccinated with a multivalent parenteral MLV vaccine at 1 to 2, 4 to 5, or 7 to 8 weeks of age had clinical and hematological evidence of protection against BVDV2 challenge 12 weeks after vaccination.[34] Also, significant disease-sparing effects were observed after BVDV2 challenge at approximately 20[41] or 35[42] weeks of age when either seropositive or seronegative calves were vaccinated at 4 to 5 weeks of age with an adjuvanted parenteral multivalent MLV vaccine containing BVDV1 and BVDV2. Even at as young as 3 days old, seropositive calves vaccinated with a multivalent MLV vaccine containing BVDV1 and BVDV2 had significantly less clinical disease and lower mortality upon BVDV2 challenge 7.5 months later.[43] Conversely, parenteral vaccination with an MLV vaccine against BRSV, BHV1, PIV3, and BVDV1 at 10 to 14 days of age in seropositive calves was ineffective at preventing disease when calves were challenged with virulent BVDV2 at 4.5 months of age, even though seronegative calves vaccinated at 10 to 14 days of age or at 4 months of age were clinically protected.[44] Similarly, Ellis and coworkers[12] found no significant difference in clinical scores and mortality between unvaccinated calves and seropositive calves vaccinated at 3 to 9 days old with a parenteral MLV containing BRSV after challenge at 11 weeks of age. In a field study that investigated the clinical effectiveness of vaccinating calves IFOMA, there was no significant effect on treatment risk when calves were vaccinated with a multivalent parenteral vaccine (BVDV1, BVDV2, BHV1, BRSV, PIV3) at 2 weeks, 5 weeks, or both.[45] However, the incidence of failed TPI was low in that population (11%), and the median age at first treatment of respiratory disease was 30 days, which was before most calves completed their assigned vaccination protocol.

A few studies that examined the efficacy of parenteral vaccination IFOMA provide support for protection against disease in small experimental pathogen challenge studies. However, these findings are not consistent and are likely influenced by the vaccine type, adjuvant, and pathogen challenge. The translations of vaccine efficacy against pathogen challenge in experimental models to vaccine effectiveness for disease protection against natural exposure remains to be clearly demonstrated.

Parenteral Vaccination in the Face of Maternal Antibodies in Clinical Practice

The interference of maternal antibodies has traditionally made the development of herd-level vaccination programs for young calves relatively challenging. Previously, the recommendation was to wait until maternal antibody concentrations had declined and the immune system of neonatal calves had matured[1] (see **Fig. 1**); thus, the optimal age for initial vaccination could range from within a week of birth up to almost a year of age. Unfortunately, this is of little use for veterinary practitioners aiming to advise their clients about when to vaccinate their calves.

The current literature on parenteral vaccination IFOMA can be summarized as the following:

- Efficacy of parenteral preweaning vaccination in seronegative calves has been repeatedly proven; however, these calves are ideally only a subgroup of the target population in clinical practice, if appropriate colostrum management practices are being used. Nonetheless, calves with suspected or confirmed failed TPI, which are by definition the population of calves most at risk of disease, are likely to respond positively to parenteral vaccination as early as the first week of life.
- In calves with high maternal antibody titers, the likelihood of seroconversion after parenteral vaccine administration is low; however, vaccination IFOMA may prolong the presence of specific antibodies in some cases. The presence of specific antibodies is associated with a reduced risk of disease after pathogen challenge. Therefore, extending the period of time when antibodies are present by vaccinating IFOMA may be beneficial for clinical protection, although this hypothesis has not been sufficiently tested.
- Few studies have investigated CMI, immunologic memory, and disease prevention after parenteral vaccination IFOMA, and the findings are variable. Some small experimental studies have shown disease-sparing effects of parenteral vaccination IFOMA. Additional studies that examine nonhumoral immunologic outcomes and clinical effectiveness in the field are required.

POTENTIAL VACCINATION STRATEGIES IN THE FACE OF MATERNAL ANTIBODIES

Although not a new area of research,[46] investigations of strategies to bypass the impacts of maternal antibodies on vaccine effectiveness have been reinvigorated by studies revealing that mucosal innoculation with a pathogen IFOMA can result in various immune responses in the bovine neonate[35,38] (see **Fig. 1**D) have reinvigorated investigation of strategies to bypass the impacts of maternal antibodies on vaccine effectiveness. Because mucosal surfaces present one of the most common entrances for pathogens in the neonate and are equipped with a variety of innate and adaptive immune mechanisms, they play a considerable role in neonatal immunology. With several new IN vaccines becoming commercially available over the last decade, opportunities have arisen to explore the circumvention of maternal antibodies via mucosal immunization. Oral vaccines also exist but are beyond the scope of this review.

Administering Parenteral Vaccines Intranasally

Before IN vaccines became commercially available, several studies investigated mucosal immunization by administering parenteral vaccines IN.

When a parenteral multivalent vaccine (BVDV1, BVDV2, BRSV, PIV3, BHV1, MH, and PM) was given IN to 3- to 8-day-old seronegative calves, they were generally protected from clinical disease after viral challenge 3 to 4 weeks later, and they generated higher antibody titers and shed fewer viruses than unvaccinated seronegative calves.[47] The IN administration of an injectable BRSV vaccine twice (6 and 9 weeks of age) to seronegative calves also led to protection against disease following BRSV challenge 21 days later.[48] On the other hand, when a BRSV vaccine licensed for SC administration was given IN to seropositive 3- to 8-day-old calves and they were challenged with BRSV 4.5 months later, there were minimal clinical differences from unvaccinated controls.[40]

Unfortunately, immunologic studies that show vaccine efficacy in seronegative calves are of questionable clinical value, albeit necessary for product licensing, because they cannot be reliably translated to seropositive calves.

Intranasal Viral Vaccination in Seronegative Versus Seropositive Calves

An important difference among vaccination trials is whether calves are seronegative or seropositive to the antigen in question at the time of vaccination, with the latter obviously being more clinically relevant for vaccination IFOMA.

A series of studies investigated seronegative and seropositive calves vaccinated IFOMA at approximately 3 weeks old with an IN attenuated live viral vaccine against BRSV and PIV3 and later challenged with BRSV[49] or PIV3.[50] Vaccination of seronegative calves resulted in some disease-sparing effects, but overall the clinical signs of BRSV were mild in that study.[49] In contrast, in the study of seropositive calves, clinical symptoms of BRSV were moderate to severe, and there were no statistical differences between vaccinated and unvaccinated calves.[49] The PIV3 challenge resulted in only mild clinical disease, and only some slight differences in rectal temperature were observed between vaccinates and controls for both seropositive and seronegative calves.[50] However, viral shedding of BRSV and PIV3 was significantly reduced by IN vaccination in both seropositive and seronegative calves.[49,50] An IN MLV vaccine against BHV1, BRSV, and PIV3 was assessed for its efficacy against BRSV[11] and BHV1[51] in seronegative and seropositive calves at 3 to 8 days of age. When challenged with BRSV within 7 to 9 weeks of vaccination, all calves became ill, but vaccinated calves had less severe clinical signs, reduced lung lesions, and lower mortality.[11] Vaccination of seronegative calves resulted in increased levels of BRSV-specific antibodies and reduced nasal shedding of BRSV, but vaccination IFOMA did not. Furthermore, there was only slight clinical protection and no difference in mortality when calves were challenged 14 weeks after vaccination, indicating that the duration of protection was relatively short lived. Interestingly, seronegative and seropositive vaccinated calves had greater anamnestic antibody responses than unvaccinated calves after BRSV challenge, regardless of when that challenge occurred, suggesting that priming did occur but that vaccination IFOMA was insufficient to protect against challenge greater than 3 months after vaccination. When calves were vaccinated in the same way but were challenged with BHV1 at 4 or 28 weeks (for seronegative calves) or 15 weeks (for seropositive calves) after vaccination, vaccinated calves shed less virus than unvaccinated controls and had reduced risk (seronegative) or duration (seropositive) of clinical signs.[51] Seronegative but not seropositive vaccinated calves had higher titers than unvaccinated calves shortly after vaccination, but all vaccinated calves had higher anamnestic antibody titers than control calves after challenge.

These studies demonstrate that although the immunologic responses do vary between seronegative and seropositive calves, IN vaccination IFOMA can induce clinically relevant protection, albeit of relatively short duration and variable magnitude (see **Fig. 1**D). Furthermore, viral shedding may be reduced, and immunologic priming can occur regardless of the serologic status at the time of IN vaccination.

Comparing Intranasal and Parenteral Routes of Administration

A few studies have compared the IN and SC route of administration to help determine optimal vaccination strategies for calves IFOMA.

When route (IN and SC) and age at administration (2 and 70 days old) were compared for a 5-way (BHV1, BRSV, PIV3, BVDV1, and BVDV2) MLV vaccine, calves vaccinated SC at 70 days of age had significantly higher titers of BVDV1 antibodies after initial vaccination compared with other vaccination groups and unvaccinated controls.[37] Anamnestic responses to a booster at weaning of calves vaccinated IFOMA (IN or SC) did not differ from control calves that were vaccinated for the first time at weaning, although the BVDV1 titers were higher in IN-vaccinated calves (2 or 70 days of age) compared with SC-vaccinated calves (2 days of age only). More recently, an IN 3-way (BHV1, BRSV, PIV3) MLV vaccine given to dairy calves at 3 to 6 days and 6 weeks of age was compared with an SC 5-way (BHV1, BRSV, PIV3, BVDV1, BVDV2) MLV vaccine at 6 weeks of age or negative (placebo) controls.[52] Vaccinated calves (both IN and SC) had lower odds of lung consolidation observed via ultrasonography relative to unvaccinated calves, and IN-vaccinated calves had lower odds than SC-vaccinated calves; however, when accounting for significant covariates, there was no difference in clinical respiratory disease between groups. This field study suggests that IN or SC vaccination IFOMA may decrease subclinical but not clinical respiratory disease and that IN vaccination may be somewhat superior. When simultaneous administration of an IN 3-way (BHV1, BRSV, PIV3) MLV vaccine and SC MH bacterial leukotoxoid vaccine was compared with administration of an SC 5-way (BVDV1, BVDV2, BHV1, BRSV, PIV3) MLV vaccine and MH vaccine in beef calves at 8 to 14 weeks of age, calves vaccinated IN IFOMA had greater BRSV antibody titers after both the primary and the secondary vaccinations than calves vaccinated parenterally.[53]

Overall, it seems IN vaccination IFOMA may be a more effective vaccination strategy than parenteral vaccination IFOMA, although responses may be variable and disease protection is not complete.

Intranasal Vaccination in the Face of Maternal Antibodies in Clinical Practice

The current literature on IN vaccination IFOMA can be summarized as the following:

- Recent research has given cause to be optimistic that IN vaccination may circumvent interference by maternal antibodies; however, clinical protection is inconsistent and relatively short lived.
- Viral shedding can be decreased, and immunologic priming may be induced by IN vaccination IFOMA in seronegative and seropositive calves.

- Unfortunately, there is a paucity of field studies that explore IN vaccination in populations of colostrum-fed calves with an externally valid spectrum of maternal antibody titers. Further studies are needed to truly understand when and how IN vaccines should be used IFOMA and how they compare to parenteral vaccines.

INTEGRATING VACCINATION IN THE FACE OF MATERNAL ANTIBODIES INTO HERD-LEVEL VACCINATION PROGRAMS

One of the challenges with translating vaccination studies into on-farm vaccination protocols is that research rarely investigates integrated immunization strategies. In actual production systems, vaccination IFOMA does not occur in isolation but is impacted by factors such as replacement heifer and breeding cow herd vaccination strategies, calving and colostrum management practices, nutrition and housing, historical herd-level disease risk, potential marketing advantages, and concurrent vaccine administration. Few immunologic research projects are able to incorporate these factors into their scope, but a few recent examples demonstrate that it can and should be attempted.

Concurrent Administration of Vaccines

Rarely are single-antigen vaccines administered, and several multivalent vaccines are commonly given at the same time, particularly in beef herds where opportunities to access animals are limited. Previous work has suggested that administering multiple vaccines at once may cause a reduction in immune response to certain antigens.[54] However, it may be that strategically using different routes of administration could avoid this issue.[53,55]

Ten-to 13-week-old beef calves with low BHV1 antibody titers were vaccinated with either an SC MH leukotoxoid vaccine alone, an IN 2-way (BHV1 and PIV3) MLV vaccine and the same SC MH vaccine, or an IN 3-way (BHV1, BRSV, PIV3) MLV vaccine and the same SC MH vaccine.[55] The humoral response to MH was equivalent, regardless of whether the SC MH vaccine was administered alone or at the same time as an IN multivalent vaccine containing BHV1. Simultaneous administration of an IN 3-way (BHV1, BRSV, PIV3) MLV vaccine, SC MLV BVDV vaccine, and SC MH vaccine was compared with administration of SC administration of a combination MLV (BVDV1, BVDV2, BHV1, BRSV, PIV3) and MH vaccine in maternal colostrum-fed beef calves at 8 to 14 weeks of age.[53] There was no difference in the initial MH leukotoxoid antibody response between treatment groups after the primary vaccination, and both groups of calves vaccinated IFOMA did show an increase in MH titer after booster. However, calves that had been initially vaccinated with a single combination vaccine had better anamnestic responses than those that received 3 separate vaccines.

It is important to note that all the aforementioned recent reports[53–55] were conducted at least in part by the pharmaceutical company that produces the studied vaccines. It remains an important question that requires further investigation: what is the impact of route of administration when giving multiple concurrent vaccines to calves IFOMA?

Sequential Administration of Vaccines

Early calfhood is only 1 stage of the production cycle, so vaccination IFOMA is just 1 issue in terms of herd-level vaccination strategies. If calves are vaccinated IFOMA, it should be investigated how this fits with vaccines given at other points in the production cycle.

In a longitudinal study, dams were vaccinated with a killed glycoprotein E negative (gE)⁻ BHV1 marker vaccine 84 and 56 days before calving, resulting in high levels of gE$^-$ BHV1 antibodies in their calves that blocked humoral responses to IN vaccination at 14 days of life with an MLV BHV1 vaccine.[16] Similarly, these same calves were BRSV seropositive after colostrum ingestion and also showed no humoral response to SC vaccination at 14 and 42 days of age with an inactivated BRSV vaccine. This study illustrates that it should be considered how dams are vaccinated when deciding how and when to vaccinate preweaned calves.

Another study evaluated the efficacy of 3 typical calf vaccination protocols used on cow-calf ranches in western Canada: an IN 3-way (BHV1, BRSV, PIV3) MLV vaccine at birth followed by either an MLV or killed parenteral 5-way (BHV1, BRSV, PIV3, BVDV1, BVDV2) vaccine at 2 months of age, compared with just a 5-way (BHV1, BRSV, PIV3, BVDV1, BVDV2) MLV parenteral vaccine at 2 months of age.[56] Calves were subsequently challenged with BRSV aerosolized in an enclosed trailer at 6 to 7 months of age, similar to what might occur at weaning. The only difference in efficacy of vaccination programs was that calves that received IN at birth and a killed vaccine as booster had higher blood oxygen levels after challenge and a stronger anamnestic response. Thus, as IN vaccination IFOMA is integrated into vaccine programs, it must be also considered how and when to booster for optimal protection.

Similarly, a recent large field trial attempted to investigate various vaccination strategies within a single large cow-calf herd, including IN vaccination at birth, IN or parenteral vaccination at spring processing (approximately 60 days of age), and/or IN or parenteral vaccination preweaning (approximately 210 days of age).[57] The IN vaccine was an MLV vaccine against BHV1, BRSV, and PIV3, while the parenteral vaccines were either a BVDV and MH vaccine or a 5-way MLV (BHV1, BRSV, PIV3, BVDV1, BVDV2) and MH vaccine. Calves that were vaccinated IN at birth had significantly higher BRSV-specific IgG titers at 60 days compared with unvaccinated calves. Unfortunately, because of suspected but undiagnosed exposure to wild-type BRSV, the remaining findings in that study are difficult to interpret.

These studies attempted to investigate the complexities of integrated vaccination programs and should serve as examples of the types of clinical research that is needed to inform evidence-based herd-level vaccination recommendations.

SUMMARY

- Because of substantive herd- and calf-level variability when it comes to initial maternal antibody titers and decay of these antibodies, developing a "one-size-fits-all" recommendation regarding optimal timing for primary and secondary immunization of calves IFOMA is challenging.
- High levels of circulating maternal antibodies in the calf at the time of parenteral vaccination are likely to inhibit seroconversion and may also have relevant negative impacts on CMI, pathogen shedding, and risk of clinical disease. However, parenteral vaccination IFOMA may prolong the presence of antibodies or result in immunologic priming, which may be clinically beneficial. Furthermore, there is some evidence that parenteral vaccination IFOMA can reduce clinical symptoms after experimental pathogen challenge.
- Calves with low levels of maternal antibodies are rarely identified in the field, and the time when most calves become seronegative cannot be easily predicted. Herds with inadequate precalving vaccination or poor colostrum management may benefit from vaccinating their calves earlier in life more so than herds that consistently ensure adequate TPI. Ensuring consistent dam vaccination practices and optimal colostrum management will improve the uniformity of the age at which calves are likely to respond to vaccination IFOMA.

- Alternatively, mucosal immunization via IN vaccination may be an advisable strategy to circumvent interference by maternal antibodies and provide short-term disease-sparing effects, particularly in herds where TPI is good. Although immune protection may not be elicited in all calves that receive IN vaccination IFOMA, immunologic priming may occur so that anamnestic responses will be generated upon later vaccination. The optimal timing, route, and type (killed vs MLV) of booster vaccine to be administered following IN priming has yet to be determined.
- Specific issues that require additional clinical research include the following:
  - Effectiveness of commercial vaccines administered to seropositive calves facing natural pathogen exposure;
  - Induction of clinically relevant outcome measures, such as CMI and protection against disease from vaccination IFOMA;
  - Impacts of integrated vaccination programs (eg, dam and neonatal vaccination strategies; preweaning and postweaning vaccination strategies);
  - Interaction of various routes of administration (eg, IN and SC) and types of vaccines (eg, MLV vs killed) as used in prime-boost vaccination strategies;
  - Impacts of adjuvants on vaccination IFOMA.

ACKNOWLEDGMENTS

The authors thank Amelia Woolums, Jennifer Pearson, Bruce Stover, and Haley Silas for proofreading this article and Nicole Hawe for helping prepare the citations.

REFERENCES

1. Chase CCL, Hurley DJ, Reber AJ. Neonatal immune development in the calf and its impact on vaccine response. Vet Clin North Am Food Anim Pract 2008;24(1): 87–104.
2. Cortese VS. Neonatal immunology. Vet Clin North Am Food Anim Pract 2009; 25(1):221–7.
3. Firth MA, Shewen PE, Hodgins DC. Passive and active components of neonatal innate immune defenses. Anim Heal Res Rev 2005;6(2):143–58.
4. Barrington GM, Parish SM. Bovine neonatal immunology. Vet Clin North Am Food Anim Pract 2001;17(3):463–76.
5. McGee M, Earley B. Review: passive immunity in beef-suckler calves. Animal 2019;13(4):810–25.
6. Godden S. Colostrum management for dairy calves. Vet Clin North Am Food Anim Pract 2008. https://doi.org/10.1016/j.cvfa.2007.10.005.
7. Waldner CL, Rosengren LB. Factors associated with serum immunoglobulin levels in beef calves from Alberta and Saskatchewan and association between passive transfer and health outcomes. Can Vet J 2009;50(3):275–81.
8. Chigerwe M, Hagey JV, Aly SS. Determination of neonatal serum immunoglobulin G concentrations associated with mortality during the first 4 months of life in dairy heifer calves. J Dairy Res 2015;82(4):400–6.
9. Buczinski S, Gicquel E, Fecteau G, et al. Systematic review and meta-analysis of diagnostic accuracy of serum refractometry and Brix refractometry for the diagnosis of inadequate transfer of passive immunity in calves. J Vet Intern Med 2018. https://doi.org/10.1111/jvim.14893.
10. Raboisson D, Trillat P, Cahuzac C. Failure of passive immune transfer in calves: a meta-analysis on the consequences and assessment of the economic impact. PLoS One 2016;11(3):1–19.

11. Ellis JA, Gow SP, Mahan S, et al. Duration of immunity to experimental infection with bovine respiratory syncytial virus following intranasal vaccination of young passively immune calves. J Am Vet Med Assoc 2013;243(11):1602–8.

12. Ellis J, Gow S, Bolton M, et al. Inhibition of priming for bovine respiratory syncytial virus-specific protective immune responses following parenteral vaccination of passively immune calves. Can Vet J 2014;55(12):1180–5.

13. Windeyer MC, Leslie KE, Godden SM, et al. Association of bovine respiratory disease or vaccination with serologic response in dairy heifer calves up to three months of age. Am J Vet Res 2015;76(3):239–45.

14. Chamorro MF, Walz PH, Passler T, et al. Efficacy of multivalent, modified-live virus (MLV) vaccines administered to early weaned beef calves subsequently challenged with virulent bovine viral diarrhea virus type 2. BMC Vet Res 2015; 11(1):29.

15. Al-Alo KZK, Nikbakht Brujeni G, Lotfollahzadeh S, et al. Correlation between neonatal calf diarrhea and the level of maternally derived antibodies. Iran J Vet Res 2018;19(1):3–8. Available at: https://www.ncbi.nlm.nih.gov/pubmed/29805455.

16. Earley B, Tiernan K, Duffy C, et al. Effect of suckler cow vaccination against glycoprotein E (gE)-negative bovine herpesvirus type 1 (BoHV-1) on passive immunity and physiological response to subsequent bovine respiratory disease vaccination of their progeny. Res Vet Sci 2018;118:43–51.

17. Chamorro MF, Woolums A, Walz PH. Vaccination of calves against common respiratory viruses in the face of maternally derived antibodies (IFOMA). Anim Health Res Rev 2016;17(02):79–84.

18. Petrini S, Iscaro C, Righi C. Antibody responses to bovine alphaherpesvirus 1 (BoHV-1) in passively immunized calves. Viruses 2019;11(1):23.

19. Brar JS, Johnson DW, Muscoplat CC, et al. Maternal immunity to infectious bovine rhinotracheitis and bovine viral diarrhea viruses: duration and effect on vaccination in young calves. Am J Vet Res 1978;39(2):241–4.

20. Lemaire M, Weynants V, Godfroid J, et al. Effects of bovine herpesvirus type 1 infection in calves with maternal antibodies on immune response and virus latency. J Clin Microbiol 2000;38(5):1885–94. Available at: http://jcm.asm.org/content/38/5/1885.abstract.

21. Kirkpatrick J, Fulton R, Burge L, et al. Passively transferred immunity in newborn calves, rate of antibody decay, and effect on subsequent vaccination with modified live virus vaccine. Bov Pract 2001;35:47–54.

22. Muñoz-Zanzi CA, Thurmond MC, Johnson WO, et al. Predicted ages of dairy calves when colostrum-derived bovine viral diarrhea virus antibodies would no longer offer protection against disease or interfere with vaccination. J Am Vet Med Assoc 2002;221(5):678–85.

23. Fulton RW, Briggs RE, Payton ME, et al. Maternally derived humoral immunity to bovine viral diarrhea virus (BVDV) 1a, BVDV1b, BVDV2, bovine herpesvirus-1, parainfluenza-3 virus bovine respiratory syncytial virus, Mannheimia haemolytica and Pasteurella multocida in beef calves, antibody decline by half-life studies and effect on response to vaccination. Vaccine 2004;22(5–6):643–9.

24. Niewiesk S. Maternal antibodies: clinical significance, mechanism of interference with immune responses, and possible vaccination strategies. Front Immunol 2014;5:446.

25. Waldner CL, Parker S, Campbell JR. Vaccine usage in western Canadian cow-calf herds. Can Vet J 2019;60(4):414–22.

26. Murray CF, Fick LJ, Pajor EA, et al. Calf management practices and associations with herd-level morbidity and mortality on beef cow-calf operations. Animal 2016; 10(3):468–77.
27. Waldner C, Jelinski MD, McIntyre-Zimmer K. Survey of western Canadian beef producers regarding calf-hood diseases, management practices, and veterinary service usage. Can Vet J 2013;54(6):559–64. Available at: https://www.ncbi.nlm. nih.gov/pubmed/24155446.
28. United States Department of Agriculture National Animal Health Monitoring Sytem. Beef 2007-2008 part IV: reference of beef cow-calf management practices in the United States, 2007-08 2010.
29. United States Department of Agriculture National Animal Health Monitoring System. Beef cow/calf health & productivity audit 1993, Part III: beef cow/calf health management 1994.
30. United States Department of Agriculture National Animal Health Monitoring System. Dairy herd management practices focusing on preweaned heifer calves, April 1991-July 1992 1993.
31. United States Department of Agriculture National Animals Health Monitoring System. Dairy 2014 dairy cattle management practices in the United States, 2014 2016.
32. Van Donkersgoed J, van den Hurk JV, McCartney D, et al. Comparative serological response in calves to eight commercial vaccines against infectious bovine rhinotracheitis, parainfluenza-3, bovine respiratory syncytial, and bovine viral diarrhea viruses. Can Vet J 1991;32(12):727–33. Available at: https://www.ncbi. nlm.nih.gov/pubmed/17423913.
33. Woolums AR. Vaccinating calves: new information on the effects of maternal immunity. Proc 40th Annu Conf Am Assoc Bov Pract. Vancouver, BC, Canada, 2007;40. p. 10–7.
34. Platt R, Widel PW, Kesi LD, et al. Comparison of humoral and cellular immune responses to a pentavalent modified live virus vaccine in three age groups of calves with maternal antibodies, before and after BVDV type 2 challenge. Vaccine 2009;27:4508–19.
35. Endsley JJ, Roth JA, Ridpath J, et al. Maternal antibody blocks humoral but not T cell responses to BVDV. Biologicals 2003;31(2):123–5.
36. Van Anne TR, Rinehart CL, Buterbaugh RE, et al. Cell-mediated and humoral immune responses to bovine herpesvirus type 1 and bovine viral diarrhea virus in calves following administration of a killed-virus vaccine and bovine herpesvirus type 1 challenge. Am J Vet Res 2018;79(11):1166–78.
37. Woolums AR, Berghaus RD, Berghaus LJ, et al. Effect of calf age and administration route of initial multivalent modified-live virus vaccine on humoral and cell-mediated immune responses following subsequent administration of a booster vaccination at weaning in beef calves. Am J Vet Res 2013;74(2):343–54.
38. Ridpath JE, Neill JD, Endsley J, et al. Effect of passive immunity on the development of a protective immune response against bovine viral diarrhea virus in calves. Am J Vet Res 2003;64(1):65–9.
39. Woolums AR, Berghaus RD, Smith DR, et al. Producer survey of herd-level risk factors for nursing beef calf respiratory disease. J Am Vet Med Assoc 2013; 243(4):538–47. Available at: http://search.proquest.com/docview/1417529934/.
40. Ellis JA, Gow SP, Goji N. Response to experimentally induced infection with bovine respiratory syncytial virus following intranasal vaccination of seropositive and seronegative calves. J Am Vet Med Assoc 2010;236(9):991–9.

41. Zimmerman AD, Boots RE, Walli JL, et al. Evaluation of protection against virulent bovine viral diarrhea virus type 2 in calves that had maternal antibodies and were vaccinated with a modified-live vaccine. J Am Vet Med Assoc 2006;228(11): 1757–61.

42. Zimmerman AD, Buterbaugh RE, Schnackel JA, et al. Efficacy of a modified-live virus vaccine administered to calves with maternal antibodies and challenged seven months later with a virulent bovine viral diarrhea type 2 virus. Bov Pract 2009;43(1):35–43.

43. Stevens ET, Brown MS, Burdett WW, et al. Efficacy of a non-adjuvanted, modified-live virus vaccine in calves with maternal antibodies against a virulent bovine viral diarrhea virus type 2a challenge seven months following vaccination. Bov Pract 2011;45(1):23–31.

44. Ellis J, West K, Cortese V, et al. Effect of maternal antibodies on induction and persistence of vaccine-induced immune responses against bovine viral diarrhea virus type II in young calves. J Am Vet Med Assoc 2001;219(3):351–6.

45. Windeyer MC, Leslie KE, Godden SM, et al. The effects of viral vaccination of dairy heifer calves on the incidence of respiratory disease, mortality, and growth. J Dairy Sci 2012;95(11):6731–9.

46. Todd JD. Intranasal vaccination of cattle against IBR and PI3: field and laboratory observations in dairy, beef, and neonatal calf populations. Dev Biol Stand 1976; 33:391–5.

47. Xue W, Ellis J, Mattick D, et al. Immunogenicity of a modified-live virus vaccine against bovine viral diarrhea virus types 1 and 2, infectious bovine rhinotracheitis virus, bovine parainfluenza-3 virus, and bovine respiratory syncytial virus when administered intranasally in young calves. Vaccine 2010;28(22):3784–92.

48. Ellis J, Gow S, West K, et al. Response of calves to challenge exposure with virulent bovine respiratory syncytial virus following intranasal administration of vaccines formulated for parenteral administration. J Am Vet Med Assoc 2007; 230(2):233–43.

49. Vangeel I, Antonis AFG, Fluess M, et al. Efficacy of a modified live intranasal bovine respiratory syncytial virus vaccine in 3-week-old calves experimentally challenged with BRSV. Vet J 2007;174:627–35.

50. Vangeel I, Ioannou F, Riegler L, et al. Efficacy of an intranasal modified live bovine respiratory syncytial virus and temperature-sensitive parainfluenza type 3 virus vaccine in 3-week-old calves experimentally challenged with PI3V. Vet J 2009; 179:101–8.

51. Mahan SM, Sobecki B, Johnson J, et al. Efficacy of intranasal vaccination with a multivalent vaccine containing temperature-sensitive modified-live bovine herpesvirus type 1 for protection of seronegative and seropositive calves against respiratory disease. J Am Vet Med Assoc 2016;248(11):1280–6.

52. Ollivett TL, Leslie KE, Duffield TF, et al. Field trial to evaluate the effect of an intranasal respiratory vaccine protocol on calf health, ultrasonographic lung consolidation, and growth in Holstein dairy calves. J Dairy Sci 2018;101(9):8159–68.

53. Stokka GL, Neville B, Seeger JT, et al. Serological effect of two concurrent IBRV, BVDV, BRSV, PI3V, and Mannheimia haemolytica vaccination protocols and time interval between the first and second dose on the subsequent serological response to the BRSV and M. haemolytica fractions in suckling beef calves. Bov Pract 2016;50(1):21–7.

54. Cortese VS, Seeger JT, Stokka GS, et al. Serologic response to Mannheimia haemolytica in calves concurrently inoculated with inactivated or modified-live

preparations of M. haemolytica and viral combination vaccines containing modified-live bovine herpesvirus type 1. Am J Vet Res 2011;72(11):1541–9.

55. Stoltenow C, Cortese VS, Seeger JT, et al. Immunologic responses of beef calves to concurrent application of modified-live viral vaccine (intranasal and systemic administration) and systemically administered mannheimia haemolytica bacterin-leukotoxoid. Bov Pract 2011;45(2):132–9.

56. Ellis J, Gow S, Berenik A, et al. Comparative efficacy of modified-live and inactivated vaccines in boosting responses to bovine respiratory syncytial virus following neonatal mucosal priming of beef calves. Can Vet J 2018;59:1311–9.

57. Cortese VS, Seeger JT, Trejo C, et al. The impact of neonatal intranasal vaccination for bovine respiratory syncytial virus on subsequent vaccination and responses to natural exposure. JSM Allergy Asthma 2018;3(1):1021.

Vaccination Management of Beef Cattle

Delayed Vaccination and Endotoxin Stacking

John T. Richeson, PhD[a],*, Heather D. Hughes, PhD[b],
Paul R. Broadway, PhD[c], Jeffery A. Carroll, PhD[c]

KEYWORDS

- Bovine respiratory disease • Cattle • Endotoxin • Vaccination management

KEY POINTS

- When administered under appropriate conditions, vaccines provide safe, effective, and economically important immunologic prevention of respiratory and other infectious bovine diseases.
- Modified-live virus (MLV) vaccination against respiratory pathogens in cattle on feedlot arrival has been unanimously recommended by consulting veterinarians.
- There is surprisingly limited, but emerging literature, describing the efficiency and safety of vaccination in different cattle production environments, including delayed administration of MLV vaccines in stressed, high-risk cattle.
- Stress-induced immunosuppression in cattle is likely during weaning, marketing, and relocation to a stocker or feedlot facility and should be considered when designing efficient vaccination protocols.
- Endotoxin concentration and handling of gram-negative bacterins should be considered when designing vaccination protocols for cattle to reduce the potential for adverse reactions.

INTRODUCTION

Prevention of infectious diseases in beef cattle is critically important, yet difficult because of the segmented infrastructure of the beef industry. Cattle progress through different stages of production and may experience exposure to novel pathogens, transportation and relocation stress, different management, and commingling with other animals.[1,2] Although there are many potential infectious disease challenges that beef cattle may encounter, bovine respiratory disease (BRD) remains the most

Disclosure Statement: None.
[a] Department of Agricultural Sciences, West Texas A&M University, WTAMU Box 60998, Canyon, TX 79016, USA; [b] SciWrite Consulting, PO Box 1041, Canyon, TX 79015, USA; [c] USDA-ARS Livestock Issues Unit, 1604 East FM 1294, Lubbock, TX 79403, USA
* Corresponding author.
E-mail address: jricheson@wtamu.edu

prevalent and costly disease affecting cattle production in North America, and the impact is greatest in the stocker and feedlot sectors of the beef industry.[3] Stress-induced immune dysfunction, viral infection, and bronchopneumonia caused by bacteria are interwoven within the complicated etiology of BRD. Therefore, vaccination against viral and bacterial agents involved in BRD is a vital instrument in the "animal health tool box" for cow-calf, stocker, and feedlot operators.

Some important considerations regarding vaccination of beef cattle at the cow-calf, preconditioning, stocker, and feedlot phases of beef production include the following:

- Cow-calf phase: at birth, branding, and weaning, beef calves could experience acute (short-term) rather than chronic (long-term) stress, which may result in priming of the immune system and contribute to an enhanced vaccine response in calves.[4] In general, the timing of vaccination during the cow-calf phase is most favorable because it allows sufficient time for vaccinates to develop immunologic protection before natural challenge with BRD-causative agents during and after transition to a stocker or feedlot facility.
- Preconditioning phase: calves that are vaccinated and retained on their ranch of origin after weaning for other preparatory management exhibit less morbidity and health costs at the feedlot and generate greater net return to the cow-calf producer because calf value is increased.[5–8] Despite clear health improvements for preconditioned cattle, the industry-wide adoption of this management practice is low, as only 39% of all beef operations vaccinated calves against respiratory disease before sale.[9]
- Stocker phase: most beef calves placed in stocker programs are lightweight, immunologically naïve, and stressed. Veterinary practitioners and stocker producers should consider vaccine safety and the potential for inadvertent antigenic enhancement of modified-live virus (MLV) vaccines administered to newly received stocker calves. Because subsequent disease challenge in the feedlot phase is probable, stocker calves should be administered vaccines with adequate time for immunization to occur before feedlot shipment. However, stocker producers should consider delaying MLV vaccination for 14 to 30 days after arrival, as improved health and performance outcomes have been reported in high-risk stocker calves using this strategy.[10,11]
- Feedlot phase: the adoption rate of respiratory vaccination in the feedlot is nearly 100% due to tradition, practical design, and labor structure of feedlot facilities, and the relatively low cost of vaccines.[12] However, further research is needed to understand the efficiency of vaccination against the numerous disease-causing agents that exist in the feedlot. As suggested for the stocker phase, delayed MLV vaccination may improve health outcomes in auction-derived feedlot cattle.[13]

CURRENT VACCINATION RECOMMENDATIONS

Beef cow-calf operations and feedlots across North America are frequently provided vaccine recommendations from veterinary practitioners or other sources; however, a scarcity of literature exists that summarizes and reports these recommendations at the cow-calf level.[14] In contrast, several publications exist that describe recommendations and practices for vaccination and health management at the feedlot level.[12,15,16]

Results from a US Department of Agriculture (USDA)-Animal and Plant Health Inspection Service survey[17] indicated that although vaccinating cattle is a relatively common practice in the cow-calf sector, it is not universally adopted, which leaves a significant portion of the US beef cattle population susceptible to numerous preventable diseases. Only 68.9% of cow-calf operations vaccinated cattle for any disease in 2007,[17] which is in sharp contrast to a 2016 survey of veterinary practitioners indicating that 93% of cow-calf operations in the United State have a vaccination plan in place for cattle.[14] It is possible that recommendations and/or adoption of vaccination protocols changed over the 9-year lapse between surveys; however, it is more likely that a discrepancy between veterinarian recommendations of vaccination and implementation by beef cow-calf operations exists. This is further supported by a survey indicating that only 39% of all beef operations vaccinated calves against respiratory disease before sale,[9] despite the overwhelming recommendation of veterinarians to vaccinate calves against BRD pathogens during the cow-calf production phase.

There are 3 distinct times in the cow-calf sector when veterinarians recommend initial vaccinations: at branding, before weaning, and after weaning. According to a survey,[14] the most common vaccine antigens recommended for calves vaccinated at branding were clostridial (96%), infectious bovine rhinotracheitis virus (IBRV; 94%), bovine respiratory syncytial virus (BRSV; 91%), parainfluenza-3 virus (PI-3V; 90%), and bovine viral diarrhea virus (BVDV) Type 1 and 2 (78% and 77%, respectively). Eighty percent of veterinarians recommended MLV vaccines at this time, with 12% of veterinarians recommending killed virus vaccines at branding.

When vaccinating calves for the first time before weaning, the most frequently recommended vaccine antigens were IBRV (99%), BRSV (98%), BVDV Types 1 and 2 (96%), PI-3 (93%), clostridial (77%), and Mannheimia haemolytica (77%).[14] Before weaning, most veterinarians recommended using MLV over killed virus vaccines (90% and 10%, respectively). First-time vaccination recommendations for cattle after weaning were for BVDV Type 2 (97%), IBRV (97%), BVDV Type 1 (96%), BRSV (96%), and PI-3V (91%).[14] As calf age increased (ie, preweaning vs postweaning), there was a slight increase in the percentage of veterinarians who recommended MLV vaccines versus killed virus vaccines (93% and 7%, respectively).[14]

Although the preceding information is consistent with other vaccine recommendations[18] and reports,[19–21] where most veterinarians recommended routine administration of respiratory vaccines to beef calves, the USDA reported[9] that 60.6% of beef cow-calf operations (accounting for 30% of the US cattle population) did not vaccinate calves for respiratory disease from birth until the time they were sold. This discrepancy between veterinarian recommendation and producer implementation is concerning, given that 99% of veterinarians in the United States and Canada recommend some type of vaccination protocol at the cow-calf level of production.[14]

For the feedlot sector, however, there is a stark contrast in respiratory vaccine use, as administration of a multivalent respiratory vaccine during initial feedlot processing is nearly 100%.[12] Furthermore, consulting feedlot veterinarians revealed that they unanimously recommend respiratory vaccination during initial processing of cattle considered high risk.[12] Despite a limited amount of research-based evidence to support on-arrival vaccination of high-risk cattle, it has been a routine practice in feedlots for decades. Several previous reviews have examined respiratory vaccination outcomes in the production setting and convey a general lack of evidence for vaccine efficiency in high-risk, newly received beef cattle.[22–24] Therefore, a need exists to critically examine current vaccination paradigms in the beef industry and consider the safety of vaccination under various conditions (eg, acute vs chronic stress, production phase, commingling), the types of vaccines selected (MLV vs killed virus), and timing of vaccine administration in relation to expected natural pathogen challenge.

VACCINE EFFICACY VERSUS EFFICIENCY

The distinction between vaccine efficacy and efficiency is critical for understanding vaccination management. Commercial vaccines that are deemed efficacious via USDA approval standards for biologics may not be efficient under all circumstances or in all vaccinates in the production setting.[25] Vaccine efficacy is defined as the percent reduction in disease incidence and pathology in a vaccinated group compared with an unvaccinated group. Typically, this is determined from a controlled BRD challenge model with previously vaccinated and nonvaccinated calves that have been inoculated with a respiratory virus and bacteria. A vaccine may also be considered efficacious if it has biological activity and stimulates an active immune response against the agents in the vaccine.

Vaccine efficiency may be defined as the ability of a vaccine to improve health outcomes in the production setting.[26] In commercial cattle production, vaccine efficiency translates to a significant reduction in clinical illness and/or death loss, improvement in weight gain, and a clear economic advantage.[27] Although bovine vaccines must demonstrate efficacy to receive USDA approval, the primary concern for producers is the efficiency, or effectiveness, of the vaccine under field conditions. It is important to note that vaccine efficiency is always associated with vaccine efficacy; however, vaccine efficacy does not always result in vaccine efficiency.

VACCINE SAFETY

Vaccine safety is vital to ensuring the efficiency of a vaccine. The safety of a vaccine may be compromised by several factors including the following:

- Improper time of administration of vaccine, such as during acute infection with wild-type virus and concurrent administration of MLV vaccine or in otherwise unhealthy animals
- Improper storage and/or handling of vaccine (ie, temperature, UV light, excessive shaking, expiration)
- Disrupted physiologic and immunologic status of cattle being vaccinated
- Manufacturing errors that may compromise safety of a particular lot group of vaccine[28]

Based on the segmented structure of the beef industry, millions of cattle annually enter the feedlot considered high-risk; however, the USDA approval process does not require examining the safety of vaccination in highly stressed, immunosuppressed cattle.[28] In fact, the USDA CVM Web site states, "Products are shown to be effective in healthy animals. A protective immune response may not be elicited if animals are incubating an infectious disease, are malnourished or parasitized, are stressed due to shipment or environmental conditions, are otherwise immunocompromised, or the vaccine is not administered in accordance with label directions."[29] The new single claim vaccine label amended by USDA in 2019 states, "This product has been shown to be effective for the vaccination of healthy cattle against (antigen)." For a vaccine to "work," it must stimulate the immune system; therefore, mild local and systemic reactions to vaccines are not uncommon.[30] It is widely accepted that physiologic stress has an impact on the bovine immune system and newly arrived feedlot cattle are often highly stressed; therefore, it is prudent to consider the interaction of stress and vaccination when providing vaccine recommendations to cattle producers.

STRESS AND VACCINE EFFICIENCY

Stress stimulates the hypothalamic-pituitary-adrenal axis (**Fig. 1**) and may be differentiated into 2 types: (1) acute stress, that is, short-term (<24 hours), and (2) chronic stress that occurs when a stressor(s) is imposed on an animal for days or even weeks. The importance of this distinction is due to the differential impact that acute or chronic stress may have on vaccine response. It is postulated that acute stress has the ability to prime the immune system, and possibly potentiate the vaccine response[4]; whereas, chronic stress is known to inhibit the humoral immune response to vaccination.[31] However, these phenomena are difficult to evaluate in research and are rarely explored in the bovine model.

Stress and vaccine interactions in cattle are also poorly understood. Nevertheless, a different humoral response to killed versus MLV respiratory antigens in immunosuppressed cattle may exist. An inhibited antibody response against killed *Salmonella dublin* vaccination was observed when calves were concurrently administered cortisol.[32] An opposing antibody response was noted when replicating MLV vaccine antigens (bovine herpesvirus-1 [BHV-1] and BVDV) were administered concurrent with increased stress-induced cortisol concentrations; the antibody response to these viruses was enhanced in stress-challenged cattle.[32] These findings are likely due to increased cortisol causing immunosuppression that allowed increased antigenicity of MLV vaccine antigens and a subsequently enhanced antibody titer response. Cattle treated with an "acute," "chronic," or "control" stress model, induced by dexamethasone treatment and vaccinated with a multivalent combination respiratory vaccine-bacterin, generated different antibody titer responses depending on the antigen-specific antibody evaluated.[33] The leukotoxin-specific antibody response from a *M haemolytica* toxoid was least in the chronic dexamethasone-challenged steers, intermediate for acute, and greatest for control steers.[33] Conversely, both the BHV-1- and

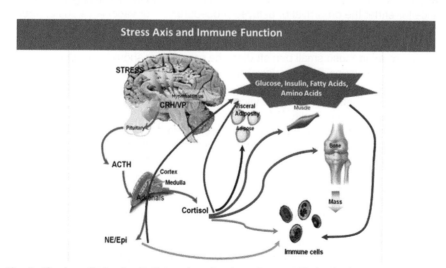

Fig. 1. The hypothalamic-pituitary-adrenal axis and some of the biological components affected by cortisol and epinephrine. ACTH, adrenocorticotropic hormone; CRH/VP, corticotropin-releasing hormone/vasopressin.

BVDV-specific antibody response from the MLV fraction of the combination vaccine was greatest for chronic dexamethasone-challenged steers, intermediate for acute, and least for control steers.[33] The greater antibody titer for dexamethasone-treated cattle administered MLV is probably a result of much greater replication of the live-attenuated vaccine agents in the immunosuppressed host. Therefore, MLV vaccination in high-risk cattle that are immunosuppressed may not be safe, which is a primary rationale for delayed vaccination recommendations.

DELAYED VACCINATION

Almost all stocker and feedlot facilities administer a parenteral multivalent MLV respiratory vaccine during initial processing with the goal of stimulating a systemic immune response against viral agents involved in BRD. However, because there is limited research to support vaccine efficiency in high-risk, newly received cattle, the practice of delaying the MLV vaccine for a time has been considered to allow the immune system to return to a homeostatic state and postpone replicating antigen exposure during the time of arrival when stress-induced immunosuppression is greatest. A previous review[34] summarized important considerations for vaccinating high-risk calves and indicated that existing literature for vaccine efficiency in newly received feedlot cattle is inconsistent. The multitude of vaccine products and regimens, random variation of population dynamics between studies or pens within a study, difficulties with clinical BRD diagnosis, and sample size limitations of research were noted as possible reasons for inconsistent findings.[34]

In a study with 528 high-risk stocker calves,[10] a delayed (14 days) MLV administration procedure was evaluated against the traditional on-arrival (day 0) MLV administration; calves receiving the delayed procedure had improved performance and numerically less BRD-associated morbidity, relapse, and mortality. A large pen study[13] with 5179 auction-derived heifers observed a decrease in the number of heifers treated twice for BRD and numerically less morbidity, mortality, and case fatality rate for those receiving their initial MLV at 30 days after feedlot arrival compared with on-arrival. However, other small studies suggest no difference in health or performance for either the on-arrival or delayed procedure[35–37] or vaccine versus control[38] in high-risk cattle. It is valuable to mention that in smaller studies it can be problematic to analyze proportional data means while avoiding a statistical type II error; therefore, when interpreting these small pen studies, the practitioner should consider evidence of biological relevance that may exist in the absence of statistical significance. In another study comparing MLV respiratory vaccination or control (no MLV vaccine) during the stocker receiving period, the vaccinated calves had significantly greater odds of BRD morbidity and mortality.[11] Ultimately, difficulty arises when assessing the current literature with regard to the benefits, or lack thereof, of vaccinating cattle immediately on feedlot arrival, due to the variation of cattle conditions (eg, immune status, marketing channels used, age, breed) and the complex nature of BRD. Therefore, it is also important to consider the biological implications of vaccine components, such as endotoxins, on the immune system.

IMMUNITY AGAINST ENDOTOXIN

In general, bacteria produce 2 primary types of toxins that are classified as either endotoxins or exotoxins. Endotoxin was first defined in 1892 as a heat-stable toxic substance released when the cell membrane of a microorganism is disrupted.[39] Endotoxins are a major component of the outer cell wall of the gram-negative bacteria[40] and are not secreted by live bacteria but released from bacterial cells when the cell is killed or lysed. The term endotoxin is most commonly associated with the lipopolysaccharide (LPS) cell membrane fractions of bacteria; however, endotoxins include peptidoglycans, lipoproteins, and other bacterial components.[39] In general, endotoxins are considered to be moderate in their toxicity and antigenicity,[40] but bovines are particularly sensitive to endotoxin[41] and differences in endotoxin reactivity, or endotoxigenicity, between bacterial antigens exist (**Table 1**).

Exotoxins, such as leukotoxins, are diffusible proteins that are primarily produced and actively released from bacteria during log-phase growth. Unlike endotoxins, exotoxins are heat-liable, highly antigenic proteins that are also considered highly toxic. However, similar to endotoxins, exotoxins may be released when bacterial cells are lysed. In 1959, Sambhu Nath De[42] discovered the first exotoxin by isolating the toxin that causes cholera. This seminal work led to subsequent research on immunologic responses to toxins and the development of vaccines, or toxoids containing attenuated toxin, and antitoxins.[43] Exotoxins are often used for vaccine development via chemical or heat inactivation of the exotoxin to create a toxoid. Although the resulting toxoid antigen maintains immunogenicity, the biological properties associated with exotoxin-related toxicity are disabled. The bacterial exotoxins can be classified threefold according to their mode of action: Type I are membrane-acting toxins that bind surface receptors and stimulate transmembrane signals; type II are membrane-damaging toxins that directly affect cell membranes by forming pores or disrupting the lipid bilayers of the cell membranes; type III toxins modify an intracellular target molecule by translocating an active enzymatic component into the cell.[44]

The innate immune system does not distinguish every possible antigen within the host, rather a few highly conserved structures present in many different microorganisms. These conserved structures are known as pathogen-associated molecular patterns[45] (PAMPs) and interact with receptors on the surface of the immune cells.[46] For example, the lipid A domain in LPS represents a specific PAMP associated with infection of gram-negative bacteria[47,48] and PAMP recognition by the innate immune system is mediated through a diverse group of receptors known as pattern-recognition receptors[49] (PRRs). The PRRs are divided into 3 functional groups: (1) circulating humoral proteins, such as the endotoxin receptor CD14 and complement proteins, (2) endocytic receptors that are expressed on the cell surface and mediate endocytosis, and (3) signaling receptors, such as toll-like receptors, that are expressed on the surface of the cell.[50]

Endotoxin exposure in cattle results in a rather predictable and conserved set of physiologic and immunologic responses known as the acute-phase response, primarily mediated by the innate immune system.[51,52] Some of the more commonly

Table 1	
Endotoxigenicity of common bacterial antigens used in cattle production	
Antigen (Primary Bovine Disease)	**Endotoxigenicity of Antigen**
Escherichia coli (mastitis)	High
Moraxella bovis (pinkeye)	High
Histophilus somni (bronchopneumonia)	High
Salmonella spp. (salmonellosis)	Moderate
E coli (scours)	Moderate
Mannheimia haemolytica (bronchopneumonia)	Moderate
Pasteurella multocida (bronchopneumonia)	Moderate
Leptospira spp. (leptospirosis)	Low

recognized inflammatory reactions include increased production of proinflammatory cytokines, fever, increases in circulating white blood cells, increased production of acute-phase proteins (APPs) by hepatocytes, and behavioral changes (**Fig. 2**). Behavioral changes can be unambiguous and varied, including lethargy, anorexia, decreased social and sexual behavior, decreased aggressive behavior, and hyperalgesia. The mechanisms by which proinflammatory cytokines, such as tumor necrosis factor-α, interleukin (IL)-1, and IL-6 induce sickness behaviors such as anorexia and depression remain to be fully elucidated; however, it has been suggested that cytokines directly act on the organum vasculosum laminae terminalis region of the brain, perhaps via intermediate messengers such as prostaglandins. Stimulation of prostaglandins could have a direct effect on the central nervous system and/or stimulate local production of cytokines in the brain.[53]

A group of APPs are also released during endotoxin exposure, inflammation, bacterial infection, or physical injury. These APPs become an integral component of proper immunologic function and restoration of homeostasis. In addition, APPs are associated with alterations in plasma iron, zinc, and copper which may play an important role in overall immune function and modulation of bacterial growth in the animal. In cattle, some primary APPs include haptoglobin, serum amyloid A, fibrinogen, α1-acid glycoprotein, ceruloplasmin, α1-antitrypsin, α1-antichymotrypsin, α2-macroglobulin,

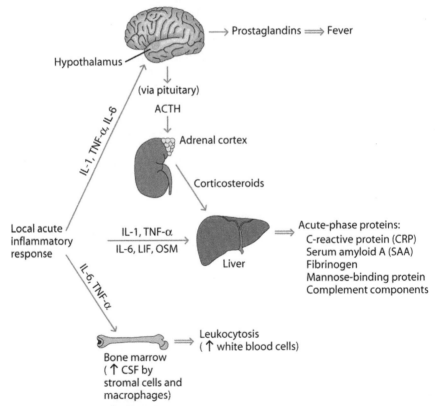

Fig. 2. Diagram of the inflammatory response. ACTH, adrenocorticotropic hormone; CSF, cerebrospinal fluid; LIF, leukemia inhibitory factor; OSM, outer surface membrane; TNF, tumor necrosis factor. (*From* R. Goldsby, T. Kindt, B. Osborne, J. Kuby. Immunology, 5th Edition. W. H. Freeman; 2002; with permission.)

and fetuin.[54] As an indicator of inflammation and/or disease, haptoglobin, α1-acid glycoprotein, fibrinogen, and serum amyloid A are the most commonly evaluated APPs in bovines.[51,55–57]

ENDOTOXIN IN VACCINES

Vaccines against gram-negative bacteria may contain endotoxins such as peptidoglycans, lipoproteins, and LPS. Commonly used vaccines against gram-negative bacteria and the associated diseases in cattle production are indicated in **Table 2**. Use of bacterins began when a physician named William Coley began treating patients with both live- and heat-killed *Serratia marcescens* and streptococci to treat sarcomas. This practice, known as Coley toxins, was used for more than 30 years with much success, despite occasionally inducing severe adverse effects, such as extreme fever and toxic shock.[58] Today, most gram-negative vaccines contain whole cell modified and/or killed bacteria, with relatively small amounts of free endotoxin, thus resulting in less risk for severe adverse effects after use. Endotoxins in each of these vaccines have different antigenicity based on the bacterium used to produce the vaccine and the structure of the endotoxin molecule present. For example, the LPS molecule can vary structurally between *Escherichia coli* vaccines depending on the strain used to develop the vaccine, and thus the antigenicity of the LPS present in a vaccine can vary. Although free endotoxin concentrations are generally low, mishandling of vaccines can increase free endotoxin released from the cell wall membrane due to killing or lysis of the bacteria, thereby increasing the antigenicity of the vaccine. Therefore, it is critical that vaccines are handled appropriately to reduce the risk of endotoxicity in vaccinated cattle. Factors that may constitute mishandling of gram-negative bacterins include the following:

- Improper temperature during storage or use leading to increased endotoxin concentration (for example, exposing bacterins to high heat or freezing temperatures can rupture bacterial cells, thus causing the release of endotoxin from the outer cell wall membrane)
- Excessive shaking of bacterins before use, resulting in lysis of the bacterial whole cells or fragments leading to the release of LPS and other endotoxins or exotoxins
- Exposure to UV light (direct sunlight) that may result in cellular degradation and release of free endotoxin

ENDOTOXIN STACKING

Adverse events associated with endotoxin-containing bacterins occur due to a phenomenon known as endotoxin stacking (ie, giving multiple gram-negative endotoxin-containing vaccines at one time). Due to the potential for endotoxins in bacterins to produce a synergistic or additive response, endotoxin stacking can lead to toxicity that could be fatal.[59] As previously mentioned, the mechanism by which endotoxins such as LPS create an immunologic response is via a cytokine cascade. This cascade is influenced by the amount of endotoxin present, whether the endotoxin is bound or free, and host factors that can make an animal more vulnerable to endotoxin. A report noted that endotoxin from multiple bacterial sources resulted in more drastic physiologic and immunologic responses than that of the same endotoxin concentration from a single source. Estimating the frequency with which endotoxin stacking occurs in beef production and the impact on cattle health and performance is difficult, as cattle vaccination protocols differ depending on the

Table 2
Licensed veterinary biological products containing bacterins, bacterial extracts, and/or toxoids approved for use in cattle

Product and Form	Licensed Producers
Autogenous vaccine, killed virus, autogenous bacterin	SolidTech Animal Health
Autogenous vaccine-autogenous bacterin	Biomune Company, Cambridge Technologies, Colorado Serum Company, Elanco US, Hennessy Research Associates, Huvepharma, Kennebec River Biosciences, Newport Laboratories, Phibro Animal Health, Texas Vet Lab
Bovine rhinotracheitis vaccine-*Haemophilus somnus-Mannheimia haemolytica-Pasteurella multocida-Salmonella typhimurium* bacterin-toxoid	Texas Vet Lab
Bovine rhinotracheitis vaccine-*Leptospira hardjo-pomona* bacterin	Boehringer Ingelheim Vetmedica
Bovine rhinotracheitis vaccine-*Leptospira pomona* bacterin	Diamond Animal Health
Bovine rhinotracheitis-virus diarrhea vaccine-*Campylobacter fetus-Leptospira canicola-grippotyphosa-hardjo-icterohaemorrhagiae-pomona* bacterin	Zoetis
Bovine rhinotracheitis-virus diarrhea-parainfluenza 3 vaccine-*Leptospira canicola-grippotyphosa-hardjo-icterohaemorrhagiae-pomona* bacterin	Colorado Serum Company, Diamond Animal Health
Bovine rhinotracheitis-virus diarrhea-parainfluenza 3-respiratory syncytial virus vaccine-*Campylobacter fetus-Haemophilus somnus-Leptospira canicola-grippotyphosa-hardjo-icterohaemorrhagiae-pomona* bacterin	Elanco US
Bovine rhinotracheitis-virus diarrhea-parainfluenza 3-respiratory syncytial virus vaccine-*Campylobacter fetus-Leptospira canicola-grippotyphosa-hardjo-icterohaemorrhagiae-pomona* bacterin	Boehringer Ingelheim Vetmedica, Elanco US, Intervet, Zoetis
Bovine rhinotracheitis-virus diarrhea-parainfluenza 3-respiratory syncytial virus vaccine-*Haemophilus somnus* bacterin	Boehringer Ingelheim Vetmedica
Bovine rhinotracheitis-virus diarrhea-parainfluenza 3-respiratory syncytial virus vaccine-*Haemophilus somnus-Leptospira canicola-grippotyphosa-hardjo-icterohaemorrhagiae-pomona* bacterin	Boehringer Ingelheim Vetmedica, Elanco US
Bovine rhinotracheitis-virus diarrhea-parainfluenza 3-respiratory syncytial virus vaccine-*Leptospira canicola-grippotyphosa-hardjo-icterohaemorrhagiae-pomona* bacterin	Boehringer Ingelheim Vetmedica, Diamond Animal Health, Elanco US, Intervet, Zoetis
Bovine rhinotracheitis-virus diarrhea-parainfluenza 3-respiratory syncytial virus vaccine-*Leptospira canicola-grippotyphosa-hardjo-icterohaemorrhagiae-pomona-Mannheimia haemolytica* bacterin	Boehringer Ingelheim Vetmedica, Elanco US

(*continued on next page*)

Table 2 (*continued*)	
Product and Form	**Licensed Producers**
Bovine rhinotracheitis-virus diarrhea-parainfluenza 3-respiratory syncytial virus vaccine-*Leptospira hardjo* bacterin	Zoetis
Bovine rhinotracheitis-virus diarrhea-parainfluenza 3-respiratory syncytial virus vaccine-*Mannheimia haemolytica* bacterin	Boehringer Ingelheim Vetmedica, Elanco US
Bovine rhinotracheitis-virus diarrhea-parainfluenza 3-respiratory syncytial virus vaccine-*Mannheimia haemolytica* toxoid	Boehringer Ingelheim Vetmedica, Zoetis
Bovine rhinotracheitis-virus diarrhea-parainfluenza 3-respiratory syncytial virus vaccine-*Mannheimia haemolytica-Pasteurella multocida* bacterin-toxoid	Diamond Animal Health
Bovine rhinotracheitis-virus diarrhea-respiratory syncytial virus vaccine-*Leptospira pomona* bacterin	Diamond Animal Health
Bovine rotavirus-coronavirus vaccine-*Clostridium perfringens* type C-*Escherichia coli* bacterin-toxoid	Elanco US, Zoetis
Bovine rotavirus-coronavirus vaccine-*Clostridium perfringens* types C and D-*Escherichia coli* bacterin-toxoid	Intervet
Bovine rotavirus-coronavirus vaccine-*Escherichia coli* bacterin	Zoetis
Bovine virus diarrhea vaccine-*Campylobacter fetus-Leptospira canicola-grippotyphosa-hardjo-icterohaemorrhagiae-pomona* bacterin	Zoetis
Bovine virus diarrhea vaccine-*Leptospira canicola-grippotyphosa-hardjo-icterohaemorrhagiae-pomona* bacterin	Zoetis
Bovine virus diarrhea vaccine-*Mannheimia haemolytica* toxoid	Zoetis
Trichomonas foetus vaccine, killed protozoa-*Campylobacter fetus-Leptospira canicola-grippotyphosa-hardjo-icterohaemorrhagiae-pomona* bacterin	Boehringer Ingelheim Vetmedica, Elanco US
Clostridium botulinum type C bacterin-toxoid	United Vaccines
Clostridium chauvoei-septicum-haemolyticum-novyi-sordellii-perfringens types C and D bacterin-toxoid	Boehringer Ingelheim Vetmedica, Intervet, Zoetis
Clostridium chauvoei-septicum-haemolyticum-novyi-sordellii-perfringens types C and D-*Haemophilus somnus* bacterin-toxoid	Intervet
Clostridium chauvoei-septicum-haemolyticum-novyi-sordellii-perfringens types C and D-*Mannheimia haemolytica* bacterin-toxoid	Zoetis
Clostridium chauvoei-septicum-haemolyticum-novyi-sordellii-tetani-perfringens types C and D bacterin-toxoid	Intervet
Clostridium chauvoei-septicum-haemolyticum-novyi-tetani-perfringens types C and D bacterin-toxoid	Intervet
Clostridium chauvoei-septicum-novyi bacterin-toxoid	Colorado Serum Company

(*continued on next page*)

Table 2
(continued)

Product and Form	Licensed Producers
Clostridium chauvoei-septicum-novyi-sordellii bacterin-toxoid	Colorado Serum Company
Clostridium chauvoei-septicum-novyi-sordellii-perfringens types C and D bacterin-toxoid	Boehringer Ingelheim Vetmedica, Elanco US, Intervet, Zoetis
Clostridium chauvoei-septicum-novyi-sordellii-perfringens types C and D-*Haemophilus somnus* bacterin-toxoid	Boehringer Ingelheim Vetmedica, Intervet, Zoetis
Clostridium chauvoei-septicum-novyi-sordellii-perfringens types C and D-*Mannheimia haemolytica* bacterin-toxoid	Zoetis
Clostridium chauvoei-septicum-novyi-sordellii-perfringens types C and D-*Moraxella bovis* bacterin-toxoid	Boehringer Ingelheim Vetmedica, Intervet
Clostridium perfringens type C-*Escherichia coli* bacterin-toxoid	Elanco US, Intervet, Zoetis
Clostridium perfringens types C and D bacterin-toxoid	Elanco US, Intervet, Zoetis
Clostridium perfringens types C and D-*tetani* bacterin-toxoid	Intervet
Clostridium tetani-perfringens type D-*Corynebacterium pseudotuberculosis* bacterin-toxoid	Colorado Serum Company
Corynebacterium pseudotuberculosis bacterin-toxoid	Boehringer Ingelheim Vetmedica, Colorado Serum Company
Escherichia coli bacterin-toxoid	Merial
Haemophilus somnus-Mannheimia haemolytica-Pasteurella multocida bacterin-toxoid	Texas Vet Lab
Haemophilus somnus-Mannheimia haemolytica-Pasteurella multocida-Salmonella typhimurium bacterin-toxoid	Texas Vet Lab
Mannheimia haemolytica bacterial extract-toxoid	Elanco US
Mannheimia haemolytica bacterin-toxoid	Zoetis
Mannheimia haemolytica-Pasteurella multocida bacterin-toxoid	American Animal Health, Merial
Pasteurella multocida bacterial extract-*Mannheimia haemolytica* toxoid	Boehringer Ingelheim Vetmedica
Salmonella typhimurium bacterin-toxoid	Immvac
Staphylococcus aureus bacterin-toxoid	Hygieia Biological Laboratories
Clostridium botulinum type B toxoid	Neogen
Clostridium perfringens type A toxoid	Elanco US, Intervet
Clostridium perfringens type C toxoid	Colorado Serum Company
Clostridium perfringens type D toxoid	Colorado Serum Company
Clostridium perfringens type D-tetanus toxoid	Colorado Serum Company
Clostridium perfringens types C and D toxoid	Boehringer Ingelheim Vetmedica, Colorado Serum Company
Clostridium perfringens types C and D-tetanus toxoid	Boehringer Ingelheim Vetmedica, Colorado Serum Company

(continued on next page)

Table 2 (continued)	
Product and Form	**Licensed Producers**
Crotalus atrox toxoid	Hygieia Biological Laboratories
Mannheimia haemolytica toxoid	Boehringer Ingelheim Vetmedica, Elanco US, Zoetis
Tetanus toxoid	Boehringer Ingelheim Vetmedica, Colorado Serum Company, Intervet, Zoetis

Data from United States Department of Agriculture, Animal and Plant Health Inspection Service, Veterinary Services, Center for Veterinary Biologics, Veterinary Biological Products; 2019.

producer, veterinarian, and geographic location. However, 2 or more gram-negative vaccines are often administered simultaneously in production settings, and often these bacterins or toxoids are administered concurrent with MLV vaccines and other biological or pharmaceutical products (ie, antimicrobials, anthelmintics) and negative interactions could occur in some cattle, but the interaction of the various animal health products used in cattle is poorly understood.

The physiologic and immunologic status of cattle also should be considered before vaccination with endotoxin-containing products. Sick cattle or cattle exposed to stressful conditions for an extended period should not be vaccinated with endotoxin-containing vaccines, as these cattle may have an altered immune system and be more susceptible to the negative effects of endotoxin. Endotoxins are well known for their pyrogenic properties; therefore, endotoxin vaccination during times of heat stress also should be avoided, as this could potentially increase the overall heat load in the animal. It is again noteworthy to mention that vaccine labels stipulate use in healthy animals. In addition, the hydration and nutritional status of the animal may influence the effectiveness of a vaccine. Generating an adequate immune response to a vaccine requires a significant amount of energy and nutrients and under-nourished and/or dehydrated cattle may not be physiologically capable of mounting an appropriate response to the vaccine. The conundrum of these scenarios is that most producers and veterinarians vaccinate juxtaposed to other processes, such as weaning, branding, or arrival at a new location. To further complicate vaccination pro-tocols and cattle-processing procedures, with respect to endotoxin overloading, pro-ducers often administer metaphylactic antimicrobials at processing in conjunction with vaccination. Many antimicrobials target gram-negative pathogens, resulting in endotoxin release after the targeted action of the antimicrobial results in killing or lysis of bacteria. Different antimicrobial classes, and different antimicrobials within classifi-cation, vary with respect to their impact on cell wall morphology and the subsequent amount of endotoxin released.[60]

POTENTIAL BENEFITS AND CONSEQUENCES

The amount, type, and structure of the endotoxin, and whether or not endotoxins are introduced from multiple sources (endotoxin stacking) combined with the physiologic and immunologic status of the host animal, affect the magnitude of the endotoxin response that may have positive or negative outcome. Exposure to structurally altered or lesser amounts of endotoxin may initiate a small immunologic response that could enhance the effectiveness of bacterins and result in immunologic memory against gram-negative bacteria. In fact, the low concentrations of endotoxins in a bacterin may indeed exert beneficial actions similar to the proposed immune-priming effects of acute stress and some commercial MLV vaccines contain very small quantities of endotoxin for this very reason. Furthermore, low concentrations of LPS will lead to a mild to moderate febrile response that can aid in controlling bacterial proliferation in the host.[40] Endotoxin exposure also stimulates B-cell differentiation and enhances phagocytic activity, thus helping the host animal immune system to recognize and eliminate invading pathogens more rapidly and effectively. For example, genetically altered mice that do not respond to LPS have been reported to be more susceptible to bacterial infections.[61] Therefore, exposure to small quantities of LPS typically aids immune function and may be beneficial in eliminating pathogens by increasing effector capacities of macrophages and other leukocytes.

Conversely, when greater endotoxin exposure occurs because of, for example, mishandling of vaccines or endotoxin stacking, the effect can be detrimental due to varying degrees of sepsis related to bacteremia and endotoxemia.[59,62,63] Exposure to high concentration of endotoxin can elicit a severe febrile and hypotensive response that rapidly leads to multiorgan failure, septic shock, and death. Interestingly, it has been reported that gram-negative bacterial endotoxins are responsible for almost half of septic cases in humans.[64] In addition to the potential for inducing lethal septic shock, endotoxin exposure stimulates the release of the proinflammatory cytokines as previously discussed. Increased cytokine production leads to vasodilation that can inadvertently increase bacterial translocation and dissemination throughout the body[65] and may lead to increased proliferation of virulent strains of bacteria, such as *Escherichia coli*.[66] Compounding this problem is the inhibited bacterial clearance invoked by endotoxicity and the impaired function of immune cells, such as monocytes.[67] Thus, although the release of proinflammatory cytokines is essential for maintaining homeostasis within the animal, there exists a "catch-22" scenario in that the permissive effects of these cytokines on bacterial proliferation leads to a perpetuating cycle of increased cytokine production and subsequent increased risk of sepsis.

SUMMARY

Vaccines provide immunologic protection against economically important cattle diseases. However, vaccine efficiency may not be realized if the timing of vaccination is inappropriate, vaccinates are immunosuppressed, and/or if the infectious challenge is greater than the immunologic protection afforded by vaccination. Vaccine recommendations in cattle often rely on anecdotal evidence and tradition, rather than scientific evidence, because there is a dearth of randomized, controlled field studies that evaluate vaccine efficiency, and some vaccination practices disregard vaccine label instructions. Veterinary practitioners should consider emerging research on the efficiency of on-arrival versus delayed vaccination in newly received stocker and feedlot cattle monitored under field conditions. Furthermore, endotoxicity risk is increased when 2 or more gram-negative bacterins are administered concurrently; therefore, veterinarians and producers should avoid endotoxin stacking when designing cattle vaccination protocols.

ACKNOWLEDGMENTS

The article cited was prepared by a USDA employee as part of his or her official duties. Copyright protection under US copyright law is not available for such works. Accordingly, there is no copyright to transfer. The fact that the private publication in which the article appears is itself copyrighted does not affect the material of the US government, which can be freely reproduced by the public.

Mention of trade names or commercial products in this article is solely for the purpose of providing specific information and does not imply recommendation or endorsement by the USDA.

The USDA prohibits discrimination in all its programs and activities on the basis of race, color, national origin, age, disability, and, where applicable, sex, marital status, familial status, parental status, religion, sexual orientation, genetic information, political beliefs, reprisal, or because all or part of an individual's income is derived from any public assistance program. (Not all prohibited bases apply to all programs.) Persons with disabilities who require alternative means for communication of program information (eg, Braille, large print, audiotape) should contact USDA's TARGET Center at (202) 720-2600 (voice and TDD). To file a complaint of discrimination, write to USDA, Director, Office of Civil Rights, 1400 Independence Avenue, SW, Washington, DC 20250-9410, or call (800) 795-3272 (voice) or (202) 720-6382 (TDD). USDA is an equal opportunity provider and employer.

REFERENCES

1. Taylor JD, Fulton RW, Lehenbauer TW, et al. The epidemiology of bovine respiratory disease: what is the evidence for predisposing factors? Can Vet J 2010;51: 1095–102.

2. Ives SE, Richeson JT. Use of antimicrobial metaphylaxis for the control of bovine respiratory disease in high-risk cattle. Vet Clin North Am Food Anim Pract 2015; 31:341–50.

3. Griffin D. Economic impact associated with respiratory disease in beef cattle. Vet Clin North Am Food Anim Pract 1997;13:367–77.

4. Hughes HD, Carroll JA, Burdick Sanchez NC, et al. Natural variations in the stress and acute phase response of cattle. Innate Immun 2013;20:888–96.

5. Dhuyvetter KC, Bryan AM, Blasi DA. Case study: preconditioning beef calves: are expected premiums sufficient to justify the practice? Prof Anim Sci 2005;21: 502–14.

6. King ME, Salman MD, Wittum TE, et al. Effect of certified health programs on the sale price of beef calves marketed through a livestock videotape auction service from 1995 through 2005. J Am Vet Med Assoc 2006;229(9):1389–400.

7. Step DL, Krehbiel CR, DePra HA, et al. Effects of commingling beef calves from different sources and weaning protocols during a forty-two-day receiving period on performance and bovine respiratory disease. J Anim Sci 2008;11:3146–58.

8. Hilton WM, Olynk NJ. Profitability of preconditioning: lessons learned from an 11-year case study of an Indiana beef herd. Bov Pract (Stillwater) 2011;45:40–50.

9. USDA. Vaccination of calves for respiratory disease on U. S. beef cow-calf operations. Info Sheet. Fort Collins (CO): USDA – Anim Plant Health Insect Serv-Vet Serv, Ctr Epidemiol Anim Health; 2009. Available at: https://www.aphis.usda.gov/animal_health/nahms/beefcowcalf/downloads/beef0708/Beef0708_is_CalfVacc.pdf. Accessed April 01, 2019.

10. Richeson JT, Beck PA, Gadberry MS, et al. Effects of on-arrival versus delayed modified live virus vaccination on health, performance, and serum infectious bovine rhinotracheitis titers of newly received beef calves. J Anim Sci 2008;86: 999–1005.

11. Griffin CM, Scott JA, Karisch BB, et al. A randomized controlled trial to test the effect of on-arrival vaccination and deworming on stocker cattle health and growth performance. Bov Pract (Stillwater) 2018;52:26–33.

12. Terrell SP, Thomson DU, Wileman BW, et al. A survey to describe current feeder cattle health and well-being program recommendations made by feedlot veterinary consultants in the United States and Canada. Bov Pract (Stillwater) 2011; 45:140–8.

13. Rogers KC, Miles DG, Renter DG, et al. Effects of delayed respiratory viral vaccine and/or inclusion of an immunostimulant on feedlot health, performance, and carcass merits of auction-market derived feeder heifers. Bov Pract (Stillwater) 2016;50:154–62.

14. Fike GD, Simroth JC, Thomson DU, et al. A survey of recommended practices made by veterinary practitioners to cow-calf operations in the United States and Canada. Prof Anim Sci 2017;33:716–28.

15. Terrell SP, Thomson DU, Reinhardt CD, et al. Perception of lameness management, education, and effects on animal welfare of feedlot cattle by consulting nutritionists, veterinarians, and feedlot managers. Bov Pract (Stillwater) 2014;48: 53–60.

16. Lee TL, Terrell SP, Bartle SJ, et al. Current feedlot cattle health and well-being program recommendations in the United States and Canada: the 2014 feedlot veterinary consultant survey. Bov Pract (Stillwater) 2015;49:124–31.

17. USDA. Beef 2007-08. Part IV: reference of beef cow-calf management practices in the United States, 2007-08. #523.0210. Fort Collins (CO): USDA – Anim Plant Health Insect Serv-Vet Serv, Ctr Epidemiol Anim Health; 2010.

18. Comerford JW, Greaser GL, Moore HL, et al. Beef cow-calf production. Agricultural alternatives. Penn State Coop Ext, The Pennsylvania State Univ, University Park (PA); 2013.

19. Waldner CM, Jelinski D, McIntyre-Zimmer K. Survey of western Canadian beef producers regarding calf-hood diseases, management practices, and veterinary service usage. Can Vet J 2013;54:559–64.

20. Woolums AR, Berghaus RD, Smith DR, et al. A survey of veterinarians in 6 US states regarding their experience with nursing beef calf respiratory disease. Bov Pract (Stillwater) 2014;48:26–35.

21. USDA. Vaccine usage in U.S. feedlots. No. 672.0513. Fort Collins (CO): USDA, Animal and Plant Health Inspection Service, Veterinary Services, Centers for Epidemiology and Animal Health; 2013.

22. Martin SW. Vaccination: is it effective in preventing respiratory disease of influencing weight gains in feedlot calves? Can Vet J 1983;24:10–9.

23. Perino LJ, Hunsaker BD. A review of bovine respiratory disease vaccine field efficacy. Bov Pract (Stillwater) 1997;31:59–66.

24. Tripp HM, Step DL, Krehbiel CR, et al. Evaluation of outcomes in beef cattle comparing preventive health protocols utilizing viral respiratory vaccines. Bov Pract (Stillwater) 2013;47:54–64.

25. Larson BL. A new look at reducing infectious disease in feedlot cattle. Proc Plains Nutr Coun 2005;AREC05-20:9–17.

26. Weinberg GA, Szilagyi PG. Vaccine epidemiology: efficacy, effectiveness, and translational research roadmap. J Infect Dis 2010;201:1607–10.

27. Richeson JT, Beck PA, Poe KD, et al. Effects of administration of a modified-live virus respiratory vaccine and timing of vaccination on health and performance of high-risk beef stocker calves. Bov Pract (Stillwater) 2015;49:37–42.

28. Rashid A, Rasheed K, Asim M, et al. Risks of vaccination: a review. J Venom Anim Toxins Incl Trop Dis 2009;15:19–27.

29. USDA, APHIS. Licensed veterinary biological product information. Available at: https://www.aphis.usda.gov/aphis/ourfocus/animalhealth/veterinary-biologics/CT_Vb_licensed_products. Accessed March 29, 2019..

30. Roth JA. Mechanistic bases for adverse vaccine reactions and vaccine failures. Adv Vet Med 1999;41:681–700.

31. Cohen S, Miller GE, Ravin BS. Psychological stress and antibody response to immunization: a critical review of the human literature. Psychosom Med 2001; 63:7–18.

32. Roth JA. Cortisol as mediator of stress-associated immunosuppression in cattle. In: Animal stress. New York: Springer; 1985. p. 225–43.

33. Richeson JT, Carroll JA, Burdick Sanchez NC, et al. Dexamethasone treatment differentially alters viral shedding and the antibody and acute phase protein response after multivalent respiratory vaccination in beef steers. J Anim Sci 2016;94:3501–9.

34. Richeson JT. Vaccinating high-risk calves against BRD. Proc Am Assoc Bov Pract 2015;48:169–72.

35. Richeson JT, Kegley EB, Gadberry MS, et al. Effects of on-arrival versus delayed clostridial or modified live respiratory vaccinations on health, performance, bovine viral diarrhea virus type I titers, and stress and immune measures of newly received beef calves. J Anim Sci 2009;87:2409–18.

36. Poe KD, Beck PA, Richeson JT, et al. Effects of respiratory vaccination timing and growth-promoting implant on health, performance, and immunity of high-risk, newly received stocker cattle. Prof Anim Sci 2013;29:413–9.

37. Hagenmaier JA, Terhaar BL, Blue K, et al. A comparison of three vaccine programs on the health, growth performance, and carcass characteristics of high-risk feedlot heifers procured from auction markets. Bov Pract (Stillwater) 2018; 52:120–30.

38. Duff GC, Malcolm-Callis KJ, Walker DA, et al. Effect of intranasal versus intramuscular modified live vaccines and vaccine timing on health and performance by newly received beef cattle. Bov Pract (Stillwater) 2000;34:66–71.

39. Pfeiffer R. Untersuchungen über das Choleragift. Med Microbiol Immunol 1892; 11(1):393–412.

40. Woltmann A, Hamann L, Ulmer AJ, et al. Molecular mechanisms of sepsis. Langenbecks Arch Surg 1998;383:2–10.

41. Carroll JA, Reuter RR, Chase CC, et al. Profiling of the bovine acute phase response following an intravenous lipopolysaccharide challenge. Innate Immun 2009;15:81–9.

42. De SN. Enterotoxicity of bacteria-free culture filtrate of *Vibrio cholerae*. Nature 1959;183:1533–4.

43. Nairv GB, Narainv JP. From endotoxin to exotoxin: De's rich legacy to cholera. Bull World Health Organ 2010;88(3):161–240.

44. Ala'Aldeen DAA, Wooldridge KG. Medical microbiology. 18th edition 2012.

45. Janeway CA Jr, Travers M, Walport M, et al. Immunobiology, the immune system in health and disease. New York: Garland Science Publishing; 2005.

46. Takeda K, Kaisho T, Akira S. Toll-like receptors. Annu Rev Immunol 2003;21: 335–76.

47. Mackay IR, Janeway C Jr. Innate immunity. N Engl J Med 2000;343:338–44.

48. Janeway CA Jr, Medzhitov R. Innate immune recognition. Annu Rev Immunol 2002;20:197–216.

49. Medzhitov R, Janeway J. Innate immunity: the virtues of a nonclonal system of recognition. Cell 1997;91:295–8.

50. Mann DL. Tumor necrosis factor and viral myocarditis: the fine line between innate and inappropriate immune responses in the heart. Circulation 2001;103: 626–9.

51. Bishop RE. Fundamentals of endotoxin structure and function. Contrib Microbiol 2005;12:1–27.

52. Peterson JW. Bacterial pathogenesis. In: Baron S, editor. Medical microbiology. 4th edition. Galveston (TX): University of Texas Medical Branch at Galveston; 1996 [Chapter: 7].

53. Exton MS. Infection-induced anorexia: active host defense strategy. Appetite 1997;29:369–83.

54. Godson DL, Baca-Estrada ME, Van Kessel AG, et al. Regulation of bovine acute phase responses by recombinant interleukin-1β. Can J Vet Res 1995;59(4): 249–55.

55. Kahl S, Elsasser TH. Exogenous testosterone modulates tumor necrosis factor- and acute phase protein responses to repeated endotoxin challenge in steers. Domest Anim Endocrinol 2006;31:301–11.

56. McSherry BJ, Horney FD, deGroot JJ. Plasma fibrinogen levels in normal and sick cows. Can J Comp Med 1970;34:191–7.

57. Eckersall PD, Conner JG. Bovine and canine acute phase proteins. Vet Res Commun 1988;12:169–78.

58. Alexander C, Rietschel ET. Bacterial lipopolysaccharides and innate immunity. J Endotoxin Res 2001;7:167–202.

59. Ellis JA, Yong C. Systemic adverse reactions in young Simmental calves following administration of a combination vaccine. Can Vet J 1997;38:45–7.

60. Crosby HA, Bion JF, Penn CW, et al. Antibiotic induced release of endotoxin from bacteria in vitro. J Med Microbiol 1994;40:23–30.

61. von Jeney N, Günther E, Jann K. Mitogenic stimulation of murine spleen cells: relation to susceptibility to *Salmonella* infection. Infect Immun 1977;15:26–33.

62. Zhang FX, Kirschning CJ, Mancinelli R, et al. Bacterial lipopolysaccharide activates nuclear factor-κB through interleukin-1 signaling mediators in cultured human dermal endothelial cells and mononuclear phagocytes. J Biol Chem 1999; 274:7611–4.

63. Muzio M, Bosisio D, Polentarutti N, et al. Differential expression and regulation of toll-like receptors (TLR) in human leukocytes: selective expression of TLR3 in dendritic cells. J Immunol 2000;164:5998–6004.

64. Jones G, Lowes J. The systemic inflammatory response syndrome as a predictor of bacteraemia and outcome from sepsis. QJM 1996;89:515–22.

65. Haziot A, Ferrero E, Köntgen F, et al. Resistance to endotoxin shock and reduced dissemination of gram-negative bacteria in CD14-deficient mice. Immun 1996;4: 407–14.

66. Porat R, Clark BD, Wolff SM, et al. Enhancement of growth of virulent strains of *Escherichia coli* by interleukin-1. Science 1991;254:430–2.

67. Koch T, Duncker HP, Axt R, et al. Alterations of bacterial clearance induced by endotoxin and tumor necrosis factor. Infect Immun 1993;61:3143–8.

Herd Immunity

David R. Smith, DVM, PhD

KEYWORDS

- Herd immunity • Contagious disease • Basic reproductive number • Infectiousness
- Immune • Susceptible

KEY POINTS

- Herd immunity is an important concept of epidemic theory regarding the population-level effect of individual immunity to prevent contagious transmission of pathogens.
- Understanding herd immunity requires consideration of the factors that affect infectiousness, agent transmission, and immunity, as well as an understanding of the human and animal behaviors that result in undesirable outcomes.
- The basic reproductive number is a measure of contagion in a population that helps to predict the proportion of immune individuals needed to prevent an epidemic.
- Vaccination programs to eliminate or eradicate pathogens from a population require that the threshold level of herd immunity be achieved.
- Some age-associated epidemics of disease, such as pneumonia in calves before weaning, may be explained by the loss of herd immunity caused by waning maternal antibodies.

INTRODUCTION

Herd immunity is an important concept of epidemic theory regarding the population-level effect of individual animal immunity to prevent transmission of pathogens. Herd immunity exists when sufficient numbers of animals in a group or population have immunity against an agent such that an outbreak fails to materialize when the agent has been introduced by an infected individual, because the likelihood of an effective contact between diseased and susceptible individuals has been reduced.[1] Herd immunity applies to a restrictive set of conditions that are discussed later. When these conditions apply, methods to achieve herd immunity serve an important role in preventing disease epidemics and are an important component of programs for disease elimination or eradication.[1] Loss of herd immunity may also explain age-associated epidemics of disease related to loss of passively acquired maternal immunity.[2] Herd immunity is not just about the immunization process. Understanding herd immunity requires consideration of infection dynamics, modes of transmission, as well as the acquisition of immunity by individuals in the population.

Disclosure: A contribution of the Beef Cattle Population Health and Reproduction Program at Mississippi State University. Supported by the Mikell and Mary Cheek Hall Davis Endowment for Beef Cattle Health and Reproduction.
Department of Pathobiology and Population Medicine, Mississippi State University College of Veterinary Medicine, PO Box 9100, 240 Wise Center Drive, Mississippi State, MS 39762, USA
E-mail address: david.smith@msstate.edu

INFECTION DYNAMICS

Infection dynamics considers the state of infectiousness of individuals, rather than whether or not the animal is infected, the stage of the disease process, or even whether disease ever manifests clinically.[3] Diseases are not transmitted, but pathogens are. Infection refers to the invasion and replication of an agent in a host. Infectiousness, or the state of being infective, refers to the capability of an infected individual to transmit the agent to others. Being infected is not the same as being infectious, because the state of infectiousness does not necessarily coincide with the entire period of the infection process. The expression of clinical signs of disease is a poor correlate of infectiousness because:

- The state of infectiousness may occur before, after, or during the period of clinical signs, depending on the agent
- Infection may not be apparent clinically (eg, subclinical infections)
- Similar clinical signs may be caused by more than 1 infectious agent
- Clinical signs of disease commonly require not only infection with the agent but also the occurrence of other component causes[4,5]

Therefore, in this article, the discussion about factors leading to herd immunity largely considers infected individuals who are infectious without regard to their current state of health.

The Risk of Infection Given Exposure

Infectious agents are acquired by a host during contact with a reservoir in a manner that facilitates infection. The reservoir can be environmental sources, animals, insect or other vectors, or humans. Infectious agents can invade a host through inhalation, ingestion, or direct penetration of skin or mucous membranes. Once exposure occurs, the factors that influence the transition to infection are related to the dose, the agent, and the host. Exposure to a larger number of organisms increases the likelihood of infection. Methods to decrease the number of organisms or their vectors, such as washing pen surfaces, using disinfectants, or applying insecticides, help to reduce the probability of infection. Agent-related factors, or infectivity factors, are characteristics of the agent that typically enhance its ability to invade the host by attachment of the pathogen to host cells. One of the most important host-related factors, or susceptibility factors, is immunity acquired after vaccination or prior infection with the pathogen. Immunity may be complete or partial, and may wane with immunosuppression; for example, because of malnutrition, chemotherapy, or some viral infections, such as bovine viral diarrhea virus (BVDV). Other susceptibility factors include whether or not hosts express receptors that pathogens use for invasion, or whether hosts have physiologic factors that affect host clearance of microorganisms. For example, impaired mucus clearing of the lungs may increase the risk of respiratory bacterial pathogens.[3]

The Risk of Infectiousness Given Infection

The degree and duration of infectiousness are essential parameters for describing an infectious process, and critical for explaining or predicting the spread of an infectious agent within a population. The degree of infectiousness depends on characteristics of the agent and host. There may be variation in the number of organisms produced by an infected individual. The dose load of agent may wax and wane with the stage of infection or by the disease state of the host. For example, individuals infected with a respiratory disease agent may be minimally infectious until they begin to cough.

Similarly, individuals infected with an enteric agent may be more infectious during the time when they have diarrhea, partly because they may be shedding more organisms and partly because there may be more opportunities for fecal-oral contact. The duration of infectiousness may be caused by characteristics of the agent, the nature of the infection, and the various host-pathogen interactions that affect the host's ability to eliminate the infection.[3]

Some infected individuals present a greater risk for transmission of infectious agents than others. Many infectious diseases show transmission heterogeneity, a superspreading effect whereby many of the infections are transmitted by a minority of individuals.[6-8] This heterogeneity of transmission may occur because of behaviors of the host or because spatial relationships lead to greater opportunities for effective contacts.[8] In some cases, superspreading occurs because of the large infectious dose produced, termed supershedding.[9] Sometimes superspreading is caused by characteristics unique to certain individuals; for example, because of genetics,[8] or persistent infection, as with BVDV.[10] Transmission heterogeneity has been observed with enterohemorrhagic *Escherichia coli* O157 (EHEC O157) infection of cattle. At a given point in time, cattle infected with EHEC O157 shed the organism at varying concentrations in feces.[9,11,12] Therefore, at any point in time, some infected cattle may be contributing vastly more EHEC organisms into the environment, and possibly to other cattle, than others.[13]

Duration of Infectiousness

The possible outcomes following infection are resolution of the infection, persistence of infection, or death caused by disease. These factors also influence the duration of infectiousness. The resolution of infectiousness depends on many factors, including the pathogenicity of the organism, host immunity, and the use of antimicrobial therapy. Pathogens that are highly virulent may paradoxically reduce duration of infectiousness by killing the host. Some pathogens, such as BVDV, have bimodal distributions of infectiousness because most hosts have a brief transient period of infection, whereas other infected hosts have prolonged, sometimes persistent, states of infectiousness. For some agents, a single host may have multiple periods of being in an infective state. Hosts infected with agents with a latent state (eg, the herpes viruses) may have recurrent periods of infectiousness between latent periods.[3] The immune response following exposure to a pathogen may be sterilizing, partial, or it may wane with time. Sterilizing immunity is not accomplished with most pathogens and may not be essential for population-level protection against transmission of infection.[14]

QUANTIFYING CONTAGION IN POPULATIONS
Secondary Attack Rate

The secondary attack rate is a statistic sometimes calculated in outbreak investigations. The secondary attack rate is the probability of infection among susceptible individuals in contact with an infectious host, and is a function of the factors affecting infectiousness and transmission given infectiousness.[3] This approach is used for quantifying the contagiousness or transmissibility of pathogens from infected individuals to susceptible individuals.

Basic Reproductive Number

Similar in concept to the secondary attack rate, the basic reproductive number, R_0, is the average, or expected, number of secondary cases that occur in a completely susceptible population following introduction of a single infectious case. The term case refers to an infectious individual regardless of disease status. R_0 is a fundamental statistic in epidemiology for the purpose of studying infectious disease dynamics to summarize a complex set of factors affecting the rate of transmission in a population. The simplest interpretation of R_0 is that if the value is greater than 1, then an outbreak of disease will occur; if R_0 is less than 1, then an outbreak is unlikely or expected to be of low magnitude. The value of R_0 is used to model the potential size of an outbreak and to estimate the proportion of the population that must be immunized to eliminate an infection from the population.

R_0 is a function of biological, behavioral, and environmental factors that affect the rate of contagion. R_0 is a dimensionless statistic, not a rate over time or a measure of disease severity. Neither is its value modified through vaccination. The basic reproductive number is rarely calculated directly. Estimations of R_0 are often modeled as a function of:

- The duration of infectiousness after infection
- The likelihood of infection given contact between an infectious and susceptible host (or vector)
- The contact rate[15]

Because of its complexity, R_0 is sometimes misunderstood and misapplied. One of the most common errors is the belief that R_0 represents a constant value for a given pathogen. Some pathogens are more contagious than others in exactly the same setting. However, the characteristics of the pathogen that favor transmission is only 1 of several factors explaining contagion of any particular pathogen. Any factor that changes the contact rate affects the value of R_0, including population density, seasonality, or social organization.[15] For example, the R_0 value for BVDV in susceptible calves housed in a feedyard drylot is likely to be higher compared with similar calves living in extensive range conditions because of the difference in population density.

Reproductive Ratio

Similar in concept to R_0 is the reproductive ratio, R, also known as the effective reproductive number.[4] The reproductive ratio is the average number of transmissions of infection that occur from each infectious case.[3] In contrast with R_0, which refers to contagion in a completely susceptible population, R can vary over time as immunity changes in a population, and it is sometimes estimated from population-based data. If the susceptible individuals are added to the population, then R increases. If the proportion of susceptible individuals decreases because of immunity from vaccination or exposure, then R decreases. In circumstances in which R is less than 1, transmission cannot be sustained and transmission of infection wanes. If R is greater than 1, then transmission is sustained and major or minor epidemics occur until the proportion of susceptible individuals decreases to the point that R becomes less than 1 and the epidemic of infectiousness wanes.[3,4]

Threshold Level

The threshold level is a concept that incorporates the effects of transmission dynamics with the geographic distribution of animals to determine the minimum density of susceptible animals that would support an outbreak of disease, or, correspondingly, the density of susceptible animals required to prevent a disease outbreak.[16] The threshold level is defined mathematically by Kendall's pandemic threshold theorem. At greater than the threshold density, 1 infected animal can, on average, infect more than 1 susceptible animal and an outbreak can occur.[16] The threshold level has not commonly been applied to animal diseases. However, as an example, it has been estimated that a minimum density of 12 dogs/km^2 is required for an epidemic of canine parvovirus to occur.[16]

Dissemination Rate

Livestock animals are typically managed as subpopulations (ie, groups of animals that cluster within farms that may be more or less biosecure against pathogen introductions). However, animals, people, and equipment may move from farm to farm, or the wind or water might work to disseminate pathogens from one place to another. The dissemination rate describes the risk for pathogens to move from one farm to infect animals on another farm. The dissemination rate depends on:

- Characteristics of the environment, including weather, animal density, and geography
- The type of farming operation, such as the species, class of animal, and opportunities for fomite transmission
- Animal movement, such as for marketing, or from one pasture to another
- The behavior of the farmer, including decisions that affect biosecurity or their own movements, or contact with animals from other sources
- Disease control strategies beyond the farm, such as requirements for quarantine, inspection, or movement restrictions
- Host factors, including their level of immunity, presence of other concurrent diseases, age, breed, and pregnancy status
- Characteristics of the pathogen that affect its survival in the environment and contagion between hosts[16]

Large, multifarm epidemics of disease are often brought under control by taking efforts to manage the factors that decrease the dissemination rate, such as changing behaviors of farmers by creating awareness, and modifying the factors that facilitate farm-to-farm transmission, such as preventing the mixing of animals at markets. The estimated dissemination rate is calculated by dividing the number of farm outbreaks in the population occurring in a defined time period by the number of farm outbreaks that occurred in the time period before (**Fig. 1**).[16]

MODELING EPIDEMICS

Epidemic models help to show the relationships between factors that result in an epidemic of infective cases, as well as showing the nature of the epidemic. There are many forms of epidemic models, with differing levels of complexity. The Reed-Frost model is a simple epidemic model that is useful for demonstrating epidemic theory and herd immunity.[17] The Reed-Frost model (**Fig. 2**) uses a contact rate and the numbers of infected, susceptible, and infected individuals at intervals equivalent to the incubation period to predict the form of a propagated epidemic over time. Propagated epidemics are epidemics that proceed through secondary cases of infection, compared with common or point-source epidemics, which occur as primary cases of infection caused by exposure to a source common to all.[16] The Reed-Frost model assumes that animals move from susceptible to infected in 1 incubation period and are then immune in subsequent periods. The process of moving from susceptible to infected occurs as a chain of binomial distributions.[16]

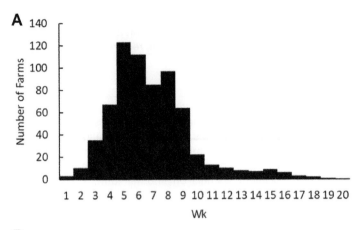

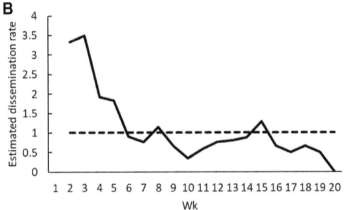

Fig. 1. (A) An epidemic curve of farms with a disease and (B) the corresponding estimated dissemination rate.

HERD IMMUNITY

The goal of vaccination programs is either to prevent the expression of clinical signs of disease following infection or to prevent the transmission of infection in the first place.[4] The strategy of vaccinating for clinical protection is useful for endemically stable pathogens that are common to many animals but only rarely cause disease. Health is improved because the probability for infected animals to show clinical signs of disease is reduced. However, the pathogen may continue to circulate in the population. For pathogens of high economic cost, such as foot and mouth disease, or important to human health, such as rabies, it may be more desirable to eliminate the agent from the population. The strategy of using vaccines to prevent transfer of infection is required to eliminate or eradicate an agent from the population. In this situation, the vaccine should be sufficient to induce herd immunity.[4] Herd immunity is the resistance of a group or population to attack by a disease to which a large proportion of the group is immune, thus lessening the likelihood of an infectious individual to make effective contact with a susceptible individual.[1] Herd immunity can function to prevent the successful introduction of infection into a population of animals or minimize the extent, or speed, of transmission after it has entered the population.[18]

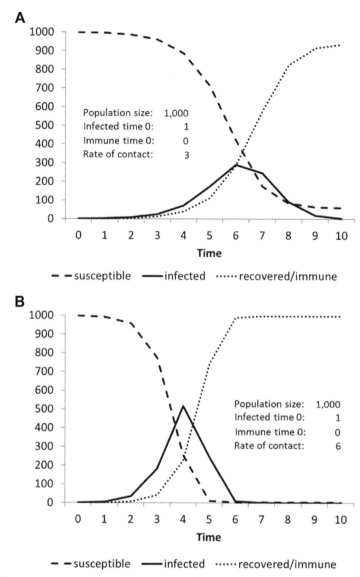

Fig. 2. (A) A Reed-Frost model of an epidemic following introduction of a single infective individual in a population of 1000 susceptible individuals with a contact rate of 3 per time period and (B) 6 per time period. Note the change in peak and duration of the epidemic depending on the contact rate.

Analogy of Herd Immunity

The following analogy is intended to help explain herd immunity and how the concept is applied to the population-level control, elimination, and eradication of disease. Where I live, the grass in my yard is lush and green in the spring. If I toss a burning match into the grass, the yard will not burn because the green grass is not susceptible to burning. In the early summer, the grass in my yard is still mostly green, but some brown, dried blades of grass are beginning to appear. If I toss a match into the grass now, a few of the dried blades might catch fire, but the yard will not burn because there are too many green blades of grass to allow the fire to spread. It is at this point that my yard is showing the value of herd immunity. Even though some of the grass is susceptible, the amount of grass immune to fire prevents the destruction of my yard. Later in the summer, the grass in my yard is dry, brown, and burnable. It has lost herd immunity. If I toss the burning match now, the grass will burn and the fire will spread because most of the grass is now susceptible to burning. The ensuing epidemic of fire might even consume my home. Eventually, everything in my yard that was susceptible to burning has been consumed and the fire burns itself out. But that is not the end of the story, because I live in a community where other people have yards. When my grass was burning, hot embers may have been disseminated to my neighbors' yards by the wind. One neighbor keeps his yard the same way I do, so his yard and house also burn. A second neighbor is worse at keeping his yard than I am. His yard has very little grass, so even though the grass he has is dry and burnable, the fire cannot spread from one blade of grass to the next. His yard and home are spared because of a low contact rate. A third neighbor keeps his yard well watered so, even though some of the grass are dry and burnable, most of the grass is still lush and green. He has maintained herd immunity and his yard is spared. Understanding this fire danger in the summer, and wanting to avoid it, the whole neighborhood could be protected by changing some risky human behaviors (such as tossing burning matches) that introduce fire, making certain that yards are less likely to burn by keeping them watered to maintain herd immunity, or by having so little grass in the yard that the basic reproductive number is less than 1.

Demonstrating Herd Immunity with the Reed-Frost Model

Fig. 3 shows what happens to the epidemic curve as the proportion of the population that is immune to the disease increases. In contrast with the circumstances represented in **Fig. 2**, with a population that is entirely susceptible at the time the pathogen is introduced, **Fig. 3**A shows that the form of the epidemic curve changes because it takes longer for the infection to spread through the population when at least part of the population is immune. The epidemic may fail to materialize if a sufficient proportion of the population is immune (see **Fig. 3**B).

The degree of contagion of the agent is a direct determinant of the proportion of immune individuals required for herd immunity. R_0 can be used to estimate the proportion of immune individuals required to reach the threshold for herd immunity. The relationship between R_0 and the proportion of immune individuals required to achieve herd immunity to the extent that an epidemic is prevented (p_c) is noted by the formula[19]:

$$p_c > (R_0 - 1)/R_0 \text{ or } 1 - 1/R_0$$

For example, if $R_0 = 5$, then the proportion of immune individuals required to achieve the threshold of herd immunity must exceed $1 - 1/5 = 80\%$. If $R_0 = 20$, then more than 95% of the population must be immune to achieve this level of herd immunity.

There are challenges to achieving herd immunity. The proportion of immune individuals in a population needed to achieve the threshold of herd immunity assumes randomness in the contacts between infected and susceptible individuals. However, heterogeneity in transmission is a reality in most human and animal populations. Highly susceptible subpopulations that sometimes experience epidemics of infection become a challenge to eliminating or eradicating important

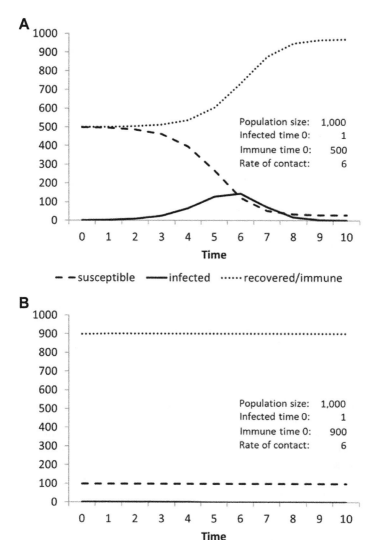

Fig. 3. (A) A Reed-Frost model of an epidemic following introduction of a single infective individual in a population of 1000 with 500 immune individuals and (B) 900 immune individuals at time 0 with a contact time of 6 individuals per time period. Note that the herd immunity threshold is exceeded when 900 of the 1000 individuals are immune and no epidemic took place.

human or animal pathogens, such as the lack of uniform distribution of vaccine in the population.[1,19–21] Further, vaccination does not ensure immunization. Even in well-executed mass-vaccination programs, immunization may only be achieved in 70% of those vaccinated once, and maybe 90% following a second round of vaccination.[21] Poor timing of vaccination, poor cooperation between farmers and veterinarians, and poor vaccine storage and preparation all contribute to lower-than-desired levels of herd immunity. Vaccination programs that result in low levels of herd immunity may even help to perpetuate the persistence of the pathogen in a population either by providing greater opportunities during the vaccination process for comingling and continued transmission, or because the vaccination program makes clinical signs of the disease less evident and therefore more tolerable to farmers, politicians, and other decision makers who become less zealous about pursuing pathogen elimination.[21]

Herd Immunity in Livestock Populations

It is not possible to achieve herd immunity against all pathogens. Herd immunity applies to restrictive circumstances such that:

- The pathogens are fairly species specific
- The pathogens are spread contagiously by fairly direct means
- Host exposure or vaccination confers fairly strong immunity[1]

For example, even though it is possible to confer strong immunity through vaccination, it is not possible to achieve herd immunity against agents such as *Clostridium tetani* or *Bacillus anthracis* because they are fairly noncontagious infections primarily spread via environmental exposure. For these diseases, there is no protection afforded to nonimmunized individuals by others in the population being immune. Because *Streptococcus agalactiae* is spread by contagion and is an obligate pathogen of the bovine mammary gland, this agent meets some of the requirements necessary to achieve herd immunity. Nevertheless, it has not been possible to induce strong immunity to this agent through either infection or vaccination.[22]

However, herd immunity still applies to many important contagious infections of cattle and small ruminants. For example, rinderpest virus, declared eradicated from the world in 2011, had the characteristics for achieving widespread herd immunity, including having a single viral immunotype and vaccine induction of long-standing protective immunity.[20,23] Rinderpest virus has additional characteristics, such as causing few inapparent infections and lacking a chronic carrier state, which helped make it an ideal candidate for eradication efforts.[20]

Vaccination has been used to achieve herd immunity in regionally targeted programs to eliminate some pathogens. For example, foot and mouth disease has been eliminated from some populations by ring vaccination around infected herds, and rabies virus has been geographically restricted by providing vaccine baits as barriers to virus transmission in wildlife.

Outbreaks of pneumonia in calves before weaning may be explained by the loss of herd immunity that occurs with the synchronous loss of passively acquired maternal immunity by calves of similar age.[2] The half-life of maternally acquired immunoglobulin G is approximately 16 days, so the remaining maternal antibodies are negligible by the time a calf is 3 to 4 months of age.[24] In herds with a short calving season, calves lose their maternally derived immunity over a similarly small window of time that seems to coincide with the period of greatest incidence of pneumonia. It is common for pneumonia to occur as sudden epidemics when most calves are 3 to 4 months of age, the age at which herd immunity might be lost.[2]

SUMMARY

Population-based vaccination programs are typically designed to either mitigate clinical signs of endemically stable diseases or to prevent transmission of important contagious pathogens for the purpose of eliminating or eradicating the organism from the population. Herd immunity in the population is required to achieve the latter strategy. Herd immunity occurs when a sufficient proportion of the population is sufficiently immune to prevent ongoing transmission of the pathogen to susceptible animals. Achieving herd immunity requires an understanding of the factors that affect infectiousness, agent transmission, and immunity as well as an understanding the human and animal behaviors that result in less-than-favorable outcomes.

REFERENCES

1. Fox JP. Herd immunity and measles. Rev Infect Dis 1983;5:463–6.
2. Smith DR. Field epidemiology to manage BRD risk in beef cattle production systems. Anim Health Res Rev 2014;15(2):180–3.
3. Horsburgh CR, Mahon BE. Infectious disease epidemiology. In: Rothman KJ, Greenland S, Lash TL, editors. Modern epidemiology. 3rd edition. Philadelphia: Lippincott Williams and Wilkins; 2008. p. 549–63.
4. De Jong MC, Bouma A. Herd immunity after vaccination: how to quantify it and how to use it to halt disease. Vaccine 2001;19:2722–8.
5. Rothman KJ. Causes. Am J Epidemiol 1976;104:587–92.
6. Galvani AP, May RM. Epidemiology: dimensions of superspreading. Nature 2005; 438:293–5.
7. Lloyd-Smith JO, Schreiber SJ, Kopp PE, et al. Superspreading and the effect of individual variation on disease emergence. Nature 2005;438:355–9.
8. Woolhouse ME, Dye C, Etard JF, et al. Heterogeneities in the transmission of infectious agents: implications for the design of control programs. Proc Natl Acad Sci U S A 1997;94:338–42.
9. Naylor SW, Gally DL, Low JC. Enterohaemorrhagic *E. coli* in veterinary medicine. Int J Mol Med 2005;295:419–41.
10. Meyling A, Houe H, Jensen AM. Epidemiology of bovine virus diarrhoea virus. Rev Sci Tech 1990;9:75–93.
11. Chase-Topping ME, McKendrick IJ, Pearce MC, et al. Risk factors for the presence of high-level shedders of *Escherichia coli* O157 on scottish farms. J Clin Monit 2007;45:1594–603.
12. Chase-Topping M, Gally D, Low C, et al. Super-shedding and the link between human infection and livestock carriage of *Escherichia coli* O157. Nat Rev Microbiol 2008;6:904–12.
13. Smith DR. Cattle production systems: ecology of existing and emerging escherichia coli types related to foodborne illness. Annu Rev Anim Biosci 2014;2:23.
14. Metcalf CJE, Ferrari M, Graham AL, et al. Understanding herd immunity. Trends Immunol 2015;36:753–5.
15. Delamater PL, Street EJ, Leslie TF, et al. Complexity of the basic reproduction number (R0). Emerg Infect Dis 2019;25:1–4.
16. Thrusfield MV. Veterinary epidemiology. 3rd edition. Oxford (United Kingdom): Blackwell Science Ltd; 2007.
17. Abbey H. An examination of the Reed-Frost theory of epidemics. Hum Biol 1952; 24:201–33.
18. Martin SW, Meek AH, Willeberg P. Theoretical epidemiology: systems analysis and modeling. Veterinary Epidemiology. 1st edition. Ames (IA): Iowa State University Press; 1987. p. 193–216.

19. Fine P, Eames K, Heymann DL. "Herd immunity": a rough guide. Clin Infect Dis 2011;52:911–6.
20. Morens DM, Holmes EC, Davis AS, et al. Global rinderpest eradication: lessons learned and why humans should celebrate too. J Infect Dis 2011;204: 502–5.
21. Roeder PL, Taylor WP. Mass vaccination and herd immunity: cattle and buffalo. Rev Sci Tech 2007;26:253–63.
22. Pereira UP, Soares SC, Blom J, et al. In silico prediction of conserved vaccine targets in Streptococcus agalactiae strains isolated from fish, cattle, and human samples. Genet Mol Res 2013;12:2902–12.
23. Plowright W. The duration of immunity in cattle following inoculation of rinderpest cell culture vaccine. J Hyg (Lond) 1984;92:285–96.
24. Cortese VS. Neonatal immunology. Vet Clin North Am Food Anim Pract 2009;25: 221–7.

Moving?

Make sure your subscription moves with you!

To notify us of your new address, find your **Clinics Account Number** (located on your mailing label above your name), and contact customer service at:

Email: journalscustomerservice-usa@elsevier.com

800-654-2452 (subscribers in the U.S. & Canada)
314-447-8871 (subscribers outside of the U.S. & Canada)

Fax number: 314-447-8029

Elsevier Health Sciences Division
Subscription Customer Service
3251 Riverport Lane
Maryland Heights, MO 63043

*To ensure uninterrupted delivery of your subscription, please notify us at least 4 weeks in advance of move.

Printed and bound by CPI Group (UK) Ltd, Croydon, CR0 4YY

03/10/2024

01040479-0006